Evidence-Based Approach to Restoring Thyroid Health

Maximizing Thyroid Patient Recovery Rates

Denis Wilson, MD

Contributing Authors:
Michaël Friedman, ND
Kent Holtorf, MD
David Brownstein, MD
Joseph Pizzorno, ND
Lara Pizzorno, MA

Evidence-Based Approach to Restoring Thyroid Health
by Denis Wilson, MD
Contributing Authors: Michaël Friedman, ND, Kent Holtorf, MD, David Brownstein, MD, Joseph Pizzorno, ND, Lara Pizzorno, MA

Muskeegee Medical Publishing Company
P.O. Box 1744
Lady Lake, FL 32158

This book is dedicated to all who are suffering from thyroid disorders and are searching for solutions that may restore vibrant good health.

ISBN: 978-0-615-97878-9

Library of Congress Control Number: 2014905958

The information in this manual is furnished for informational use only, and should not be construed as a commitment by the author or publisher. It is not recommended that patients be treated solely on the information presented here, but that physicians consider these points and the medical literature in this area in the exercise of their professional clinical judgment. The author and publisher assume no responsibility or liability for any errors or inaccuracies that may appear in this manual.

Author and Contributing Authors

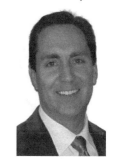

- Denis Wilson, MD identified Wilson's Temperature Syndrome as low body temperature and low thyroid symptoms with normal thyroid blood tests that often remains improved after a few months of treatment have been discontinued. He was the first doctor to use sustained-release liothyronine (in over 5000 patients), and for over twenty years he has educated over 2000 physicians about the use of sustained-release liothyronine for patients with symptoms of low thyroid and low body temperature despite having normal blood tests. His novel treatment of using sustained release T3 is now standard of care with a subsection of physicians practicing complementary and alternative medicine. He is also cofounder and vice president of Restorative Formulations (restorative.com).

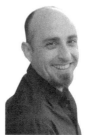

- Michaël Friedman, ND was adjunct instructor of endocrinology at the University of Bridgeport in Connecticut. He is currently the Executive Director of the non-profit Association for the Advancement of Restorative Medicine (AARM) which holds the annual Restorative Medicine Conference. He is also editor in chief of the Journal of Restorative Medicine. Dr. Friedman is the author of the medical textbook Fundamentals of Naturopathic Endocrinology and co-author or Healing Diabetes. His research on the use of SR T3 has been published by the University Puerto Rico Medical School. He is also cofounder and president of Restorative Formulations (Restorative.com).

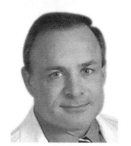

- Kent Holtorf, MD is the medical director of the Holtorf Medical Group and Holtorf Medical Group Affiliate Centers (HoltorfMed.com). He is a guest editor and peer reviewer for a number of medical journals including *Endocrine*, and he has published a number of reviews on complex and controversial topics in endocrinology. He has helped to demonstrate that much of the long-held dogma in endocrinology is inaccurate. He is founder and director of the non-profit National Academy of Hypothyroidism (NAHypothyroidism.org), which is dedicated to dissemination of new information to doctors and patients on the diagnosis and treatment of hypothyroidism.

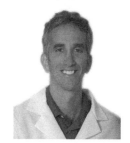

- David Brownstein, MD is a Board-Certified family physician who utilizes the best of conventional and alternative therapies. He is the Medical Director for the Center for Holistic Medicine in West Bloomfield, MI. Dr. Brownstein is a member of the American Academy of Family Physicians and the American College for the Advancement in Medicine. He has lectured internationally about his success using natural items and is the author of eleven books, including: Iodine, *Why You Need It, Why You Can't Live Without It*, and Overcoming Thyroid Disorders. Dr. Brownstein also authors a monthly health newsletter titled, Dr. Brownstein's Natural Way to Health (www.drbrownstein.com)

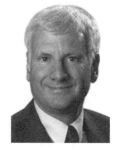

- Joseph Pizzorno, ND is one of the world's leading authorities on science-based natural medicine, a term he coined in 1978. A licensed naturopathic physician with prescriptive rights, educator, researcher and expert spokesman, he is the founding president of Bastyr University, Editor-in-Chief of *Integrative Medicine, A Clinician's Journal*, Vice-chair of the Board of Directors of the Institute for Functional Medicine, co-founder of the American Association of Naturopathic Physicians, member of the Board of Science Counselors for the Gateway for Cancer Research and Chair of the Science Board of Bioclinic Naturals. He is author of 10 books, including the *Textbook of Natural Medicine* and *Encyclopedia of Natural Medicine and the newly released, Clinical Pathophysiology, A Functional Perspective*.

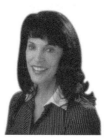

- Lara Pizzorno, MA A member of the American Medical Writers Association with 29+ years of experience writing for physicians and the public, Lara is Editor of Longevity Medicine Review (www.lmreview.com), and Senior Medical Editor for SaluGenecists, Inc., and Integrative Medicine Advisors, LLC. Recent publications include: *Your Bones*, contributing author to the *Textbook of Functional Medicine, Textbook of Natural Medicine*; lead author of *Natural Medicine Instructions for Patients*; co-author of The *Encyclopedia of Healing Foods*; and editor, *The World's Healthiest Foods Essential Guide for the healthiest way of eating*.

Restorative medicine approach to Graves' disease, Hashimoto's thyroiditis, and Wilson's Temperature Syndrome

- Clinical applications of botanical medicine, nutrition, and hormonal therapy as powerful tools to help the body heal itself and restore thyroid function.
- Too many doctors are trained to focus on what happens **upstream** from the deiodinase enzyme that converts T4 to T3, but how patients feel has everything to do with what happens **downstream** from that enzyme.
- T4 and rT3 accelerate the destruction of the deiodinase enzyme that converts T4 to T3
- T4-containing therapy can sometimes actually suppress T3 expression in the cells
- Research proves T4 replacement is often inadequate for restoring thyroid hormone levels in the tissues of the body
- Body temperature correlates with low thyroid symptoms much better than thyroid stimulating hormone does
- T3-only therapy can often turn T4-treatment-failures into treatment successes by normalizing body temperature and eliminating hypometabolic symptoms
- T3-only therapy depletes T4 and rT3 levels, reducing deiodinase suppression, setting the stage for restored T4 to T3 conversion

Hyperthyroidism

Botanical support can calm and nourish the thyroid gland to the point that patients can recover and radioactive or surgical ablation may not be necessary.

Hashimoto's Thyroiditis

Especially when caught early, some people can recover from Hashimoto's thyroiditis, with normalization of anti-TPO antibody levels. Botanicals and nutrition and T3 can be used to normalize body temperatures and help people to feel well.

Wilson's Temperature Syndrome (WTS)

Just as irregular menstrual cycles can often be completely corrected with a few months of birth control pills, so too, WTS is a reversible form of low thyroid function that can often be completely corrected with a few months of treatment that can include herbs, nutrition, and T3 therapy.

Contents

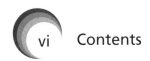

Preface

Most doctors have been trained to rely on thyroid blood tests for diagnosing thyroid disorders. However, prior to the development of the thyroid-stimulating hormone (TSH) test, doctors relied on clinical signs and symptoms as a guide for the medical management of thyroid disorders … and with good results. Back then, some doctors found triiodothyronine (T3) to be more useful than thyroxine (T4) therapy for treating patients with symptoms of low thyroid. However, as doctors began to focus more on blood tests than on signs and symptoms, T3 therapy fell out of favor. The increase in T4 popularity is probably because it is easier to manage and is less prone to side effects. However, many patients still do not feel well even when their TSH levels are normalized with T4-containing medicine. On the other hand, many of those patients do feel well when their body temperatures are normalized with T3 therapy.

Between 1988 and 1990, I found and described a form of low thyroid hormone expression I called Wilson's Temperature Syndrome (WTS). WTS presents with signs and symptoms of low thyroid (e.g., low temperature) despite normal thyroid blood tests. One notable characteristic of WTS is that it not only responds well to T3 therapy [i.e., the Wilson's T3 (WT3) protocol described in this book], but its signs and symptoms often remain improved even after the treatment has been discontinued. WTS is a form of hypothyroidism that is often completely reversible, usually within a matter of months. This can often be accomplished by resetting the thyroid hormone system by clearing out the thyroid hormone pathways, for a time, enabling the body to maintain normal body temperatures on its own again. In the last two decades, accumulating evidence in the medical literature confirms that the TSH test is not a reliable indicator of thyroid hormone expression in the cells of the body and confirms why many patients might feel better on T3 than on T4, especially when thyroid blood tests are within the normal range.

Much can be done to restore health to patients with hyperthyroidism and hypothyroidism as well. The aim of this book is to systematically present the current medical evidence in support of restorative therapies for hyperthyroidism, hypothyroidism, and WTS. This includes information supporting the use of nutritional and herbal interventions in thyroid disorders as well as the use of T3 in the treatment of WTS. By implementing this evidence-based information into your practice, I know you will be able to make a significant difference in the lives of many people suffering from untreated or inadequately treated thyroid hormone dysfunction.

1

Thyroid Physiology

Hypothalamic–Pituitary–Thyroid Axis

The hypothalamic–pituitary–thyroid axis (HPT axis), a.k.a. *thyroid homeostasis* or *thyrotropic feedback control*, is a complex web of multi-loop feedback systems that balances the body's regulatory responses in order to maintain thyroid hormone signaling under normal conditions and in the face of thyroid hormone deficiencies.[1] As its name suggests, the HPT axis depends upon the hypothalamus, pituitary gland, and thyroid gland for the ultimate purpose of regulating the body's metabolism and body temperature. This system also influences several important non-endocrine functions such as the activity of the autonomic nervous system and appetite.

The hypothalamus is considered the coordinating center of the endocrine system. It consolidates internal stimuli (e.g., cortical inputs, autonomic function, and endocrine feedback), as well as environmental cues (e.g., light and temperature) in order to deliver thyrotropin-releasing hormone (TRH) to the anterior pituitary gland. The pituitary gland in turn secretes thyroid-stimulating hormone (TSH) that binds to receptors on the surface of follicle cells in the thyroid gland. Finally, the thyroid is stimulated to secrete the thyroid hormones thyroxine (T4) and, to a lesser degree, triiodo-thyronine (T3).[1] These thyroid hormones exert negative feedback control over the hypothalamus as well as the anterior pituitary, thus controlling the release of both TRH from the hypothalamus and TSH from the anterior pituitary gland.[2]

Thyroid Cell Function

The Sodium/Iodide Symporter (NIS)

The sodium/iodide symporter (NIS), also known as sodium/iodide co-transporter, is a transmembrane glycoprotein that mediates the uptake of iodide into the follicular cells (i.e., thyrocytes) by transporting two sodium cations (Na^+) for each iodide anion (I^-) into the cell. This NIS-mediated uptake of iodide into the cells of the thyroid gland is the first step in the synthesis of thyroid hormone (i.e., T3 and T4).[3]

This active transport is driven by the electrochemical gradient of sodium, which causes the iodide concentration inside follicular cells of thyroid tissue to be 20 to 50 times higher than in the plasma. Once inside the follicular cells, the iodide is metabolically oxidized through the action of thyroid peroxidase (TPO) to iodinium (I^+), which in turn iodinates tyrosine residues of the thyroglobulin (Tg) proteins in the follicle colloid. NIS activity is regulated by TSH and iodide concentrations via transcriptional and posttranscriptional mechanisms.[3]

Organification

Organification is a biochemical process occurring in the thyroid glands, which involves the incorporation of iodine into Tg in order to produce T4 or T3, and thyroid hormones. The term "organification" comes from the fact that iodine, an inorganic chemical, is being joined to the protein Tg, which is an organic molecule.[4]

The organification of iodine occurs in the follicle and is accomplished via the enzyme TPO, which oxidizes iodide to atomic iodine (I) or iodinium (I^+), preparing the iodine for addition onto tyrosine residues on Tg.[5] TPO catalyzes both the iodination of tyrosine residues to form monoiodotyrosine (MIT) and diiodotyrosine (DIT) residues and the coupling of iodotyrosine residues in Tg, resulting in the formation of T3 and T4. TPO is well known as an autoantigen in autoimmune thyroid disease, that is targeted by anti-thyroid peroxidase antibodies (i.e., anti-TPO antibodies). These antibodies are most commonly associated with Hashimoto's thyroiditis but are also found in some patients with Graves' disease.[6]

Iodide passes through the follicular cells in its reduced form since glutathione and glutathione peroxidase (GPX) keep hydrogen peroxide levels low in the follicular cells. Under conditions of oxidative stress or nutritional deficiency, oxidative damage to the iodine transporter (NIS) can occur. This oxidative damage may contribute to autoimmune thyroid disease. Selenium deficiency can lead to low GPX (a selenoprotein). Glutathione levels may become depleted when it is used up in the detoxification of environmental toxins such as toxic metals and persistent organic pollutants (POPs) such as polychlorinated biphenyls (PCBs), organochlorine pesticides, polybrominated diphenyl ethers (PDBEs), plastics, phthalates, and polychlorinated dibenzo-p-dioxins (PCDDs). This is just one potential mechanism for how POPs can disrupt the function of the thyroid system.[7]

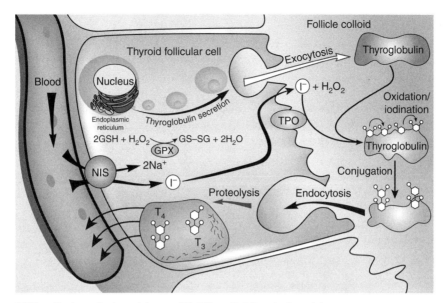

GSH = Reduced glutathione, GS-SG = Oxidized glutathione,
GPX = Glutathione peroxidase, TPO = Thyroid peroxidase

Thyroid Hormone Synthesis

The thyroid is touted as the most important gland in the body due to its ability to produce the hormones T4, T3, and calcitonin. Through the actions of TPO, iodine is covalently bound to tyrosine residues within Tg to form T4 and T3. Then lysosomal proteases sever the T4 and T3 from the Tg and the hormones are released into circulation.

Thyroid hormones have several functions including regulating metabolism, directing cellular activity, stimulating heart muscles, nerves, and brain functioning, as well as increasing utilization of carbohydrates, proteins, fats, and cholesterol. The thyroid hormones accomplish this by attaching to thyroid hormone receptors on the nuclear membranes of the cells, affecting the transcription of the DNA. Thyroid hormones regulate the rate of DNA transcription and expression, thereby regulating the rate of life, or in other words, metabolism. However, perhaps the most important effect of thyroid hormones is their regulation of mitochondrial production of ATP – the energy coin of the body that is required for almost all enzymes and body functions to work. No wonder thyroid hormones can affect so many bodily functions and symptoms.

The thyroid gland produces several immunologic factors and requires complex nutrients in order to facilitate hormone synthesis. Thyroid hormone metabolism has a step up and step down metabolism where T4 can either be stepped up to the active form, T3, or stepped down to the inactive form, reverse T3 (rT3), both of which are further converted to 3,3'-diiodothyronine.

Thyroid Support Nutrients

Iodine

Potassium iodide and T4 therapy are often used for treating thyroid disorders as they have been shown to inhibit and prevent the growth of benign thyroid nodules in 66% of patients.[8] However, caution must be exercised because prescribing iodine in the presence of a hidden hot nodule can lead to thyroid storm.

Iodine is a crucial constituent of thyroid function and is a component of T4 and T3. It is well established that the highest prevalence of thyroid disorders is seen in populations where iodine deficiency is prevalent. Goiter is usually endemic in areas where daily iodine intake is <50 mcg and congenital hypothyroidism is seen in areas where intake is <25 mcg/day. Approximately 30% of the world's population lives in areas of iodine deficiency. These areas see a prevalence of goiter as high as 80%.[9] Iodine supplementation has been reported to reduce thyroid volume with sustained effects seen through 12 months post-therapy in patients with goiter.[10] In contrast, although T4 therapy also decreases thyroid volume, these effects are reversed when therapy is removed.

In areas of iodine deficiency, when supplemented with iodine those with thyroid dysfunction (typically thyroid nodules) develop a higher prevalence of autoimmune disease. These autoimmune diseases range from Hashimoto's disease to thyrotoxicosis resulting from Graves' disease.[9]

Selenium

Selenium is an essential component of the antioxidant GPX. Reduction in selenium reduces the formation of GPX resulting in increased levels of reactive oxygen species and hydrogen peroxide, which can damage the thyroid.

A deficiency in selenium (a constituent of selenoproteins) has been implicated in autoimmune thyroiditis by increasing the duration and exacerbating the disease severity. Furthermore, its supplementation can decrease inflammatory activity among patients with autoimmune thyroiditis.[11] It is possible that supplementation increases the activity of the selenoprotein GPX leading to decreased production of hydrogen peroxide in the follicular cells. Iodothyronine selenodeiodinases D1 and D2 are another class of selenoproteins that produce active T3 through deiodination in peripheral tissues.

Selenium, a component of selenocysteine is found in all three deiodinases as well as GPX.

Selenium supplementation has consistently been shown to increase serum selenium and GPX levels by 45% and 21% respectively. It has also been reported to decrease TPO antibodies by 76%. Upon withdrawal of supplementation, a sharp decrease was seen in selenium and GPX accompanied by marked increase in TPO.[12] A healthy level of glutathione is vitally important because it modulates hydrogen peroxidase and organification of iodine. It also functions to prevent oxidation damage to the thyrocytes themselves.

The maintenance of an optimal selenium level is critical for a number of other reasons as well. For example, selenium is a critical component of selenocysteine, which is required for the synthesis of deiodinases. Furthermore, patients who are not converting T4 to T3 very well, or those with Graves', may recover faster and have significantly better outcomes when supplemented with selenium (400 mcg/day). Some experts suggest selenium supplementation may even benefit those with mild orbitopathy.[13,14]

Zinc

Zinc is a metallic chemical element essential for many biochemical processes such as cell proliferation. There are indications that zinc is also important for normal thyroid homeostasis. Its effects on thyroid hormones are complex and include both synthesis and mode of action.[15] For example, thyroid transcription factors, that are essential for modulation of gene expression, contain zinc at cysteine residues.

Zinc deficiency can influence thyroid function through its effects on TSH and thyroid hormone levels. Conversely, thyroid hormones influence zinc metabolism by affecting zinc absorption and excretion. In patients with nodular goiter, serum zinc levels were significantly negatively correlated with thyroid volume.[16]

Iron

Data from both animals and human studies have shown that iron deficiency anemia (IDA) impairs thyroid metabolism. The mechanism by which iron status influences thyroid and iodine metabolism is unclear. IDA (as indicated by an iron saturation below 25 or a ferritin below 70) decreases plasma total T4 and T3 concentrations, reduces peripheral conversion of T4 to T3, increases rT3 levels, and/or increases circulating thyrotropin (TSH). Iron deficiency may also hinder the production of thyroid hormone by reducing activity of the enzyme TPO, which in turn blocks the thermogenic (metabolism boosting) properties of thyroid hormone.[17] Other possible mechanisms include altering central nervous system control of thyroid metabolism and nuclear T3 binding.[18–24]

In one study, 15.7% of women with subclinical hypothyroidism were found to be iron deficient, compared to only 9.8% of the control group.[25] Individuals taking iodine supplementation may also benefit from iron supplementation, especially if they are iron deficient.[26,27] Subclinical hypothyroid patients with comorbid iron deficiency often require treatment with both levothyroxine (T4) and iron supplementation, as either therapy alone is often not adequate in this patient population.[28]

Deiodinases

Of the hormones secreted by the thyroid gland, about 92% is T4 and about 8% is T3. About 40% of T4 is converted to T3 but 80% of T3 comes from peripheral conversion. This is interesting because about 8% of hormone secreted by thyroid is T3. T4 to T3 conversion is kept very low in the thyroid (due to high T4 concentration, which accelerates destruction of D2 by proteosomes). Deiodinase enzymes are considered essential control points of cellular thyroid activity because they determine intracellular activation and deactivation of thyroid hormones independently from plasma hormone levels. This constitutes a potent mechanism of thyroid homeostasis. The deiodinases can locally adjust thyroid hormone levels in cases of hypothyroidism and hyperthyroidism. This local control of cellular thyroid levels is mediated by three distinct deiodinase enzymes present in different tissues in the body: type I deiodinase (D1) and type II deiodinase (D2) increase cellular thyroid activity by converting less active T4 to more active T3, while type III deiodinase (D3) reduces cellular thyroid activity by converting T4 to the inactive reverse T3. D1 can also convert T4 to rT3 albeit weakly.[29–38]

The activity of each type of deiodinase enzyme changes in response to differing physiologic conditions. This local control of intracellular T4 and T3 results in different tissue levels of T4 and T3 under different conditions. Serum thyroid hormone levels may not necessarily predict tissue thyroid levels under a variety of physiologic conditions. This is because the transport of T4 and T3 into the cell and the activity of these deiodinases determine tissue and cellular thyroid levels.

Deiodinase Type I (D1)

D1 converts less active T4 to more active T3 throughout the body, but D1 is not a significant determinant of pituitary T4 to T3 conversion, which is controlled by D2.[30,36,39] D1 is expressed especially in the liver and kidneys and is sublocated in the plasma membrane and contributes a significant fraction of T3 in the plasma. D1 conversion of T4 to T3 is increased in hyperthyroidism, which is why propylthiouracil (PTU) is effective in treating hyperthyroidism because D1 (but not D2) is inhibited by PTU. As well as activating T4 to T3 through outer ring deiodination (ORD), D1 can also deactivate T4 to RT3 through inner ring deiodination (IRD). IRD by D1 is weak; therefore, D3 is the primary deactivating deiodinase.[30]

The activity of deiodinases. IRD by D1 is weak; therefore, D3 is the primary deactivating deiodinase.[301]

D1 and D2 are suppressed and down-regulated (decreasing T4 to T3 conversion) in response to physiologic and emotional stress;[40-51] depression;[52-73] dieting;[74-79] weight gain and leptin resistance;[75-119] insulin resistance, obesity, and diabetes;[119-127] inflammation from autoimmune disease or systemic illness;[40,128-143] chronic pain;[144-148] chronic fatigue syndrome (CFS) and fibromyalgia;[149-153] and exposure to toxins and plastics.[154-162] The reduced thyroid tissue levels associated with these conditions is often quoted as a beneficial response that lowers metabolism and thus does not require treatment. However, there is significant evidence demonstrating that this response is detrimental rather than beneficial.[163-170]

Deiodinase Type II (D2)

D2 performs ORD only. As compared to D1, D2 has 1000 times the affinity for T4 and consequently performs ORD much more quickly and powerfully. D2 is sublocalized in the membrane of the endoplasmic reticulum, which is continuous with the nuclear membrane. This proximity to the nucleus makes it very easy for T3 to interact with thyroid receptors (TRs). Whereas much of the T3 that is produced by D1 on the plasma membrane can go into the plasma, most of the T3 that is produced by D2 on the endoplasmic reticulum membrane stays intracellular. It is likely that D2 is the determining factor of energy expenditure in humans, with D1 having very little impact in euthyroid subjects.

D2 is a key enzyme that controls the intracellular concentration of T3. It is under careful intracellular regulation. Different metabolic signals stimulate ubiquitin (Ub) conjugation of D2, which leads to selective uptake and proteolysis in proteasomes. This process of destruction of D2 is greatly accelerated in the presence of T4 and RT3. In fact, only 8% of T4 is converted to T3 inside the thyroid gland while 40% of T4 is converted to T3 outside the thyroid gland. It is likely that the low T4 to T3 conversion in the thyroid is due to the high concentration of T4 there that encourages proteolysis of the 5′-deiodinases. Most T4 in the body is extracellular in the plasma whereas most T3 in the body is intracellular. D2 has a very short activity half-life (40 mins) that can be reduced to about 20 mins when proteolysis is accelerated by T4 and RT3. Interestingly, D1 is not under the same control. D1 is not ubiquinated and has a half-life that is greater than 12 hours.

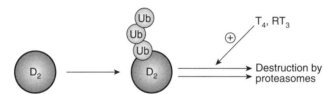

T4 and RT3 accelerate the destruction of the type II deiodinase (D2), slowing the conversion of T4 to T3.

The T3 in D1-expressing tissues equilibrates rapidly with plasma T3 suggesting D1 is under less regulation. On the other hand, D2-expressing tissues equilibrate very slowly with plasma T3. TR occupancy is 70–90% in D2-expressing tissues (as opposed to 40–50% in D1-expressing tissues) and 50–80% of the T3 occupying the TR is T3 from the intracellular conversion of T4 to T3 (not from the plasma compartment). This shows that D2 is under a great deal of regulation and that there is sophisticated local regulation of thyroid hormones that can greatly affect intracellular T3 concentrations in the absence of changes in T4 secretion.

The following diagram shows the intricate interrelationships among the deiodinases, their actions in peripheral tissues, and their role in monitoring both the prohormone T4 and active hormone T3. These interconnecting pathways show how the deiodinases can greatly affect thyroid status and T3 concentration in the cells even when T4 levels don't change.[30]

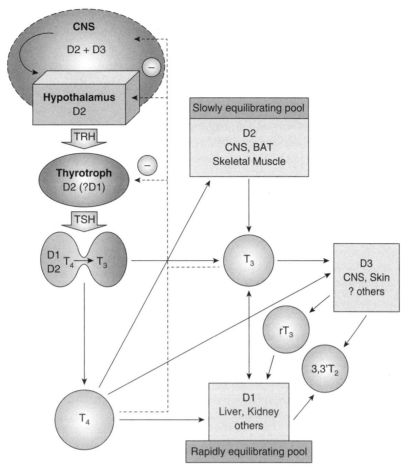

Schematic diagram of the human thyroid axis depicting the role and probable tissue location of D1, D2, and D3 in the production and inactivation of plasma T3 and in feedback regulation of thyroid function.[30]

TSH is produced in the pituitary and regulated by intra-pituitary T3 levels, which often do not correlate or provide an accurate indicator of T3 levels in the rest of the body. While TSH is often used as an indicator for the body's overall thyroid status, this theory assumes that T3 levels in the pituitary are directly correlated with that of other tissues in the body under a wide range of physiologic conditions. However, this hypothesis does not appear to be accurate, as the pituitary is different than every other tissue in the body.

T4 to T3 conversion is controlled by D2, which has been shown to be less sensitive to selenium deficiency than D1 or D3.[171] Numerous conditions can result in an increase in pituitary T3 levels while simultaneously suppressing cellular T3 levels in the rest of the body. The regulation of intracellular T3 levels by deiodinase activity occurs on a tissue-specific and time-specific basis. This means that thyroid expression can be relatively high in one area of the body and low in another at the same time. Therefore, TSH is a poor indicator of thyroid status in the tissues of the body.[172]

As opposed to the rest of the body that is also regulated by D1 and D3, the pituitary contains little D1 and no D3;[164] so pituitary T3 levels are determined solely by D2 activity.[30,36,39] In the pituitary, 80–90% of T4 is converted to T3,[33,172,173] while the peripheral tissue only converts about 30–50% of T4 to T3;[173,174] this is likely due to competition from D3 which converts T4 to rT3 in all tissues of the body but which is not present in the pituitary.[36] In addition to having a unique make-up of deiodinases, the pituitary also contains unique membrane thyroid transporters and TRs.

Given that pituitary T3 levels are under completely different physiologic control than in the rest of the body, T3 levels can be significantly higher there than elsewhere in the body.[31,175–182] Consequently, many tissues of the body may be deficient in T3 even when the TSH is normal.

Differing thyroid levels and physiologic conditions will impact T3 levels in the pituitary differently than in the rest of the body, making TSH an unreliable biomarker under a variety of circumstances. For instance, as the level of T4 declines (as it does in hypothyroidism), the activity of D2 increases in order to partially compensate for the reduction in serum

T4.[32,183–191] On the other hand, reduced T4 levels cause the activity and efficiency of D1 to decrease, resulting in a reduction in cellular T3 levels.[192–197] Meanwhile, TSH remains unchanged due to the ability of pituitary D2 to compensate for diminished T4.

As stated above, the lack of correlation between TSH and peripheral tissue levels of T3 can be exacerbated by numerous disorders. These include chronic emotional or physical stress, chronic illness, diabetes, insulin resistance, obesity, leptin resistance, depression, CFS, fibromyalgia, premenstrual syndrome (PMS), dieting, and weight gain. In such conditions, tissue levels of T3 have been shown to drop dramatically out of proportion with serum T3 levels.[37,38,128–131,198–200] While serum T3 levels may drop by 30%, which is significant but still may be in the so-called "normal range," tissue T3 may drop by 70–80%. This can result in profound cellular hypothyroidism, despite normal serum levels of TSH, T4, and T3.[37,40,128–131,198,201] Therefore, in the presence of such conditions, even a normal TSH level may not necessarily indicate that the patient is euthyroidic (normal thyroid), especially in the presence of symptoms consistent with thyroid deficiency.

Doctors in the thyroid division of the department of Medicine at Brigham and Women's Hospital and Harvard Medical School reported on the physiologic roles of the deiodinase enzymes. In their review published in *Endocrine Reviews*, the authors state, "The approximately 1000-fold lower Km of D2 than D1 [D2 is 1000 times more efficient] may give this enzyme a major advantage in terms of extrathyroidal T3 production ... The free T3 concentration in different tissues varies according to the amounts of hormone transported and the activity of the tissue deiodinases. As a result, the impact of the plasma thyroid hormones on target tissues is not the same in every tissue."[30]

Table 1.1. Human iodothyronine selenodeiodinases[30]

Parameter	Type 1 (ORD and IRD)	Type 2 (outer ring)	Type 3 (inner ring)
Physiological role	rT_3 and T_3S degradation; source of plasma T_3, especially in hyperthyroid patients	Provide intracellular T_3 in specific tissues; source of plasma T_3 (50%)	Inactivate T_3 and T_4
Tissue location	Liver, kidney, thyroid, and pituitary (but not CNS)	CNS, pituitary, BAT, placenta thyroid, skeletal muscle, heart	Placenta, CNS, fetal liver, hemangiomas
Subcellular location	Plasma membrane	ER	Not known
Molecular mass of monomer (Da)	29,000	30,500	31,500
Preferred substrates (position)	rT_3 (5′), T_3S (5)	T4, rT_3	T_3, T_4
K_m (apparent) (M)	10^{-7}, 10^{-6}	10^{-9}	10^{-9}
Active center	Sec	Sec	Sec
Susceptibility to inhibitors/mechanism			
PTU	High/competitive with thiol substrate	Very low	Very low
Gold	High/competitive with iodothyronine	Low/non-specific	Low/specific, competitive with iodothyronine
Carboxymethylation	High/competitive with iodothyronine	Low/non-specific	Not known
Specific labeling with $BrAcT_3$, T_4	Yes Competitive with iodothyronine	No	Yes Competitive with iodothyronine
Response to increased T_4			
Pretranslational mechanism Posttranslational mechanism	↑ ↑ Transcriptional ↓ ↓ (slow) Oxidation of active center	↓ ↓ Transcriptional ↓ ↓ (rapid) ↑ ubiquitination	↑ ↑ Transcriptional (not known)

In the journal *Endocrinology*, Lim et al. measured peripheral (liver) and pituitary levels of T3 in response to induced chronic illness. They found that pituitary T3 and TSH levels remained unchanged while the peripheral tissues were significantly reduced. The authors summarize their findings by stating,

> "The reduction in hepatic nuclear T3 content and T3-Cmax in the Nx2 rats is consistent with the presence of selective tissue deficiency of thyroid hormones. The pituitary, however, had normal T3 content, suggesting dissociation in thyroid hormone-dependent metabolic status between peripheral tissue (liver) and the pituitary. This explains the failure to observe an increase in serum TSH level, a manifestation of reduced intracellular rather than serum T3 concentration ... Most interesting, we found that, in contrast to the liver, the pituitary of the Nx rats was not deprived of thyroid hormone. This finding offers a convincing explanation of the failure to observe an increase of serum TSH when illness or stress-induced reduction of hepatic T4 5'-monodeiodination causes a fall in serum T3 concentration."[243]

In the *New England Journal of Medicine*, Larsen et al. concludes that the pituitary has a unique composition of deiodinases that is not present in any other tissue in the body, making the pituitary T3 levels, and thus TSH, a poor indicator for tissue T3 in the rest of the body. He also found that TSH cannot be reliably used as a marker of thyroid status in the rest of the body. The author goes on to state,

> "Changes in pituitary conversion of T4 to T3 are often opposite of those that occur in the liver and kidney under similar circumstances. The presence of this pathway of T3 production indicates that the pituitary can respond independently to changes in plasma levels of T4 and T3 ... Given these results, it is not surprising that a complete definition of thyroid status requires more than the measurement of the serum concentrations of thyroid hormones. For some tissues, the intracellular T3 concentration may only partially reflect those in the serum. Recognition that the intracellular T3 concentration in each tissue may be subject to local regulation and an understanding of the importance of this process to the regulation of TSH production should permit a better appreciation of the limitations of the measurements of serum thyroid hormone and TSH levels."[172]

Deiodinase Type III (D3)

The pituitary is the only tissue that does not contain D3,[36] which converts T4 to rT3 and competes with the ability of D1 and D2 to convert T4 to T3.[37,38,40,52,120,132,202–208] rT3 is a competitive inhibitor of T3, blocking T3 from binding to its receptor, which blocks T3's effect,[209–214] reduces metabolism,[209,212,213] suppresses D1 and D2 and T4 to T3 conversion,[210,212,215–218] and blocks T4 and T3 uptake into the cell.[208,219] All of these effects reduce intracellular T3 levels and thyroid activity. The inhibitory effects on the peripheral tissues causing hypothyroidism are not reflected by TSH testing because many tissues may have abundant D3 levels while the pituitary is uniquely devoid of D3.[36]

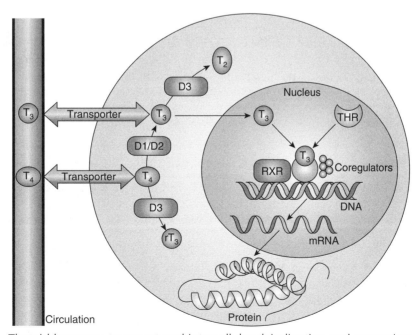

Thyroid hormone transport and intracellular deiodination and expression.

rT3 is present in varying concentrations in different tissues and with different individuals.[30,41,89,90,175,204–208,220–222] It is upregulated with chronic physiologic stress and illness,[30,221,222] and is an indicator for reduced T4 to T3 conversion as well as low intracellular T3 levels (even if the TSH is normal).[132,202–204,207,209,219,221,222]

Because increased serum and tissue levels of rT3 can result in a blocking of the TRs, even small increases in rT3 can produce a significant decrease in thyroid action and cause severe hypothyroidism that would not be detected by standard blood tests.[209–214] Because any T4 given will contribute to more rT3, T4-only preparations should not be considered optimal thyroid replacement in the presence of high or high-normal rT3 levels while T3 can be significantly beneficial.[80,81,149–152,223–241]

Since D1 can only perform inner ring deiodination weakly, D3 is the primary deactivating deiodinase. D3 is high in the developing fetus. It protects the fetus during development from too much thyroid stimulation.[30]

Stress

Chronic physiologic stress results in decreased D1 activity,[40–46] and an increase in D3 activity.[30,221,222] This decreases thyroid activity by converting T4 into rT3 instead of T3.[30,221,222,242,243] Conversely, D2 is stimulated, which results in increased T4 to T3 conversion in the pituitary and reduced production of TSH.[40,47–51,67,243] The increased cortisol levels seen with stress also contribute to the physiologic disconnect between TSH and levels of T3 in the peripheral tissue.[45,47–49] This stress-induced decrease in tissue T3 and increased rT3 results in tissue hypothyroidism and potential weight gain, fatigue, and depression.[41,42,220,244–246] This stress-related vicious cycle of weight gain, fatigue, and depression can be prevented with supplementation of time-release T3[53,54,80,149–152,225,227–241,247,248] but not T4.[80,223–225,227,249,250]

The reduced immunity from chronic stress has been thought to be due to excess cortisol production, but the associated reduction in tissue thyroid levels play a larger role, and thyroid supplementation can reverse this stress-induced reduction in immunity.[244]

As with stress, treatment with prednisone or other glucocorticoids will suppress D1 and stimulate D3, reducing the conversion of T4 to T3 and increasing conversion of T4 to rT3. This results in relative tissue hypothyroidism that is not detected by TSH testing.[41,47–50,220,245,251] This low cellular thyroid level contributes to weight gain and other associated side effects related to such treatment. Thus, stressed or corticosteroid-treated patients often experience reduced T3 levels in the tissue, which is not reflected by measuring TSH levels.

Dieting

Acute or chronic dieting can result in a significant (up to 50%) decrease in intracellular and circulating T3 levels,[74,75,79,118] which drastically reduces basal metabolic rate (number of calories burned per day) by 15–40%.[76,252,253] This appears to be an adaptive measure the body takes to conserve energy and survive starvation (a starvation mode). Even moderate dieting can lead to lower metabolic rates that persist after the dieting is over. With chronic dieting, the thyroid levels and metabolism often do not return to normal levels. This causes the body to stay in starvation mode for years with significantly reduced metabolism despite the resumption of normal food intake, ultimately making it very difficult to lose or maintain lost weight.[76]

A study by Araujo et al. published in *American Journal of Physiology, Endocrinology and Metabolism* found that 25 days of calorie restriction (dieting) significantly reduced D1, resulting in a 50% reduction in T3. This dramatic reduction in T3 was associated with an increase in D2, and a decrease in TSH from an average of 1.20 ng/ml to 0.7 ng/ml. This demonstrates that TSH is a poor marker for tissue T3 levels, especially in a chronically dieting patient.[75]

Fontana et al. found that T3 levels were significantly decreased by 25% in chronically dieting individuals compared to non-dieting individuals with no difference in TSH and T4 (thus undetected by TSH and T4 testing). TSH remained in the normal range despite the significant decline (in T3), demonstrating the weakness and unreliability of utilizing popular reference ranges that consider 95% of the population as "normal".[77] The reduced T3 associated with dieting could potentially contribute to fatigue and depression, as well as interfering with the patient's ability to lose weight, and the regaining of lost weight.

A study by Leibel and Jirsch published in the journal *Metabolism* found that individuals who had lost weight in the past had a significantly lower metabolism than those of same weight who had not gained or lost significant weight in the past.[76] The metabolism in the weight-reduced patients was 25% less than an equal weight person who did not lose or gain significant weight in the past, and equal to someone who weighed 60% less than they did. Additionally, the reduction was shown to be present years later.

This 25% reduction in metabolism equates to an approximate deficit of 500–600 cal per day. Thus, if the previous overweight person is to maintain their weight loss, he/she must either eat 600 cal per day less (compared to a person of the same weight who has not had a weight problem) or they must jog about 1½ hours per day to maintain the lost weight. This equates to approximately a pound per week of weight gain, explaining why weight is so quickly gained back without continued very strict dieting. Many people who have difficulty keeping weight off are not excessive eaters, but are continually told they are eating too much or they need to exercise more. They are made to feel it is a character issue and that nobody believes how little food they actually consume. Unless the physiologic thyroid dysfunction is corrected, any diet and exercise strategy is doomed.

Croxson and Ibbertson in *Journal of Endocrinology and Metabolism* found that individuals with a history of intense dieting had dramatic reductions in T4 to T3 conversion, which causes an intracellular deficiency of T3. The inadequacy and inaccuracy of standard TSH and T4 testing was demonstrated, as such testing failed to detect the dramatic reduction in tissue levels of T3 in all of the patients.[78]

Insulin Resistance/Diabetes/Metabolic Syndrome/Obesity

As with leptin resistance, numerous studies have shown that insulin resistance, diabetes, or metabolic syndrome are associated with a significant reduction in T4 to T3 conversion, an intracellular deficiency of T3, and an increased conversion of T4 to rT3 (further reducing intracellular T3 levels).[119,120,122,128,209–219,254] Additionally, the related elevation of insulin will increase D2 activity and suppress TSH levels, further decreasing thyroid levels and making it inappropriate to use TSH as a reliable marker for tissue thyroid levels. This is particularly true for patients with obesity, insulin resistance, or type II diabetes.[119–127,255]

Pittman et al. found that diabetics had a significantly lower rate of conversion of T4 to T3 as well as an increased T4 to rT3 rate as compared to normal controls. Improvement in glucose levels only increased T4 to T3 conversion by one percentage point.[121]

Islam et al. investigated the T4 to T3 conversion in 50 diabetic patients compared to 50 non-diabetic controls. They found no difference in TSH and free T4 levels, but the diabetic individuals had significantly decreased free T3 (FT3) levels (p = 0.0001) that averaged 46% less than controls. The FT3/FT4 ratio was 50% less in diabetic patients versus controls. TSH failed to elevate despite the fact that serum T3 was approximately half of normal.[120] Saunders et al. also found that diabetics had approximately a 50% reduction in T3 levels and significantly increased rT3 levels as well as decreased T3/rT3 ratios.[122]

In the *International Journal of Obesity*, Krotkiewski published the results of his investigation on the impact of supplemental T3 on cardiovascular risk in obese patients in order to partially reverse the reduced T4 to T3 conversion associated with obesity.[81] Seventy obese patients with "normal" standard thyroid function tests were treated with 20 mcg of straight T3 for 6 weeks. While the dose was not high enough to completely reverse the reduced T4 to T3 conversion seen with obesity, there was a significant reduction in a number of cardiovascular risk factors, including cholesterol and markers for insulin resistance. There were no side effects in any of the patients. The author concludes "T3 may be considered to ameliorate some of the risk factors associated with abdominal obesity, particularly in some subgroups of obese women with a relative resistance to thyroid hormones possibly dependent on decreased peripheral deiodination of thyroxine (T4)."[81]

Thus, supplementation with time-release T3 preparations to normalize the reduced intracellular T3 levels is appropriate in such patients despite so-called "normal" levels. However, T4-only preparations do not address the physiologic abnormalities of such patients and should be considered inappropriate for obese patients or those with insulin resistance, leptin resistance, or diabetes, as they do not address the physiologic abnormalities in this group.

Leptin

The hormone leptin is a major regulator of body weight and metabolism. The body secretes leptin as weight is gained to signal the brain (specifically the hypothalamus) that there are adequate energy (fat) stores. The hypothalamus should then stimulate metabolic processes that result in weight loss, including a reduction in hunger, an increased satiety with eating, an increase in resting metabolism, and an increase in lipolysis (fat breakdown). New research has found that this leptin signaling is dysfunctional in the majority of people who have difficultly or are unable to lose weight.[82–86] The problem is not in the production of leptin, since studies show that the majority of overweight individuals who are having difficulty losing weight actually have a leptin resistance. Among these patients, leptin is unable to elicit its normal effects to stimulate weight loss;[82–86] this leptin resistance is sensed as starvation, so multiple mechanisms are activated to increase, rather than burn fat stores.[82–111]

Leptin resistance is known to suppress D1 and stimulate D2 in the pituitary, resulting in reduced cellular T3 and serum TSH.[75,112–117] A study by Cettour-Rose et al. published in *American Journal of Physiology, Endocrinology and Metabolism* demonstrated that the physiologic reversal of leptin resistance can restore deiodinase activity except in the presence of elevated rT3.[114] Thus, elevated leptin (above 10) levels reduce cellular T3 and suppress TSH, making TSH an unreliable indicator of thyroid status, especially in the presence of elevated rT3. For those who have difficulty losing weight, a leptin level above 10 may indicate that low intracellular thyroid levels are contributing to this difficulty, especially if combined with a high normal or elevated rT3 (above 150).

Exercise

It has been shown that women or men who perform vigorous exercise, especially when associated with dieting, have reduced T4 to T3 conversion and increased rT3, which may be counteracting some of the positive effects that goes along with exercise (e.g., weight loss).[256,257] Therefore, when determining cellular thyroid function among individuals who exercise and/or diet, T3 and rT3 levels may be more diagnostic than TSH and T4 levels.

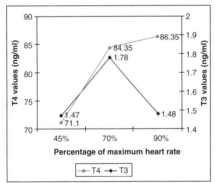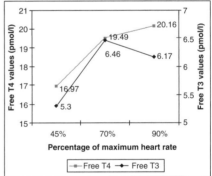

Vigorous exercise and dieting can reduce T4 to T3 conversion.[537]

Inflammation Associated with Common Conditions

The inflammatory cytokines IL-1, IL-6, C-reactive protein (CRP), and TNF-alpha will significantly decrease D1 activity and reduce tissue T3 levels.[133–141] Inflammatory conditions, such as those listed below, are associated with a decreased T4 to T3 conversion in the body and a relative tissue hypothyroidism:

Physical or emotional stress[258–263]
Obesity[263–267]
Diabetes[263,264,268]
Depression[269–272]
Menopause (surgical or natural)[273]
Heart disease[263,274,275]
Autoimmune disease (lupus, Hashimoto's, multiple sclerosis, arthritis, etc)[142,143,188,276]
Injury[277]
Chronic infection[278,279]
Cancer[280–282]

In addition, the inflammatory cytokines will increase the activity of D2 and suppress TSH despite reduced peripheral T3 levels, making a normal TSH an unreliable indicator of tissue thyroid levels.[133–141]

There is a direct inverse correlation between CRP and tissue T3,[140,283] so individuals with elevated CRP (greater than 3 mg/l) or other inflammatory cytokines will have a significant reduction in cellular T3 levels. The suppression of intracellular T3 levels corresponds to an elevation of CRP, despite serum thyroid tests being "normal".[140,283] Thus, if any inflammation is present (see the above disorders), the body will likely have inadequate cellular T3 levels for optimal functioning. In addition, the pituitary will have increased levels of T3, resulting in a suppression of TSH that could potentially be inappropriately interpreted as "normal" thyroid levels.

Due to the reduced T4 to T3 conversion induced by the inflammatory conditions mentioned above, effective treatment will likely include T3 (combination or time-release T3). Inflammation will also stimulate D3, which increases the production of RT3, further contributing to cellular hypothyroidism by suppressing the intracellular conversion of T4 to T3, and blocking the T3 receptor inside the cell.[284] Therefore, free T3 and rT3 levels along with other clinical parameters should be utilized to determine optimal thyroid treatment, rather than just using TSH alone.

Environmental Toxins

POPs have emerged as important contributors to many of today's chronic diseases, perhaps more so than many well-accepted risk factors. POPs display synergistic and low-dose effects that have allowed them to escape the closer regulatory scrutiny that is given to high dose and directly mutagenic toxins. At least part of their toxicity appears to be mediated via epigenetic mechanisms, which now appear to be on par with genetic polymorphisms for clinical importance. Unlike genetic mutations, epigenetic modifications appear to be reversible with appropriate interventions. While much remains to be determined, avoidance of exposure seems highly indicated, as does nutritional support of relevant metabolic pathways, including glutathione synthesis and methylation, particularly during crucial periods of development.[285]

The evidence base supporting a link between POP exposure and a wide spectrum of diseases continues to grow, particularly for cardiometabolic and neurological conditions. These lipophilic and stable substances include a range of substances, such as PCBs, organochlorine pesticides, PDBEs, plastics, phthalates, PCDDs, and polychlorinated dibenzofurans (PCDFs), many of which are widespread globally. PCBs resemble thyroid hormone structurally and have been shown to disrupt thyroid function *in vivo*.[286] Blood concentrations of PCBs negatively correlate with circulating thyroid hormone levels.[287,288] Immunomodulatory effects of PCBs may be responsible for increases in TPO antibodies and subsequent interference with iodide transport seen in populations with long-term exposure to PCBs. One study reported that as PBDE increased, increased subclinical hyperthyroidism was seen in pregnant women.[289]

In a large cross-sectional study of adults, part of the National Health and Nutrition Examination Survey (NHANES) 1999–2002, lipid-adjusted serum levels of six POPs were all found to have a strong positive and dose-dependent correlation with diabetes risk. Indeed, individuals with the highest levels of all six had a 38-fold increase in risk for diabetes compared to those who had serum levels below the limit of detection. Additionally, in those patients with undetectable levels of these six POPs, no association was found between obesity and diabetes, suggesting that excessive adipose tissue may contribute to the risk of diabetes primarily by enhancing the storage and/or toxicity of POPs.[290] POPs have been shown to affect several of the root causes of impaired glucose regulation, including the development of insulin resistance, dyslipidemia, inflammation, mitochondrial inhibition, and a decline in pancreatic beta-cell function, and increased risk of prediabetes and obesity.[291–293]

Numerous toxins, including plastics such as bisphenol-A, pesticides, mercury, and flame retardants (e.g., PBDE), have been shown to block tissue TRs and reduce the conversion of T4 to T3 with resultant low tissue levels of thyroid that are not detected by standard blood tests.[144–162,294] The structure of PBDE is similar to thyroid hormone and can displace T4 from serum thyroid binding protein transthyretin (TTR).[295]

D2 is up to 1000 times less sensitive to suppression by toxins and mineral or hormonal deficiencies,[30–34,251,296–298] as well as being 1000 times more efficient at converting T4 to T3.[30,296] Thus, D1 in the body is suppressed by toxins, pesticides, and plastics at levels that are hundreds to thousands times lower than are required to suppress D2 in the pituitary. This is proving to be a major problem for the population in general, as levels of plastics and other toxins commonly found in individuals (toxins that are considered "normal" exposure) result in reduced T3 levels in all tissues with the exception of the pituitary (which is resistant to the effect of toxins). Because the pituitary is relatively unaffected, the reduced tissue thyroid levels are not detected by standard TSH testing.

Toxins such as bisphenol-A are ubiquitous in the environment and can leach into food and liquids from plastic water bottles and the lining of aluminum cans. This contamination can significantly block thyroid activity in all tissues more than in the pituitary, potentially contributing to weight gain, fatigue, and depression.[156,157,160,161,299] Levels of a number of thyroid-blocking toxins (e.g., bisphenol-A and PBDEs), are significantly higher among individuals in the United States (PBDEs being especially high in California),[299,300] resulting in reduced T3 effects in all tissues that is undetected by standard thyroid testing. This is potentially a significant contributor to the epidemic of obesity and depression in the US, when compared to other regions of the world.

Cadmium and mercury toxicity can reduce T4 to T3 conversion. Cadmium and mercury can deplete levels of selenium and decreased selenium can decrease the function of the deiodinases as well as GPX, which can result in increased lipid peroxidation.[301,302] Halogens such as perchlorate, chlorine, fluorine, and bromine can also impair thyroid function in a variety of ways (see *Chapter 3: Hypothyroidism*).

Avoidance of POP exposure is primarily accomplished through dietary means. Because these toxins bioaccumulate in adipose tissue and up the food chain, an organic and largely plant-based diet may be the most effective for reducing exposure. For example, diet has been shown to be the largest source of exposure to OP pesticides in young children, and an organic diet dramatically reduces urinary metabolites levels.[303,304] Diet is not the only source of exposure to many POPs; phthalates are found in many personal care products, and bisphenol-A in many food containers. Exercise, particularly more vigorous exercise, has also shown to be helpful. Glutathione conjugation of toxins is the primary way the body has for ridding itself of POPs. Providing support for glutathione synthesis either directly or with precursors such as N-acetylcysteine may be very helpful. Also, providing adequate methyl donors, such as folic acid, betaine, B12, etc., appears to reduce the risk of conditions ranging from autism to cardiovascular disease, at least in part via epigenetic mechanisms, and may be indicated in those with high exposure and/or signs of impaired methylation capacity.[305,306]

Testosterone

Low testosterone in men will result in a lowering of D1 activity without changing pituitary D2.[307] Thus, a drop in testosterone will result in lower T3 tissue levels without producing an elevation in TSH.[307,308] Environmental factors, including pesticides, plastics, and other pollutants, have resulted in a significant decrease in the average testosterone levels for men. Therefore, many men exposed to these contaminants will experience at least a relative testosterone deficiency.[309] Unfortunately, major laboratories have reduced the "normal" range of free testosterone in order to maintain the 95 percentile. As a result, many men with abnormally low levels of testosterone will be inappropriately considered normal.

Male diabetics and those with insulin resistance are particularly susceptible to low testosterone, which further suppresses D1 and tissue T3 levels, and perpetuates the weight gain or contributes to an inability to lose weight, which in turn exacerbates the original disorder (i.e., diabetes and insulin resistance).[310–312]

Growth Hormone

Growth hormone deficiency reduces T4 to T3 conversion and increases rT3 while supplementation with growth hormone improves the conversion of T4 to T3 and reduces rT3.[220,255,313,314] Thus, the age-related decline in growth hormone contributes to reduced T3 levels and is not detected by TSH and T4 testing.

Individual Variations in Deiodinase

The relative amounts of D1, D2, and D3 vary within different tissue types among different individuals[315] and under varying conditions.[37,40–50,52–54,128–131,144–148,154–157,198–201,242,251,316] This can result in a number of possible hypothyroid symptoms, depending on the relative level of T3 in each tissue. Unfortunately, serum thyroid levels often do not accurately reflect intracellular tissue levels or levels within any particular tissue.

Signaling Pathways and Peripheral Regulation

Thyroid hormone signaling primarily results from the interaction of nuclear thyroid hormone receptors (TRs) with specific target gene promoters.[317] This process is modulated by the binding of thyroid hormone to the TRs, which results in alterations in the composition of the transcriptional complex that can either enhance or repress transcription.[318-320] This signaling pathway is not only sensitive to changes in serum thyroid hormone concentrations (e.g., Graves' hyperthyroidism or Hashimoto's thyroiditis), but is also impacted by local activation or inactivation of thyroid hormone specific to individual tissues, even as serum hormone concentrations remain normal.[321-323] This signaling via thyroid hormone is tightly regulated in both a time- and tissue-specific fashion via the expression pattern of deiodinases. For example, signals such as bile acids, sonic hedgehog, and exposure to cold can result in the regulation of the deiodinases in the tissues through activation and deactivation.

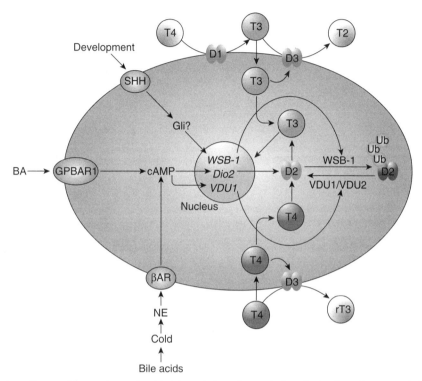

The thyroid hormone signaling pathway is under tight peripheral regulation in both a time- and tissue-specific fashion via expression of the deiodinases.[317]

Deiodinase Enzyme Summary

Based on an improved understanding of thyroid physiology that includes the local control of intracellular activation and deactivation of thyroid hormones by deiodinases, researchers now know that standard thyroid tests often do not reflect the thyroid status of various tissues in the body (other than the pituitary). This is especially true with physiologic and emotional stress, depression, dieting, obesity, leptin and insulin resistance, diabetes, CFS and fibromyalgia, inflammation, autoimmune disease, and/or systemic illness. Consequently, it is inappropriate to rely on TSH as an adequate indicator of the body's overall thyroid level status, especially in the presence of any of the above mentioned disorders.

In order to appropriately evaluate and treat thyroid dysfunction, it is important that clinicians understand the limitations of standard thyroid testing and assess potential signs and symptoms of thyroid hormone imbalance despite normal standard thyroid tests. To this end, the free T3/rT3 ratio can be valuable for evaluating potential deiodinase dysregulation. However, even patients with high T3 levels and low rT3 levels can still have low body temperatures and low thyroid symptoms that can respond well to T3 therapy and remain improved even after the treatment has been discontinued. The symptoms of poor T4 to T3 conversion correlate extremely well with the body temperature. With symptoms, the temperature is low and the symptoms frequently resolve when the temperature is normalized with treatment. Another useful method for properly assessing of tissue thyroid levels is measuring the relaxation phase of the muscle reflex, and calculating the basal metabolic rate.

Triac/Tetrac

Physiologic stress, depression, emotional stress, and chronic dieting also shunt thyroid hormones down alternate pathways resulting in reduced cellular thyroid activity but would not be detected by standard blood tests. This abnormal metabolic pathway converts T4 into a substance called tetraiodothyroacetic acid (Tetrac), and T3 into a substance called triiodothyroacetic acid (Triac).[324-328] The levels of Tetrac and Triac increase by a factor of 2–12 with dieting or physiologic stress.[325-329] Both these substances are selectively taken up by the pituitary and suppress TSH production, but have no effect on the rest of the body.[324,325,330-333] Everts et al. found that Triac is twice as potent as T3 at suppressing TSH secretion and 20 times more potent than T4 at suppressing TSH secretion.[333] Thus, with physiologic or emotional stress, chronic dieting, depression, and inflammation, the pituitary T3 levels do not correlate with T3 levels in the rest of the body (i.e., the TSH does not rise despite significant cellular hypothyroidism). The ubiquity of these conditions is yet another reason that the TSH is not a reliable or sensitive marker of an individual's true thyroid status.

Thyroid Hormone Transport

Given the clinical significance of thyroid hormone transport, any physician who evaluates or treats thyroid dysfunction must have a clear and thorough understanding of this topic. Unfortunately, only a small fraction of physicians and endocrinologists grasp even the basics of thyroid transport. When one understands the physiology involved with thyroid hormone transport, it becomes clear that standard blood tests (e.g., TSH and T4 levels) cannot be used to accurately determine intracellular and tissue thyroid levels. This is especially true in the presence of a wide range of common conditions such as chronic and acute dieting, anxiety, stress, insulin resistance, obesity, diabetes, depression and bipolar disorder, hyperlipidemia (i.e., high cholesterol and triglycerides), CFS, fibromyalgia, neurodegenerative diseases (Alzheimer's, Parkinson's, and multiple sclerosis), migraines, cardiomyopathy, and aging.

Serum thyroid levels are, of course, commonly used as an indication of cellular thyroid activity. However, in order to have biological activity, T4 and T3 must cross the cellular membrane from the serum into the target cells. It follows that the activity of these transport processes may have a significant impact on the biological activity of these thyroid hormones. For about two and a half decades, it was assumed that the uptake of thyroid into the cells occurs by simple diffusion, and that the driving force for this diffusion is the concentration of free hormones in the serum. This "free hormone" or "diffusion hypothesis" was formulated in 1960 and assumes that the concentration of free hormones (free T4 and free T3) in the serum determines the rate and extent of uptake into the cell and thus intracellular concentration of thyroid hormone.

More recent data has demonstrated that this hypothesized mechanism of thyroid uptake into the cell is completely inaccurate.[334-376] Instead, the medical literature clearly shows that the rate-limiting (and most important) step associated with thyroid hormone transport involves active (requiring energy) rather than passive transport.[334-399] Despite accumulating evidence to the contrary, this incorrect "diffusion hypothesis" continues to be taught in medical school and is believed to be true by most physicians and endocrinologists.

Conditions Associated with Abnormal Thyroid Transport

Since the transport of thyroid hormones into the cell is energy dependent, any condition associated with reduced production of the cellular energy (i.e., mitochondrial dysfunction) will also be associated with reduced transport of thyroid hormone into the cell. This can result in cellular hypothyroidism despite having standard blood tests in the "normal" range. Conditions linked with reduced mitochondrial function and impaired thyroid transport include:

Insulin resistance, diabetes, and obesity[400–404]
Chronic and acute dieting[337,383,398,405–412]
Diabetes[401,413–416]
Depression[413,417–419]
Anxiety[413,420]
Bipolar depression[413,417,421,422]
Neurodegenerative diseases[413,423–427]
Aging[413,414,428–440]
Chronic fatigue syndrome (CFS)[413,441,442]
Fibromyalgia[413,443,444]
Migraines[413]
Chronic infections[413]
Physiologic stress and anxiety[413,419]
Cardiovascular disease[413,439,444–446]
Inflammation and chronic illness[413,447–449]
High cholesterol and triglyceride levels[390,392,404,405,450]

Thus, standard blood tests can be very unreliable if any of these common conditions are present.[334–405,413–445,450]

The exact cause of the inhibition of thyroid hormone transport is unknown, but it is clear that there are a number of substances that are produced by the body in response to dieting and physiologic stress that negatively affect this transport process.[338,374] For instance, studies clearly show that cell cultures incubated with serum from physiologically stressed or dieting individuals exhibit a dramatic reduction in the uptake of T4 into cells. This reduction correlates with the degree of stress.[374,375]

It has also been demonstrated that there are a variety of distinct and specific transporters that are necessary for the transport of T4 and T3 into the cell. The transporter for T4 is much more energy dependent than the transporter for T3 (see figure).[338,373,374,381,384,385,398] Even slight reductions in cellular energy (i.e., mitochondrial function) can result in a dramatic reduction in the uptake of T4 while the uptake of T3 is much less affected.[338,374,394,399] Thus, the conditions listed above are particularly linked with impaired T4 transport, resulting in cellular hypothyroidism. When a dysfunctional transport system leaves the interior of the cell low in T4, it can in turn cause serum T4 to be high or high-normal. This is why cellular hypothyroidism is not routinely detected by serum T4 levels. The TSH level will also not identify cellular hypothyroidism because the pituitary has completely different transporters that are not energy dependent. Therefore, while the rest of body has impaired thyroid transport, the pituitary experiences increased transport activity.

Pituitary Thyroid Transport Determines TSH Levels

As discussed previously, the pituitary is different than every cell in the body with different deiodinases and different high affinity TRs. It is also shown to have unique thyroid transporters that are also distinct from those in the rest of the body.[334,350,376,382,384,387,391–393] The pituitary thyroid hormone transporters are not energy dependent and can maintain or even increase the uptake of T4 and T3 during low energy states. This stands in stark contrast to transporters found in other parts of the body that would experience significantly reduced transport under similar circumstances.[334,350,355,376,380,384,387,391–393]

The pituitary T4 and T3 transporters are also somewhat immune to numerous environmental toxins and other substances produced by the body during physiologic stress and calorie reduction that would inhibit thyroid transport into other cells of the body (e.g., bilirubin and fatty acids). Since thyroid hormone uptake in the pituitary is relatively unaffected by outside factors, intracellular hypothyroidism is not reflected by TSH testing. Thus, TSH is a poor marker for cellular thyroid function in any tissue other than the pituitary.[334,376,387] Even common medications including benzodiazepines such as diazepam (Valium®), lorazapam (Atavan®), and alprazolam (Xanax®) are shown to inhibit T3 uptake into the cells of the body but have no effect on transport of T3 into the pituitary.[393]

This difference in pituitary thyroid transport was investigated by St Germain and Galton. They demonstrated that the pituitary does not respond to calorie restriction (i.e., dieting) in the same way as the rest of the body. The dramatically reduced serum T4 and T3 levels that accompany dieting are associated with an increase in pituitary T3 receptor saturation (i.e., percent of activated T3 receptors), which results in a decrease in TSH even when serum levels were reduced by 50%.[387]

Studies show that numerous conditions are associated with reduced transport of thyroid hormone into the cells, which can lead to dramatic cellular hypothyroidism that may not be detected by standard blood tests. This is because TSH will be normal and serum T4 may actually increase due to reduced uptake into the cells.[386] Most physicians and endocrinologists are unaware of the functional differences in cellular thyroid activity between the pituitary and the rest of the body. Physicians are often quick to declare a person with numerous symptoms of low thyroid as having "normal" thyroid function based solely on a normal TSH and T4 level.

In the *Journal of Endocrinology*, Wassen et al. concludes that "thyroid hormone transport into the pituitary is regulated differently than that in the liver."[382] Therefore, a high-normal T4 and low-normal TSH often leads an endocrinologist to erroneously make a diagnosis of "normal" or "high-normal" thyroid level, when in fact, the patient is suffering from low cellular thyroid levels.

Stress

Chronic emotional or physiologic stress can cause a significant reduction in T4 levels within the cells of the body while the pituitary remains relatively unaffected. A study published in the *Journal of Clinical Endocrinology and Metabolism* examined the effect of adding serum from different groups of individuals to cell cultures and measuring the amount of T4 uptake into the cell. Their data suggests that the serum from those with significant physiologic stress inhibits the uptake (transport) of T4 into the cell, while the serum from non-physiological stress has no effect. This shows that serum T4 levels are artificially elevated in physiologically stressed individuals and are thus poor markers for tissue thyroid levels in this patient population.[337]

A number of studies have shown that significant physiologic stress reduces cellular uptake of T4 and T3 by nearly 50%.[395,396,447–449] Arem et al. found that with significant physiological stress, tissue levels of T4 and T3 were dramatically reduced by up to 79% without a corresponding increase in TSH. It is also important to note that significant inter-patient variability exists with respect to T4 and T3 levels among different tissues in the body, which may explain the wide range of symptoms caused by tissue-specific hypothyroidism. Furthermore, this variation is not reflected by TSH or serum T4 and T3 levels.[388]

Another study published in the *Journal of Clinical Endocrinology and Metabolism* also confirmed that serum from physiologically stressed individuals is linked with an up to 44% reduction in T4 uptake into the cell. Data from this study suggests that the ratio of free T3 to rT3 was the most accurate marker for reduced cellular uptake of T4 in this patient population.[375]

A number of substances produced in response to physiologic stress or calorie reduction have been identified, and include 3-carboxy-4-methyl-5-propyl-2-furan-propanoic acid (CMPF), indoxyl sulfate, bilirubin, and fatty acids.[334,336,389,390,392] When these substances are added to cell cultures in concentrations comparable to those normally seen in patients, it results in a 27–42% reduction in cellular uptake of T4, but has no effect on T4 or T3 uptake into the pituitary.[334,350,389,390,392]

Dieting

In a highly controlled study, Brownell et al. found that after repeated cycles of dieting, weight loss occurred at half the rate and weight gain occurred at three times the rate compared to controls with the same calorie intake.[412] Chronic and yo-yo dieting, which is an extremely common practice, has been shown to reduce cellular T4 uptake by 25–50%.[336,381,406,408–410] This decrease in cellular uptake of T4 is generally not detected by standard laboratory testing, and can make successful weight loss exceedingly difficult. Experts recommend measuring the free T3/rT3 ratio in order to appropriately identify this clinical problem. Many physicians that treat WTS feel that the disposition for prolonged depression of metabolism from chronic dieting can often be reversed by resetting the thyroid hormone pathways by reducing T4 and RT3 levels for a time with T3 therapy.

In a study published in the *American Journal of Physiology-Endocrinology and Metabolism*, van der Heyden et al. investigated the effect of calorie restriction (dieting) on the transport of T4 and T3 into the cell.[381] They found that obese individuals in the process of dieting exhibited a 50% reduction of T4 into the cell and a 25% reduction of T3 into the cell. This is thought to be due to the reduced cellular energy stores, demonstrating that in such patients standard thyroid blood tests are not accurate indicators of intracellular thyroid levels. This also explains why it is so difficult for obese patients to lose weight because, as calories are decreased, thyroid utilization is reduced and metabolism drops. Again, this type of thyroid hormone transport dysfunction (resulting in intracellular hypothyroidism) is not detected by standard TSH, T4, and T3 testing. Among these patients, assessing the free T3/rT3 ratio can aid in the diagnosis of reduced uptake of thyroid hormones (although even patients with high T3 and low rT3 levels can sometimes respond well to empiric T3 therapy). Additionally, there are increased levels of free fatty acids in the serum with chronic dieting, which further suppresses T4 uptake into the cells and exacerbates cellular hypothyroidism.[389,390,404,405,408]

Many overweight individuals fail to lose weight with dieting. While many assume these people are doing a poor job of dieting, it has been shown, however, that chronic dieting in overweight individuals results in increased levels of non-esterified fatty acids (NEFAs), which suppresses T4 uptake into the cells.[336] This suppressed T4 uptake can cause a reduction in intracellular T4 levels and subsequent T4 to T3 conversion as well as reducing metabolism.[336,406,408–410]

rT3

TSH and serum T4 levels do not correlate well with intracellular thyroid levels. Additionally, free T3 will also tend to appear to be higher in the blood than it actually is in the cells in the presence of reduced cellular energy due to its reduced uptake into the cell. Also, the transporter for rT3 is similar to that of T4, in that it is energy dependent and has the same kinetics as the T4 transporter.[339,374,377,394,398,399] Thus, rT3 can be a useful indicator of diminished transport of T4 into the cell.[377]

Thus, a high rT3 demonstrates that there is either an inhibition of rT3 uptake into the cell and/or there is increased conversion of T4 to rT3. These always occur together in a wide range of physiologic conditions, and both can cause reduced intracellular T4 and T3 levels as well as cellular hypothyroidism. Thus, rT3 is an excellent marker for identifying reduced cellular T4 and T3 levels that would not normally be detected by TSH or serum T4 and T3 tests. Since increased rT3 is a marker for reduced uptake of T4 and reduced T4 to T3 conversion, any increase (high or high normal) in rT3 is not only suggestive of tissue hypothyroidism but also suggests that T4-only replacement would not be considered optimal therapy.

The free T3/rT3 ratio is proving to be the next best physiologic marker of intracellular thyroid levels, next to the body temperature. Some patients with high free T3/rT3 ratios may still have low body temperatures and low thyroid symptoms that respond well to T3 therapy. Researchers are finding that the most accurate measure of the adequacy of thyroid levels and treatment in the tissues of the body is the signs and symptoms of the effects of thyroid. There are many signs and symptoms, but one key sign is the body temperature. Even patients with hyperthyroidism (or excessive T4 therapy) can have high rT3 levels, low body temperatures, and hypothyroid symptoms.

Treatment

T4-only replacement with products such as Synthroid® and Levoxyl® are the most widely accepted forms of thyroid replacement. This is based on a widely held assumption that the body will convert what it needs to the biologically active form (T3). Based on this theory, most physicians and endocrinologists believe that the normalization of TSH with a T4 preparation demonstrates adequate tissue levels of thyroid. This assumption, however, had never been directly tested until two studies were published.[451,452] The first study investigated whether or not giving T4-only preparations will provide adequate T3 levels in varying tissues. Plasma TSH, T4, and T3 levels and 10 different tissue levels of T4 and T3 were measured after the infusion of 12–13 days of T4. This study demonstrated that the normalization of plasma TSH and T4 levels with T4-only preparations provide adequate tissue T3 levels to only a few tissues, including the pituitary (hence the normal TSH), but almost every other tissue was deficient. The study demonstrated that it is often impossible to achieve normal tissue levels of T3 by giving T4-only preparations unless supra-physiological levels of T4 are given. The authors conclude: "It is evident that neither plasma T4 nor plasma T3 alone permit the prediction of the degree of change in T4 and T3 concentrations in tissues … the current replacement therapy of hypothyroidism [giving T4] should no longer be considered adequate …"[453]

The second study compared plasma TSH, T4, and T3 levels and 13 different tissue levels of T4 and T3 when T4 or T4/T3 treatments were utilized.[451] This study found that a combination of T4/T3 is required to normalize tissue levels of T3. The study found that the pituitary was able to maintain normal levels of T3 despite the rest of the body being hypothyroid on T4-only preparations. Under normal conditions it was shown that the pituitary will have 7 to 60 times the concentration of T3 of other tissues of the body; and when thyroid levels drop, the pituitary was shown to have 40 to 650 times the concentration of T3 of other tissues. Thus, the pituitary is unique in its ability to concentrate T3 in the presence of diminished thyroid levels, whereas other tissues in the body cannot. Consequently, pituitary levels of T3 and the subsequent level of TSH are poor measures of tissue hypothyroidism, as almost the entire body can be severely hypothyroid despite having a normal TSH level.[451]

These studies add to the large body of medical literature demonstrating that pituitary thyroid levels are not indicative of other tissues in the body. They also show that the TSH level is a poor indicator of a proper thyroid dose. These studies also demonstrate that it is impossible to achieve normal tissue thyroid levels with T4 preparations such as Synthroid® and Levoxyl®. Given this data, it is no surprise that the majority of patients on T4 preparations will continue to suffer from symptoms of hypothyroidism despite being told their levels are "normal." Patients on T4-only preparations should seek out a physician who is well versed in the medical literature and understands the physiologic limitations and inadequacy of commonly used thyroid preparations.

The dramatic reduction of T4 cellular uptake associated with a wide variety of conditions (T3 being less affected) also explains why T4 preparations are often associated with poor clinical response and continued residual symptoms. This also sets up a situation where the ordering physician unwittingly assumes that the residual symptoms are unrelated to low thyroid, because serum levels look "good", and the physician is unaware of the inner workings of thyroid hormone transport. As stated by Hennemann et al. in *Endocrine Reviews*: "Even a small decrease in cellular ATP concentration results in a major reduction in the transport of T4 (and rT3) but only slightly affects T3 uptake."[338] This makes it inappropriate to use T4-only preparations if treating any condition associated with reduced mitochondrial function or ATP production, such as:

Insulin resistance, diabetes, and obesity[400–404]
Chronic and acute dieting[337,383,398,406–412]
Diabetes[401,413–416]
Depression[413,417–419]
Anxiety[413,420]
Bipolar depression[413,417,421,422]
Neurodegenerative diseases[413,423–427]
Aging[413,414,428–440]
Chronic fatigue syndrome (CFS)[413,441,442]
Fibromyalgia[413,443,444]
Migraines[413]
Chronic infections[413]
Physiologic stress and anxiety[413,419]
Cardiovascular disease[413,439,444,445,446]
Inflammation and chronic illness[413,447–449]

In addition to the above conditions, high levels of cholesterol, fatty acids, or triglyceride can selectively inhibit T4 (as opposed to T3) transport into the cell,[389–392,404,405,408,450] making T4-only preparations physiologically inappropriate for individuals with high cholesterol or triglycerides. This is also the case with chronic dieting, which dramatically increases serum free fatty acids.[405] Given this evidence, it should not be surprising that T3 has been shown to be superior in such patient populations.

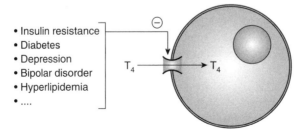

Conditions that decrease thyroid hormone transport.

Fraser et al. investigated the correlation between tissue thyroid activity and serum blood tests (i.e., TSH, free T4, and T3) and published their results in the *British Medical Journal*. The authors concluded that "The serum concentration of thyroid stimulation hormone is unsatisfactory as the thyrotrophs in the anterior pituitary are more sensitive to changes in the concentration of thyroxin in the circulation than other tissues, which rely more on triiodothyronine (T3)." They found that a suppressed or undetectable TSH was not an indication or a reliable marker of over-replacement or hyperthyroidism. They state,

> "It is clear that serum thyroid hormone and thyroid stimulating hormone concentrations cannot be used with any degree of confidence to classify patients as receiving satisfactory, insufficient, or excessive amounts of thyroxine replacement ... The poor diagnostic sensitivity and high false positive rates associated with such measurements render them virtually useless in clinical practice ... Further adjustments to the dose should be made according to the patient's clinical response."[452]

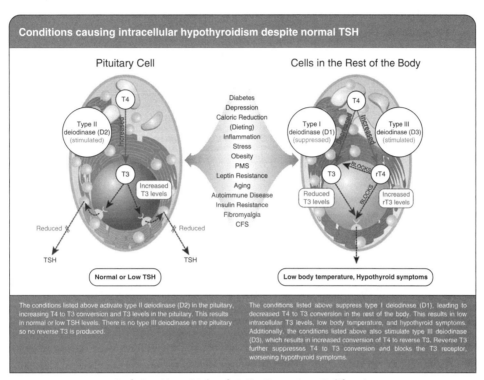

Ref: Dr. Kent Holtorf, MD: Torrance, California

The likelihood that a suppressed TSH actually indicates over-replacement or hyperthyroidism has been determined to be only 16%, making it an inaccurate and inappropriate marker for determining an appropriate thyroid replacement dose. TSH becomes an even worse indicator under the following conditions:

Insulin resistance or obesity[400–404]
Chronic dieting[337,383,398,405,406–412]
Diabetes[401,413–416]
Depression[413,417–419]
Bipolar depression[413,417,421,422]
Neurodegenerative diseases[413,423–427]
Older age[413,414,428–440]
Chronic fatigue syndrome (CFS)[413,441,442]
Fibromyalgia[413,443,444]
Migraines[413]
Chronic infections[413]
Stress or anxiety[413,419,420]
Heart failure or cardiovascular disease[413,439,444–446]
Migraines[413]
Inflammation or a chronic illness[413,447–449]
High cholesterol or triglyceride levels[389,390,392,404,405,408,450]

In a study published in the *British Medical Journal*, Meir et al. also investigated the correlation between TSH and tissue thyroid effect. It was shown that the TSH level had no correlation with tissue thyroid levels and could not be used to determine a proper or optimal thyroid replacement dose. The authors concluded that "TSH is a poor measure for estimating the clinical and metabolic severity of primary overt thyroid failure .... We found no correlations between the different parameters of target tissues and serum TSH." They stated that signs and symptoms of thyroid effect and not the TSH should be used to determine the proper replacement dose.[454]

Alevizaki et al. also studied the accuracy of using TSH to determine the proper thyroid replacement dose in T4-treated individuals. The study found that such a practice, although common, results in the majority of tissues being hypothyroid, except for the pituitary. They conclude, "TSH levels used to monitor substitution, mostly regulated by intracellular T3 in the pituitary, may not be such a good indicator of adequate thyroid hormone action in all tissues."[455]

In a study published in the *Journal of Clinical Endocrinology and Metabolism*, Zulewski et al. also investigated the accuracy of TSH to determine proper thyroid replacement. The study found that the TSH was not a useful measure of optimal or proper thyroid replacement, as there was no correlation between the TSH and tissue thyroid levels. Serum T4 and T3 levels had some correlation, with T3 being a better indicator than T4. In contrast, a thorough assessment of signs and symptoms of hypothyroidism was shown to be the most accurate method to determine proper replacement dosing. The authors also agreed that it is improper to use TSH as the major determinant of the optimal thyroid replacement dose, stating "The ultimate test of whether a patient is experiencing the effects of too much or too little thyroid hormone is not the measurement of hormone concentration in the blood but the effect of thyroid hormones on the peripheral tissues [symptoms]."[456]

Thyroid Hormone Transport Summary

The most important determinant of thyroid activity is the intracellular level of T3, and the most important determinant of the intracellular T3 level is the activity of the cellular thyroid transporters.[334-399] Reduced thyroid transport into the cell is seen with a wide range of common conditions, including insulin resistance, diabetes, depression, bipolar disorder, hyperlipidemia (high cholesterol and triglycerides), CFS, fibromyalgia, neurodegenerative diseases (Alzheimer's, Parkinson's, and multiple sclerosis), migraines, stress, anxiety, chronic dieting, and aging.[334-376,378,381,383-385,390,392,398,400,404-450]

This high incidence of reduced cellular thyroid transport seen with these conditions makes standard thyroid tests a poor indicator of cellular thyroid levels. The pituitary has different transporters than every other tissue in the body, and is not very energy dependent, unlike the thyroid transporters in the rest of the body. Furthermore, the pituitary is much more resilient in the face of such conditions. Because the pituitary remains relatively unaffected, there is no elevation in TSH despite widespread tissue hypothyroidism, making the TSH an inaccurate marker for tissue T3 levels.[334,336,337,350,355,376,382,384,387,391-393]

The reduced thyroid transport caused by these conditions results in an artificial elevation in serum thyroid levels (especially T4), making T4 a poor marker for tissue thyroid levels as well.[338,373,374,381,384,385,394,398,399] Based on the most current knowledge, an elevated or high-normal rT3 appears to be the best blood test marker for reduced thyroid hormone transport and an indication that a person has low cellular thyroid levels, despite standard thyroid test results such as TSH, free T4, and free T3 being normal.[339,365,374,377,394,398,399,457-504] However, researchers are now rediscovering what many practitioners have known for years, that the best indicators for thyroid status and response to thyroid treatment are the symptoms and signs (such as body temperature).

The intracellular T3 deficiency seen with these conditions often results in a vicious cycle of worsening symptoms that usually goes untreated, especially when standard thyroid tests look normal. It should not come as a surprise that T4 preparations are generally ineffective in the presence of such conditions, while T3 replacement is shown to be beneficial, with potentially dramatic results.[403,414-416,420-422,426,437,440-445,505-529] In the presence of such conditions, it should be understood that significant intracellular hypothyroidism may exist and go undiagnosed by standard blood tests. This is why the free T3/rT3 ratio is recommended in order to aid in such a diagnosis. Thus, assessments that go beyond standard thyroid function tests should be considered, and appropriate supplementation with T3 is also suggested in these patient populations.

Thyroid Resistance

In addition to thyroid hormone conversion dysfunction, evidence suggests that thyroid resistance might well be a secondary response to the initial trigger causing CFS. Although the concept of fatigue in the face of euthyroid was recognized by conventional medicine in the 1950s, it was not until recently that it has gained acceptance again in the medical literature. For example, current case studies and clinical trials are identifying euthyroid patients who exhibit hypothyroid symptoms as having "thyroid resistance." Thyroid resistance shares many of the same symptoms as CFS, including headaches, anxiety, fatigue, and recurring sore throats.

One postulated mechanism for thyroid hormone resistance found in WTS/CFS might be due to a dysregulation in the type I interferon (IFN-alpha/beta) pathway. This results in a sustained upregulation of 2′-5′-oligoadenylate synthetases (2-5OAS). Patients treated with IFN-alpha/beta therapy usually complain of severe fatigue as a limiting side effect, perhaps due to the same effect. The IFN-alpha/beta stimulates the 2-5OAS to make more of three closely related proteins. The amino acid sequences of the 2-5OASL proteins display 96% identity with the partial sequence of the thyroid receptor interacting protein (TRIP). It is hypothesized that the 2-5OASL proteins are TRIP's mechanism of suppressing the TR transactivation and/or possibly destroying the TR by the proteasome. This is perhaps how CFS/WTS patients might have normal TSH values yet have a clinical hypothyroid state in CFS/WTS.[530]

One other mechanism of thyroid resistance found in CFS might be due to a chronic consumptive coagulopathy, which itself might be associated with chronic infections, such as mycoplasmids, and other microbes. It is suggested that supraphysiological doses of thyroid hormone or anti-coagulants and anti-infective agents might be effective treatment options. Current research has not found any clear association between an infectious agent and CFS.[531] However, based on a multi-causal model, it is possible that some infectious agents might contribute to these symptoms for a certain subset of patients, or that it might be a trigger for CFS even after the infection is gone.[532]

Immune system dysfunction might also be involved in a certain amount of CFS cases, as there is evidence of inappropriate cytokine response.[533] While the etiological cause is still not known, it is hypothesized that it might be due to decreased thyroid function. Thyroid resistance has been associated with increased infections, such as chronic sore throats.[532]

Stress stimulates the HPA axis, which leads to increased levels of cortisol, in turn inhibiting thyroid function.[534] Moreover, low thyroid function has been shown to affect cortisol levels.[532] However, the data surrounding this subject is conflicting since some research suggests that hypothyroidism increases cortisol levels, while other studies have found that it decreases cortisol levels.[535] Given that some CFS studies have found cortisol levels to be lower than healthy controls,[536] there is no conclusive evidence that cortisol replacement is an effective treatment for these CFS symptoms. Therefore, cortisol deficiency does not appear to be the main cause of CFS.

In conclusion, CFS/WTS might have a variety of causative factors that compromise the immune system through stress or other insults that upset the body's normal functioning (e.g., viruses, bacteria, toxins, or other triggering agents). After the initial insult to the body, CFS/WTS symptoms remain, perhaps due to thyroid hormone resistance or peripheral thyroid hormone conversion problems. Regardless of the mechanism, WT3 therapy seems to restore metabolism to the vast majority of patients.

[1]   Zoeller RT, Tan SW, Tyl RW. General background on the hypothalamic-pituitary-thyroid (HPT) axis. Crit Rev Toxicol 2007;37(1–2):11–53.
[2]   Dietrich JW, Landgrafe G, Fotiadou EH. TSH and thyrotropic agonists: key actors in thyroid homeostasis. J Thyroid Res 2012;351864(10):30.
[3]   Bizhanova A, Kopp P. Minireview: the sodium-iodide symporter NIS and pendrin in iodide homeostasis of the thyroid. Endocrinology 2009;150(3):1084–90.
[4]   Molina PE. Endocrine physiology. 3rd ed. McGraw-Hill; New York City, USA, p. 81.
[5]   Ruf J, Carayon P. Structural and functional aspects of thyroid peroxidase. Arch Biochem Biophys 2006;445(2):269–77.
[6]   Chardes T, Chapal N, Bresson D, et al. The human anti-thyroid peroxidase autoantibody repertoire in Graves' and Hashimoto's autoimmune thyroid diseases. Immunogenetics 2002;54(3):141–57.
[7]   Lee DH, Jacobs DR Jr, Porta M. Hypothesis: a unifying mechanism for nutrition and chemicals as lifelong modulators of DNA hypomethylation. Environ Health Perspect 2009;117:1799–802.
[8]   Grineva EN, Malakhova TV, Tsoi UA, Smirnov BI. [Efficacy of thyroxine and potassium iodide treatment of benign nodular thyroid lesions]. Ter Arkh 2003;75:72–5.
[9]   Vanderpump MP. The epidemiology of thyroid disease. Br Med Bull 2011;99:39–51.
[10]   Kahaly GJ, Dienes HP, Beyer J, Hommel G. Iodide induces thyroid autoimmunity in patients with endemic goitre: a randomised, double-blind, placebo-controlled trial. Eur J Endocrinol 1998;139:290–7.

11   Gartner R, Gasnier BC, Dietrich JW, Krebs B, Angstwurm MW. Selenium supplementation in patients with autoimmune thyroiditis decreases thyroid peroxidase antibodies concentrations. J Clin Endocrinol Metab 2002;87(4):1687–91.

12   Zagrodzki P, Ratajczak R. Selenium supplementation in autoimmune thyroiditis female patient–effects on thyroid and ovarian functions (case study). Biol Trace Elem Res 2008;126:76–82.

13   Drutel A, Archambeaud F, Caron P. Selenium and the thyroid gland: more good news for clinicians. Clin Endocrinol (Oxf) 2013;78(2):155–64.

14   Berger MM, Reymond MJ. Influence of selenium supplements on the post-traumatic alterations of the thyroid axis: a placebo-controlled trial. Intensive Care Med 2001;27(1):91–100.

15   Arthur JR, Beckett GJ. Thyroid function. British Medical Bulletin 1999;55:658–68.

16   Ertek S, Cicero AF, Caglar O, Erdogan G. Relationship between serum zinc levels, thyroid hormones and thyroid volume following successful iodine supplementation. Hormones 2010;9(3):263–8.

17   Hess SY, Zimmermann MB, Arnold M, Langhans W, Hurrell RF. Iron deficiency anemia reduces thyroid peroxidase activity in rats. J Nutr 2002;132(7):1951–5.

18   Beard JL, Brigham DE, Kelley SK, Green MH. Plasma thyroid hormone kinetics are altered in iron-deficient rats. J Nutr 1998;128(8):1401–8.

19   Smith SM, Finley J, Johnson LK, Lukaski HC. Indices of in vivo and in vitro thyroid hormone metabolism in iron-deficient rats. Nutrition Research 1994;14(5):729–39.

20   Dillman E, Gale C, Green W, et al. Hypothermia in iron deficiency due to altered triiodothyronine metabolism. Am J Physiol 1980;239(5):R377–81.

21   Smith SM, Johnson PE, Lukaski HC. In vitro hepatic thyroid hormone deiodination in iron-deficient rats: effect of dietary fat. Life Sci 1993;53(8):603–9.

22   Eftekhari MH, Keshavarz SA, Jalali M. The relationship between iron status and thyroid hormone concentration in iron-deficient adolescent Iranian girls. Asia Pac J Clin Nutr 2006;15(1):50–55.

23   Zimmermann MB, Köhrle J. The impact of iron and selenium deficiencies on iodine and thyroid metabolism: biochemistry and relevance to public health. Thyroid 2002;12(10):867–78.

24   Beard J, Tobin B, Green W. Evidence for thyroid hormone deficiency in iron-deficient anemic rats. J Nutr 1989;119:772–778.

25   Duntas LH, Papanastasiou L, Mantzou E, Koutras DA. Incidence of sideropenia and effects of iron repletion treatment in women with subclinical hypothyroidism. Exp Clin Endocrinol Diabetes 1999;107(6):356–60.

26   Zimmermann MB. The influence of iron status on iodine utilization and thyroid function. Annu Rev Nutr 2006;26:367–89.

27   Zimmermann MB, Kohrle J. The impact of iron and selenium deficiencies on iodine and thyroid metabolism: biochemistry and relevance to public health. Thyroid 2002;12(10):867–78.

28   Cinemre H, Bilir C, Gokosmanoglu F, Bahcebasi T. Hematologic effects of levothyroxine in iron-deficient subclinical hypothyroid patients: a randomized, double-blind, controlled study. J Clin Endocrinol Metab 2009;94(1):151–6.

29   Moreno M, Berry MJ, Horst C, et al. Activation and inactivation of thyroid hormone by type I iodothyronine deiodinase. FEBS Lett 1994;344 (2-3):143–6.

30   Bianco AC, Salvatore D, Gereben B, Berry MJ, Larsen PR. Biochemistry, cellular and molecular biology, and physiological roles of the iodothyronine selenodeiodinases. Endocrine Reviews 2002;23(1):38–89.

31   Silva JE, Larsen PR. Pituitary nuclear 3,5,3'-triiodothyronine and thyrotropin secretion: an explanation for the effect of thyroxine. Science 1977;198:617–620.

32   Koenig RJ, Leonard JL, Senator D, Rappaport N. Regulation of thyroxine 5'-deiodinase activity by 3,5,3'-triiodothyronine in cultured rat anterior pituitary cells. Endocrinology 1984;115(1):324–329.

33   Silva JE, Dick TE, Larsen PR. The contribution of local tissue thyroxine monodeiodination to the nuclear 3,5,3'-triiodothyroinine in pituitary, liver and kidney of euthyroid rats. Endocrinology 1978;103:1196. Location of D2.

34   Visser TJ, Kaplau MM, Leonard JL, Larsen PR. Evidence for two pathways of iodothyroinine 5'-deiodination in rat pituitary that differ in kinetics, propylthiouracil sensitivity, and response to hypothyroidism. J Clin Invest 1983;71:992.

35   Larsen PR, Silva JE, Kaplan MM. Relationship between circulation and intracellular thyroid hormones: physiological and clinical implications. Endocr Rev 1981;2:87.

36   Kaplan MM. The role of thyroid hormone deiodination in the regulation of hypothalamo-pituitary function progress in neuroendocrinology. Neuroendocrinology 1984;38:254–260.

37   Peeters RP, Geyten SV, Wouters PJ, et al. Tissue thyroid hormone levels in critical illness. J Clin Endocrinol Metab 2005;12:6498–507.

38   Peeters RP, Wouters PJ, Toor HV, et al. Serum 3,3',5-triiodothyronine (rT3) and 3,5,3'-triiodothyronine/rT3 are prognostic markers in critically ill patients and are associated with postmortem tissue deiodinase activities. J Clin Endocrinol Metab 2005;90(8):4559–4565.

39   Campos-Barros A, Hoell T, Musa A, et al. Phenolic and tyrosyl ring iodothyronine deiodination and thyroid hormone concentrations in the human central nervous system. J Clin Endocrinol Metab 1996;81:2179–2185.

40   Chopra IJ, Chopra U, Smith SR, et al. Reciprocal changes in serum concentrations of 3,3',5-triiodothyronine (T3) in systemic illnesses. J Clin Endocrinol Metab 1975;41:1043–9.

41   Chopra IJ, Williams DE, Orgiazzi J, Solomon DH. Opposite effects of dexamethasone on serum concentrations of 3,3',5'-triiodothyronine (reverse T3) and 3,3',5-triiodothyronine (T3). J Clin Endocrinol Metab 1975;41:911–920.

42   Duick DS, Warren DW, Nicoloff JT, Otis CL, Croxson MS. Effect of single dose dexamethasone on the concentration of serum triiodothyronine in man. J Clin Endocrinol Metab 1974;39:1151–1154.

43   Cavalieri RR, Castle JN, McMahon FA. Effects of dexamethasone on kinetics and distribution of triiodothyronine in the rat. Endocrinology 1984;114:215–221.

44   Bianco AC, Nunes MT, Hell NS, Maciel RMB. The role of glucocorticoids in the stress-induced reduction of extrathyroidal 3,5,3'-triiodothyronine generation in rats. Endocrinology 1987;120:1033–1038.

45   DeGroot LJ. Non-thyroidal illness syndrome is functional central hypothyroidism, and if severe, hormone replacement is appropriate in light of present knowledge. J Endocrinol Invest 2003;26:1163–1170.

46   Reed HL, Brice D, Shakir KM, et al. Decreased free fraction of thyroid hormones after prolonged Antarctic residence. J Applied Physiol 1990;69:1467–1472.

47   Forhead AJ, Curtis K, Kaptein E, Visser TJ, Fowden AL. Developmental control of iodothyronine deiodinases by cortisol in the ovine fetus and placenta near term. Endocrinology 2006;147:5988–5994.

48   Nicoloff JT, Fisher DA, Appleman MD. The role of glucocorticoids in the regulation of thyroid function in man. J Clin Invest 1970;49(10): 1922–1929.

49   Brabant G, Brabant A, Ranft U, et al. Circadian and pulsatile thyrotropin secretion in euthyroid man under the influence of thyroid hormone and glucocorticoid administration. J Clin Endocrinol Metab 1987;65:83–88.

50   Benker G, Raida M, Olbricht T, et al. TSH secretion In Cushing's syndrome: relation to glucocorticoid excess, diabetes, goitre, and the "Sick Euthyroid Syndrome". Clin Endocrinol 1990;33(6):777–86.

51   Mebis L, Langouche L, Visser TJ, Van den Berghe G. The type II iodothyronine is up-regulated in skeletal muscle during prolonged critical illness. J Endocrinol Metab 2007;92(8):3330–3333.

52   Linnoila M, Lamberg BA, Potter WZ, Gold PW, Goodwin FK. High reverse T3 levels in manic and unipolar depressed women. Psychiatry Research 1982;6:271–276.

53   Jackson I. The thyroid axis and depression. Thyroid 1998;8(10):951–956.

54   Gitlin M, Altshuler LL, Frye MA, et al. Peripheral thyroid hormones and response to selective serotonin reuptake inhibitors. J Psychiatry Neurosci 2004;29(5):383–386.

55   Clausen P, Mersebach H, Nielsen B, et al. Hypothyroidism is associated with signs of endothelial dysfunction despite 1-year replacement therapy with levothyroxine. Clinical Endocrinology 2009;70:932–937.

56   Duval F, Mokrani MC, Bailey P, et al. Thyroid axis activity and serotonin function major depressive episode. Psychoneuroendocrinology 1999;24:695–712.

57   Unden F, Ljunggren JG, Kjellman BF, Beck-Friis J, Wetterberg L. Twenty-four-hour serum levels of T4 and T3 in relation to decreased TSH serum levels and decreased TSH response to TRH in affective disorders. Acta Psychiatr Scand 1986;73:358–365.

58   Linnoila M, Lamberg BA, Rosberg G, Karonen SL, Welin MG. Thyroid hormones and TSH, prolactin and LH responses to repeated TRH and LRH injections in depressed patients. Acta Psychiat Scand 1979;59:536–544.

59   Kirkegaard C, Faber J. Altered serum levels of thyroxine, triiodothyronines and diiodothyronines in endogenous depression. Acta Endocrinologica 1981;96:199–207.

60   Sintzel F, Mallaret M, Bougerol T. Potentializing of tricyclics and serotoninergics by thyroid hormones in resistant depressive disorders. Encephale 2004;30(3):267–75.

61   Panicker V, Evans J, Bjoro T, Asvold BO. A paradoxical difference in relationship between anxiety, depression and thyroid function in subjects on and not on T4: findings from the Hunt study. Clinical Endocrinology 2009;71:574–580.

62   Thompson FK. Is there a thyroid-cortisol-depression axis? Thyroid Science 2007;2(10):1.

63   Forman-Hoffman V, Philibert RA. Lower TSH and higher T4 levels are associated with current depressive syndrome in young adults. Acta Psychiatry Scand 2006;114:132–139.

64   Cole DP, Thase ME, Mallinger AG, et al. Slower treatment response in biolar depression predicted by lower pretreatment thyroid function. Am J Psychiatry 2002;159:116–121.

65   Premachandra1 BN, Kabir MA, Williams IK. Low T3 syndrome in psychiatric depression. J Endocrinol Invest 2006;29:568–572.

66   Isogawa K, Haruo Nagayama H, Tsutsumi T, et al. Simultaneous use of thyrotropin-releasing hormone test and combined dexamethasone/-corticotropine-releasing hormone test for severity evaluation and outcome prediction in patients with major depressive disorder. J Psych Res 2005;39:467–473.

67   Sullivan GM, Hatterer JA, Herbert J, Chen X, Rosse SP. Low levels of transthyretin in CSF of depressed patients. Am J Psych 1999;156:710–715.

68   Hatterer JA, Herbert J, Jidaka C, Roose SP, Gorman JM. CSF transthyretin in patients with depression. Am J Psychiatry 1993;150:813–815.

69   Whybrow PC, Coppen A, Prange AJ, Noguera R, Bailey JE. Thyroid function and the response to liothyronine in depression. Arch Gen Psychiatry 1972;26:242–245.

70   Kirkegaard C, Faber J. Free thyroxine and 3,3′,5′-triiodothyronine levels in cerebrospinal fluid in patients with endogenous depression. Acta Endocrinol 1991;124:166–172.

71   Kirkegaard C. The thyrotropin response to thyrotropin-releasing hormone in endogenous depression. Psychoneuroendocrinology 1981;6:189–212.

72   Baumgartner A, Graf KJ, Kurten I, Meinhold H. The hypothalamic-pituitary-thyroid axis in psychiatric patients and healthy subjects. Psychiatry Research 12988;24:271–332.

73   Stipcevic T, Pivac N, Kozaric-Kovacic D, Muck-Seler D. Thyroid activity in patients with major depression. Coll Antropol 2008;32(3):973–976.

74   Cheron RG, Kaplan MM, Larsen PR. Physiological and pharmacological influences on thyroxine to 3,5,3′-triiodothyronine conversion and nuclear 3,5,3′-triiodothyronine binding in rat anterior pituitary. J Clin Invest 1979;64:1402–1414.

75   Araujo RL, Andrade BM, da Silva ML, et al. Tissue-specific deiodinase regulation during food restriction and low replacement dose of leptin in rats. Am J Physiol Endocinol Metab 2009;296:E1157–E1163.

76   Leibel RL, Jirsch J. Diminished energy requirements in reduced-obese patients. Metabolism 1984;33(2):164–170.

77   Fontana L, Klein S, Holloszy JO, Premachandra BN. Effect of long-term calorie restriction with adequate protein and micronutrients on thyroid hormones. J Clin Endocrinol Metab 2006;91(8):3232–3235.

78   Croxson MS, Ibbertson HK. Low serum triiodothyronine (T3) and hypothyroidism. J Clin Endocrinol Metab 1977;44:167–174.

79   Silva JE, Larsen PR. 1986. Hormonal regulation of iodothyronine 5-deiodinase in rat brown adipose tissue. Am J Physiol 251:E639–E643.

80   Krotkiewski M, Holm G, Shono N. Small doses of triiodothyronine can change some risk factors associated with abdominal obesity. Inter J Obesity 1997;21:922–929.

81   Krotkiewski M. Thyroid hormones and treatment of obesity. Int J Obes Relat Metab Disord 2000;24(2):S116–S119.

82   Dagogo-Jack S. Human leptin regulation and promise in pharmacotherapy. Current Drug Targets 2001;2:181–195.

83   Considine RV, Sinha MK, Heiman ML, Kriauciunas A, et al. Serum immunoreactive-leptin concentrations in normal-weight and obese humans. New England Journal of Medicine 1996;334:292–295.

84   Dagogo-Jack S, Fanelli C, Paramore D, Brothers J, Landt M. Plasma leptin and insulin relationships in obese and nonobese humans. Diabetes 1996;45:695–698.

85   Maffei M, Halaas J, Ravussin E, et al. Leptin levels in human and rodent: measurement of plasma leptin and ob NAN in obese and weight-reduced subjects. Nature Medicine 1995;1:1155–1161.

86   Hassink SG, Sheslow DV, de Lancey E, et al. Serum leptin in children with obesity: relationship to gender and development. Pediatrics 1996;98:201–203.

87   Kozlowska L, Rosolowska-Huszcz D. Leptin, thyrotropin, and thyroid hormones in obese/overweight women before and after two levels of energy deficit. Endocrine 2004;24(2):147–153.

88   Fekete C, Singru PS, Sanchez E, et al. Differential effects of central leptin, insulin, or glucose administration during fasting on the hypothalamic-pituitary-thyroid axis and feeding-related neurons in the arcuate 84 nucleus. Endocrinology 2006;147(1):520–529.

89 Ahima RS, Prabakaran D, Mantzoros C, et al. Role of leptin in the neuroendocrine response to fasting. Nature 1996;382:250–252.

90 Legradi G, Emerson CH, Ahima RS, Flier JS, Lechan RM. Leptin prevents fasting-induced suppression of prothyrotropin-releasing hormone messenger ribonucleic acid in neurons of the hypothalamic paraventricular nucleus. Endocrinology 1997;138:2569–2576.

91 Zimmermann-Belsing T, Brabant G, Holst JJ, et al. Circulating leptin and thyroid dysfunction. Eur J Endocrinol 2003;149:257–271.

92 Schwartz MW, Woods SC, Porte D, Seeley RJ, Baskin DG. Central nervous system control of food intake. Nature 2000;404;61–671.

93 Mantzoros CS, Moschos SJ. Leptin: in search of role(s) in human physiology and pathophysiology. Clinical Endocrinology 1998;49:551–567.

94 Fruhbeck G, Jebb SA, Prentice AM. Leptin: physiology and pathophysiology. Clin Physiol 1998;18(5):399–419.

95 Flier JS, Harris M, Hollenber A. Leptin, nutrition and the thyroid: the why, the wherefore and the wiring. J Clin Invest 2000;105(7):859–861.

96 Gon DW, He Y, Karas M, Reitman M. Uncoupling protein-3 is a mediator of thermogenesis regulated by thyroid hormone, beta 3-adrenergic agonists and leptin. J Biol Chem 1997;272:24129–24132.

97 Cusin I, Rouru J, Visser T, Burger AG, Rohner-Jeanrenaud F. Involvement of thyroid hormones in the effect of intracerebroventricular leptin infusion on uncoupling protein-3 expression in rat muscle. Diabetes 2000;49:1101–1105.

98 Rosenbaum M, Goldsmith R, Bloomfield D, et al. Low-dose leptin reverses skeletal muscle, autonomic, and neuroendocrine adaptations to maintenance of reduced weight. J Clin Invest 2005;115:3579–3586.

99 Rosenbaum M, Murphy EM, Heymsfield SB, et al. Low dose leptin administration reverses effects of sustained weight-reduction on energy expenditure and circulation concentration of thyroid hormones. JCEM 2002:87(5):2391–2394.

100 Leibel RL, Rosenbaum M, Hirsch J, et al. Changes in energy expenditure resulting from altered body weight. N Eng J Med 1995;332:621–28.

101 Rosenbaum M, Hirsch J, Murphy E, et al. Effects of changes in body weight on carbohydrate metabolism, catecholamine excretion, and thyroid function. Am J Clin Nutr 2000;71:1421–32.

102 Ahima RS, Prabakaran D, Mantzoros C, et al. Role of leptin in the neuroendocrine response to fasting. Nature 1996;382:250–52.

103 Rosenbaum M, Nicolson M, Hirsch J, et al. Effects of weight change on plasma leptin concentrations and energy expenditure. J Clin Endocrinol Metab 1997;82:3647–54.

104 Légrádi G, Emerson CH, Ahima RS, et al. Leptin prevents fasting-induced suppression of prothyrotropin-releasing hormone messenger ribonucleic acid in neurons of the hypothalamic paraventricular nucleus. Endocrinology 1998;138:2569–76.

105 Boozer CN, Leibel RL, Love RJ, et al. Synergy of sibutramine and low-dose leptin in treatment of diet-induced obesity in rats. Metabolism 2001;50:889–93.

106 Campfield LA, Smith FJ, Guisez Y, et al. Recombinant mouse OB protein: evidence for a peripheral signal linking adiposity and central neural networks. Science 1995;269:546–48.

107 Farooqi IS, Jebb SA, Langmack G, et al. Effects of recombinant leptin therapy in a child with congenital leptin deficiency. N Eng J Med 1999;341:879–84.

108 Chehab F. Leptin as a regulator of adipose tissue mass and reproduction. Trends Pharmacol Sci 200;21:309–14.

109 Rosenbaum M, Leibel RL. The role of leptin in human physiology. N Eng J Med 1999;341:913–15.

110 Näslund E, Andersson I, Degerblad M, et al. Associations of leptin, insulin resistance and thyroid function with long-term weight loss in dieting reduced-obese men. J Int Med 2000;248:299–308.

111 Doucet E, Imbeault P, St-Pierre S, et al. Appetite after weight-loss by energy restriction and a low-fat diet-exercise follow up. Int J Obesity 2000;24:906–14.

112 Lisboa PC, Oliveira KJ, Cabanelas A, et al. Acute cold exposure, leptin, and somatostatin analog (octreotide) modulate thyroid 5'-deiodinase activity. Am J Physiol Endocrinol Metab 2003;284:E1172–E1176.

113 Cabanelas A, Lisboa PC, Moura EG, Pazos-Moura CC. Leptin acute modulation of the 5'-deiodinase activities in hypothalamus, pituitary and brown adipose tissue of fed rats. Horm Metab Res 2006;38(8):481–5.

114 Cettour-Rose P, Burger AG, Meier CA, et al. Central stimulatory effect of leptin on T3 production is mediated by brown adipose tissue type II deiodinase. Am J Physiology Endocrinol Metab 2002;283(5):E980–7.

115 Fekete C, Kelly J, Mihaly E, et al. Neuropeptide Y has a central inhibitory action on the hypothalamic–pituitary–thyroid axis. Endocrinology 2001;142:2606–2613.

116 Fekete C, Legradi G, Mihaly E, et al. a-Melanocyte-stimulating hormone is contained in nerve terminals innervating thyrotropin-releasing hormone-synthesizing neurons in the hypothalamic paraventricular nucleus and prevents fasting-induced suppression of prothyrotropin-releasing hormone gene expression. J Neurosci 2000;20:1550–1558.

117 Legradi G, Emerson CH, Ahima RS, et al. Arcuate nucleus ablation prevents fasting-induced suppression of ProTRH mRNA in the hypothalamic paraventricular nucleus. Neuroendocrinology 1998;68:89–97.

118 Vignati L, Finley RJ, Hagg S, Aoki TT. Protein conservation during prolonged fast: a function of triiodothyronine levels. Trans Assoc Am Physicians 1978;91:169–179.

119 Katzeff HL, Selgrad C. Impaired peripheral thyroid hormone metabolism in genetic obesity. Endocrinology 1993;132(3):989–995.

120 Islam S, Yesmine S, Khan SA, Alam NH, Islam S. A comparative study of thyroid hormone levels in diabetic and non-diabetic patients. SE Asian J Trop Med Public Health 2008;39(5):913–916.

121 Pittman CS, Suda AK, Chambers JB, McDaniel HG, Ray GY. Abnormalities of thyroid hormone turnover in patients with diabetes mellitus before and after insulin therapy. JCEM 1979;48(5):854–60.

122 Saunders J, Hall SHE, Sonksen PH. Thyroid hormones in insulin requiring diabetes before and after treatment. Diabetologia 1978;15:29–32.

123 Chamras H, Hershman JM. Effect of diabetes mellitus on thyrotropin release from isolated rat thyrotrophs. Am J Med Sci 1990;300(1):16–21.

124 Ortiga-Carvalho TM, Curty FH, Nascimento-Saba CC, et al. Pituitary neuromedin B content in experimental fasting and diabetes mellitus and correlation with thyrotropin secretion. Metabolism 1997;46(2):149–153.

125 Jolin T, Gonzalez C. Thyroid iodine metabolism in streptozotocin-diabetic rats. Acta Endocrinologica 1978;88:506–516.

126 Montoya E, Gonzalez C, Lamas L, Jolin T. Changes of the hypothalamus-pituitary-thyroid axis in streptozotocin-diabetic rats during adaptation to a low iodine diet. Acta Endocrinologica 1978;88:721–728.

127 Pericas I, Jolin T. The effect of streptozotocin-induced diabetes on the pituitary-thyroid axis in goitrogen-treated rats. Acta Endocrinologica 1977;86:128–139.

128 Docter R, Krenning EP, de Jong M, et al. The sick euthyroid syndrome: changes in thyroid hormone serum parameters and hormone metabolism. Clin Endocrinol (Oxf) 1993;39:499–518.

129 Fliers E, Alkemade A, Wiersinga WM. The hypothalamic-pituitary-thyroid axis in critical illness. Best Practice & Research Clinical Endocrinology & Metabolism 2001;15(4):453–64.

130 Chopra IJ. Euthyroid sick syndrome: is it a misnomer? J Clin Endocrinol Metab 1997;82(2):329–34.

131 Nagaya T, Fujieda M, Otsuka G, et al. A potential role of activated NF-Kappa B in the pathogenesis of euthyroid sick syndrome. J Clin Invest 2000;106(3):393–402.

132 Chopra IJ, Solomon DH, Hepner GW, et al. Misleadingly low free thyroxine index and usefulness of reverse triiodothyronine measurement in nonthyroidal illnesses. Ann Intern Med 1979;90(6):905–12.

133 Van der Poll T, Romijn JA, Wiersinga WM, et al. Tumor necrosis factor: a putative mediator of the sick euthyroid syndrome in man. J Clin Endocrinol Metab 1990;71(6):1567–72.

134 Stouthard JM, van der Poll T, Endert E, et al. Effects of acute and chronic interleukin-6 administration on thyroid hormone metabolism in humans. J Clin Endocrinol Metab 1994;79(5):1342–6.

135 Corssmit EP, Heyligenberg R, Endert E, et al. Acute effects of interferon-alpha administration on thyroid hormone metabolism in healthy men. Clin Endocrinol Metab 1995;80(11):3140–4.

136 Nagaya T, Fujieda M, Otsuka G, et al. A potential role of activated NF-Kappa B in the pathogenesis of euthyroid sick syndrome. J Clin Invest 2000;106(3):393–402.

137 Zoccali C, Tripepi G, Cutrupi S, et al. Low triiodothyronine: a new facet of inflammation in end-stage renal disease. J Am Soc Nephrol 2005;16:2789–95.

138 Chopra IJ, Sakane S, Teco GNC. A study of the serum concentration of tumor necrosis factor-α in thyroidal and nonthyroidal illnesses. J Clin Endocrinol Metab 1991;72:1113–1116.

139 Boelen A, Platvoet-Ter Schiphorst MC, Wiersinga WM. Association between serum interleukin-6 and serum 3,5,3′-triiodothyronine in nonthyroidal illness. J Clin Endocrinol Metab 1993;77:1695–1699.

140 Hashimoto H, Igarashi N, Yachie A, et al. The relationship between serum levels of interleukin-6 and thyroid hormone in children with acute respiratory infection. J Clin Endocrinol Metab 1994;78:288–291.

141 van der Poll T, Romijn JA, Wiersinga WM, Sauerwein HP. Tumor necrosis factor: a putative mediator of the sick euthyroid syndrome in man. J Clin Endo Metab 1990;71:1567–1572.

142 Altomonte L, Zoli A, Mirone L, et al. Serum levels of interleukin-1alpha, tumor necrosis factor-alpha and interleukin-2 in rheumatoid arthritis. Correlation with disease activity. Clin Rheumatol 1992;11(2):202–205.

143 Espersen GT, Vestergaard M, Ernst E, et al. Tumor necrosis factor-alpha and interleukin-2 in plasma from rheumatoid arthritis patients in relation to disease. Clin Rheumatol 1991;10(4):374–376.

144 Morley JE. The endocrinology of the opiates and opioid peptides. Metabolism 1981;30(2):195–209.

145 Krulich L, Giachetti A, Marchlewska-Koj A, et al. On the role of central norandrenergic and dopaminergic systems in the regulation of TSH secretion in the rat. Endocrinology 1977;100:496–505.

146 Lomax P, Kokka N, George R. Thyroid activity following intracerebral injection of morphine in the rat. Neuroendocrinolgoy 1970;6(146):152.

147 Morley JE, Yamada T, Shulkes A, et al. Effects of morphine addiction and withdrawal on thyrotropin releasing hormone (TRH), somatostatin (SLI) and vasoactive intestinal peptide (VIP). Clin Res 1979;27:75A.

148 Dons RF. Changes in triiodothyronine mark severe pain syndrome: a case report. Military Medicine 1994;159(6):465.

149 Lowe JC, Garrison RL, Reichman AJ, et al. Effectiveness and safety of T3 (triiodothyronine) therapy for euthyroid fibromyalgia: a double-blind placebo-controlled response-driven crossover study. Clin Bull Myofascial Ther 1997;2(2/3):31–58.

150 Lowe JC, Reichman AJ, Yellin J. The process of change during T3 treatment for euthyroid fibromyalgia: a double-blind placebo-controlled crossover study. Clin Bull Myofascial Ther 1997;2(2/3):91–124.

151 Lowe JC, Garrison RL, Reichman AJ, et al. Triiodothyronine (T3) treatment of euthyroid fibromyalgia: a small-n replication of a double-blind placebo-controlled crossover study. Clin Bull Myofascial Ther 1997;2(4):71–88.

152 Yellin BA, Reichman AJ, Lowe JC. The process of change during T3 treatment for euthyroid fibromyalgia: a double-blind placebo-controlled crossover study. The metabolic treatment of fibromyalgia. Clin Bull Myofascial Ther 1996;2(2–3):91–124.

153 Neeck G, Riedel W. Thyroid function in patients with fibromyalgia syndrome. J Rheumatol 1992;19(7):1120–1122.

154 Watanabe C, Yoshida K, Kasanuma Y, Kun Y, Satoh H. In utero methylmercury exposure differentially affects the activities of selenoenzymes in the fetal mouse brain. Environ Res 1999;80(3):208–14.

155 Ellingsen DG, Efskind J, Haug E, Thomassen Y, Martinsen I, Gaarder PI. Effects of low mercury vapour exposure on the thyroid function in chloralkali workers. J Appl Toxicol 2000;20(6):483–9.

156 Moriyama K, Tagami T, Akamizu T, et al. Thyroid hormone action is disrupted by bisphenol A as an antagonist. J Clin Endocrin Metab 2002;87(11):5185–5190.

157 Zoeller RT, Bansal R, Parris C. Bisphenol-A, an environmental contaminant that acts as a thyroid hormone receptor antagonist in vitro, increases serum thyroxine, and alters RC3/neurogranin expression in the developing rat brain. Endocrinology 2005;146(2):607–12.

158 Santini F, Mantovani A, Cristaudo A, et al. Thyroid function and exposure to styrene. Thyroid 2008;18(10):1065–1069.

159 Meeker JD, Calafat AM, Hauser R. Di(2-ethylhexyl) phthalate metabolites may alter thyroid hormone levels in men. Environ Health Perspect 2007;115:1029–1034.

160 Massart F, Massai G, Placidi G, Saggese G. Child thyroid disruption by environmental chemicals. Minerva Pediatrica 2004;58(1):47–53.

161 Heimeier RB, Buchholz DR, Shi YB. The xenoestrogen bisphenol A inhibits postembryonic vertebrate development by antagonizing gene regulation by thyroid hormone. Endocrinology 2009;150(6):2964–2973.

162 Lema, SC, Dickey JT, Schulz IR, Swanson P. Dietary exposure to 2,2′,4,4′-tetrabromodiphenyl ether (PBDE 47) alters thyroid status and thyroid hormone-regulated gene transcription in the pituitary and brain. Environmental Health Perspectives 2008;116:1694–1699.

163 De Groot LJ. Non-thyroidal illness syndrome is a manifestation of hypothalamic-pituitary dysfunction, and in view of current evidence, should be treated with appropriate replacement therapies. Crit Care Clin 2006;22:57–86.

164 Schilling JU, Zimmermann T, Albrecht S, et al. Low T3 syndrome in multiple trauma patients–a phenomenon or important pathogenetic factor? Medizinische Klinik 1999;3:66–9.

165 Schulte C, Reinhardt W, Beelen D, et al. Low T3-syndrome and nutritional status as prognostic factors in patients undergoing bone marrow transplantation. Bone Marrow Transplant 1998;22:1171–8.

166 Girvent M, Maestro S, Hernandez R, et al. Euthyroid sick syndrome, associated endocrine abnormalities, and outcome in elderly patients undergoing emergency operation. Surgery 1998;123:560–7.

167 Maldonado LS, Murata GH, Hershman JM, et al. Do thyroid function tests independently predict survival in the critically ill? Thyroid 1992;2:119–23.

168 Vaughan GM, Mason AD, McManus WF, et al. Alterations of mental status and thyroid hormones after thermal injury. J Clin Endocrinol Metab 1985;60:1221–5.

169 De Marinis L, Mancini A, Masala R, et al. Evaluation of pituitary-thyroid axis response to acute myocardial infarction. J Endocrinol Invest 1985;8:507–11.

170 Kantor MJ, Leef KH, Bartoshesky L, et al. Admission thyroid evaluation in very-low-birthweight infants: association with death and severe intraventricular hemorrhage. Thyroid 2003;13:965–9.

171 Köhrle J. Thyroid hormone deiodinases--a selenoenzyme family acting as gate keepers to thyroid hormone action. Acta Medica Austriaca 1996;23(1-2):17–30.

172 Larsen PR. Thyroid-pituitary interaction: feedback regulation of thyrotropin secretion by thyroid hormones. NEJM 1982;306(1):23–32.

173 Silva JE, Larsen PR. Pituitary nuclear 3,5,3′-triiodothyronine and thyrotropin secretion: an explanation for the effect of thyroxine. Science 1977;198(4317):617–620.

174 Schimmel M, Utiger RD. Thyroidal and peripheral production of thyroid hormones: review of recent finding and their clinical implications. Ann Intern Med 1977;87:760–8.

175 Silva JE, Leonard JL, Crantz FR, Larsen PR. Evidence for two tissue specific pathways for in vivo thyroxine 5′-deiodination in the rat. J Clin Invest 1982;69:1176–1184.

176 Silva JE, Larsen PR. Contributions of plasma triiodothyronine and local thyroxine monodeiodination to triiodothyronine to nuclear triiodothyronine receptor saturation in pituitary, liver, and kidney of hypothyroid rats: further evidence relating saturation of pituitary nuclear triiodothyronine receptors and the acute inhibition of thyroid-stimulating hormone release. J Clin Invest 1978;61:1247–1259.

177 Silva JE, Dick TE, Larsen PR. The contribution of local tissue thyroxine monodeiodination to the nuclear 3,5,3′-triiodothyronine in pituitary, liver, and kidney of euthyroid rats. Endocrinology 1978;103:1196–1207.

178 Bianco AC, Silva JE. Nuclear 3,5,3′-triiodothyronine (T3) in brown adipose tissue: receptor occupancy and sources of T3 as determined by in vivo techniques. Endocrinology 1987;120:55–62.

179 van Doorn JD, Roelfsema F, van der Heide D. Contribution from local conversion of thyroxine to 3,5,3′-triiodothyronine to cellular 3,5,3′-triiodothyronine in several organs in hypothyroid rats at isotope equilibrium. Acta Endocrinol (Copenh) 1982;101:386–406.

180 van Doorn JD, van der Heide D, Roelfsema F. Sources and quantity of 3,5,3′-triiodothyronine in several tissues of the rat. J Clin Invest 1983;72:1778–1892.

181 van Doorn JD, Roelfsema F, van der Heide D. Concentrations of thyroxine and 3,5,3′-triiodothyronine at 34 different sites in euthyroid rats as determined by an isotopic equilibrium technique. Endocrinology 1985;117:1201–1208.

182 Eales JG, McLeese JM, Holmes JA, Youson JH. Changes in intestinal and hepatic thyroid hormone deiodination during spontaneous metamorphosis of the sea lamprey, Petromyzon marinus. J Exp Zool 2000;286:305–312.

183 Croteau W, Davey JC, Galton VA, St. Germain DL. Cloning of the mammalian type II iodothyronine deiodinase. A selenoprotein differentially expressed and regulated in human and rat brain and other tissues. J Clin Invest 1996;98:405–417.

184 Gereben B, Bartha T, Tu HM, Harney JW, Rudas P, Larsen PR. Cloning and expression of the chicken type 2 iodothyronine 5′-deiodinase. J Biol Chem 1999;274:13768–13776.

185 Tu HM, Kim SW, Salvatore D, et al. Regional distribution of type 2 thyroxine deiodinase messenger ribonucleic acid in rat hypothalamus and pituitary and its regulation by thyroid hormone. Endocrinology 1997;138:3359–3368.

186 Leonard JL, Kaplan MM, Visser TJ, Silva JE, Larsen PR. Cerebral cortex responds rapidly to thyroid hormones. Science 1981;214:571–573.

187 Burmeister LA, Pachucki J, St. Germain DL. Thyroid hormones inhibit type 2 iodothyronine deiodinase in the rat cerebral cortex by both pre- and posttranslational mechanisms. Endocrinology 1997;138:5231–5237.

188 Salvatore D, Bartha T, Harney JW, Larsen PR. Molecular biological and biochemical characterization of the human type 2 selenodeiodinase. Endocrinology 1996;137:3308–3315.

189 Hosoi Y, Murakami M, Mizuma H, et al. Expression and regulation of type II iodothyronine deiodinase in cultured human skeletal muscle cells. J Clin Endocrinol Metab 1999;84:3293–3300.

190 Riskind PN, Kolodny JM, Larsen PR. The regional hypothalamic distribution of type II 5′-monodeiodinase in euthyroid and hypothyroid rats. Brain Res 1987;420:194–198.

191 Guadano-Ferraz A, Obregon MJ, St. Germain DL, Bernal J. The type 2 iodothyronine deiodinase is expressed primarily in glial cells in the neonatal rat brain. Proc Natl Acad Sci USA 1997;94:10391–10396.

192 Berry MJ, Banu L, Larsen PR. Type I iodothyronine deiodinase is a selenocysteine-containing enzyme. Nature 1991;349:438–440.

193 Maia AL, Berry MJ, Sabbag R, Harney JW, Larsen PR. Structural and functional differences in the dio1 gene in mice with inherited type 1 deiodinase deficiency. Mol Endocrinol 1995;9:969–980.

194 Kaplan MM, Utiger RD. Iodothyronine metabolism in liver and kidney homogenates from hypothyroid and hyperthyroid rats. Endocrinology 1978;103:156–161.

195 Harris ARC, Fang SL, Vagenakis AG, Braverman LE. Effect of starvation, nutrient replacement, and hypothyroidism on in vitro hepatic T4 to T3 conversion in the rat. Metabolism 1978;27:1680–1690.

196 Berry MJ, Kates AL, Larsen PR. Thyroid hormone regulates type I deiodinase messenger RNA in rat liver. Mol Endocrinol 1990;4:743–748.

197 Maia AL, Harney JW, Larsen PR. Pituitary cells respond to thyroid hormone by discrete, gene-specific pathways. Endocrinology 1995;136:1488–1494.

198 van der Poll T, Romijn JA, Wiersinga WM, et al. Tumor necrosis factor: a putative mediator of the sick euthyroid syndrome in man. J Clin Endocrinol Metab 1990;71(6):1567–72.

199 Stouthard JM, van der Poll T, Endert E, et al. Effects of acute and chronic interleukin-6 administration on thyroid hormone metabolism in humans. J Clin Endocrinol Metab 1994;79(5):1342–6.

200 Corssmit EP, Heyligenberg R, Endert E, et al. Acute effects of interferon-alpha administration on thyroid hormone metabolism in healthy men. Clin Endocrinol Metab 1995;80(11):3140–4.

201 Leonard JL. Dibutyryl cAMP induction of type II 5′-deiodinase activity in rat brain astrocytes in culture. Biochem Biophys Res Commun 1988;151:1164–1172.

202 Annewieke W, van den Beld AW, Visser TJ, et al. Thyroid hormone concentrations, disease, physical function and mortality in elderly men. J Clin Endocrinol Metab 2005;90(12):6403–9.

203 Chopra IJ, Williams DE, Orgiazzi J, Solomon DH. Opposite effects of dexamethasone on serum concentrations of 3,3′,5′-triiodothyronine (reverse T3) and 3,3′,5′-triiodothyronine (T3). JCEM 1975;41:911–920.

[204] Danforth EJ, Desilets EJ, Jorton ES, et al. Reciprocal serum triiodothryronine (T3) and reverse (rT3) induced by altering the carbohydrate content of the diet. Clin Res 1975;23:573.

[205] Palmbald J, Levi J, Burger AG, et al. Effects of total energy withdrawal (fasting) on the levels of growth hormone, thyrotropin, cortisol, noradrenaline, T4, T3 and rT3 in healthy males. Acta Med Scand 1977;201:150.

[206] De Jong F, den Heijer T, Visser TJ, et al. Thyroid hormones, dementia, and atrophy of the medical temporal lobe. J Clin Endocrinol Met 2006;91(7):2569–73. High reverse t3 with brain atrophy.

[207] Goichot B, Schlienger JL, Grunenberger F, et al. Thyroid hormone status and nutrient intake in the free-living elderly. Interest of reverse triiodothyronine assessment. Eur J Endocrinol 1994;130:244–52.

[208] Visser TJ, Lamberts WJ, Wilson JHP, Docter WR, Hennemann G. Serum thyroid hormone concentrations during prolonged reduction of dietary intake. Metabolism 1978;27(4):405–409.

[209] Okamoto R, Leibfritz D. Adverse effects of reverse triiodothyronine on cellular metabolism as assessed by 1H and 31P NMR spectroscopy. Res Exp Med (Berl) 1997;197(4):211–7.

[210] Tien ES, Matsui K, Moore R, Negishi M. The nuclear receptor constitutively active/androstane receptor regulates type 1 deiodinase and thyroid hormone activity in the regenerating mouse liver. J Pharmacol Exp Ther 2007;320(1):307–13.

[211] Benvenga S, Cahnmann HJ, Robbins J. Characterization of thyroid hormone binding to apolipoprotein-E: localization of the binding site in the exon 3-coded domain. Endocrinology 1993;133:1300–1305.

[212] Sechman A, Niezgoda J, Sobocinski R. The relationship between basal metabolic rate (BMR) and concentrations of plasma thyroid hormones in fasting cockerels. Follu Biol 1989;37(1–2):83–90.

[213] Pittman JA, Tingley JO, Nickerson JF, Hill SR. Antimetabolic activity of 3,3',5'-triiodo-dl-thyronine in man. Metabolism 1960;9:293–5.

[214] Santini F, Chopra IJ, Hurd RE, Solomon DH, Teco GN. A study of the characteristics of the rat placental iodothyronine 5-monodeiodinase: evidence that is distinct from the rat hepatic iodothyronine 5-monodeiodinase. Endocrinology 1992;130:2325–2332.

[215] Silva JE, Gordon MB, Crantz FR, Leonard JL, Larsen PR. Qualitative and quantitative differences in pathways of extrathyroidial triiodothyronine generation between euthyroid and hypothyroid rats. J Clin Invest 1984;73:898–907.

[216] Silva JE, Leonard JL. Regulation of rat cerebrocortical and adenophypophyseal type II 5'-deidodinase by thyroxinem triiodothyronine, and reverse triiodothyronine. Endocrinology 1985;116(4):1627–1635.

[217] Obregon MJ, Larsen PR, Silva JE. The role of 3,3',5'-triiodothyroinine in the regulation of type II iodothyronin 5'-deiodinase in the rat cerebral cortex. Endocrinology 1986;119(5):2186–2192.

[218] Chopra IJ. A study of extrathyroidal conversion of thyroxine (T4) to 3,3',5-triiodothyronine (T3) in vitro. Endocrinology 1977;101(2):453–63.

[219] Mitchell AM, Manley SW, Rowan KA, Mortimer RH. Uptake of reverse T3 in the human choriocarcinoma cell line Jar. Placenta 1999;20:65–70.

[220] Van der Geyten S, Buys N, Sanders JP, et al. Acute pretranslational regulation of type III iodothyronine deiodinase by growth hormone and dexamethasone in chicken embryos. Mol Cell Endocrinol 1999;147:49–56.

[221] Peeters RP, Wouters PJ, van Toor H, et al. Serum 3,3',5'-triiodothyronine (rT3) and 3,5,3'-triiodothyronine/rT3 are prognostic markers in critically ill patients and are associated with postmortem tissue deiodinase activities. J Clin Endocrinol Metab 2005;90(8):4559–65.

[222] Peeters RP, Wouters PJ, Kaptein E, et al. Reduced activation and increased inactivation of thyroid hormone in tissues of critically ill patients. J Clin Endocrinol Metab 2003;88:3202–11.

[223] Brent GA, Hershman JM. Thyroxine therapy in patients with severe nonthyroidal illnesses and low serum thyroxine concentration. J Clin Endocrinol Metab 1986;63(1):1–8.

[224] Escobar-Morreale HF, Obregon MJ, Escobar del Rey F, Morreale de Escobar G. Replacement therapy for hypothyroidism with thyroxine alone does not ensure euthyroidism in all tissues. J Clin Invest 1995;96(6):2828–2838.

[225] Lomenick JP, El-Sayyid M, Smith WJ. Effect of levo-thyroxine treatment on weight and body mass index in children with acquired hypothyroidism. J Pediatrics 2008;152(1):96–100.

[226] Acker CG, Singh AR, Flick RP, et al. A trial of thyroxine in acute renal failure. Kidney Int 2000;57:293–8.

[227] Samuels MH, Schuff KG, Carlson NE, Carello P, Janowsky JS. Health status, psychological symptoms, mood, and cognition in L-thyroxine-treated hypothyroid subjects. Thyroid 2007;17(3):249–58.

[228] Cooke RG, Joffe RT, Levitt AJ. T3 augmentation of antidepressant treatment in T4-replaced thyroid patients. J Clin Psychiatry 1992;53(1):16–8.

[229] Bettendorf M, Schmidt KG, Grulich-Henn J, et al. Tri-iodothyronine treatment in children after cardiac surgery: a double-blind, randomized, placebo-controlled study. Lancet 2000;356:529–34.

[230] Pingitore A, Galli E, Barison A, et al. Acute effects of triiodothyronine replacement therapy in patients with chronic heart failure and low-T3 syndrome: a randomized placebo-controlled study. J Clin Endocrin Metab 2008;93(4):1351–8.

[231] Meyer T, Husch M, van den Berg E, et al. Treatment of dopamine-dependent shock with triiodothyronine: preliminary results. Deutsch Med Wochenschr 1979;104:1711–14.

[232] Dulchavsky SA, Hendrick SR, Dutta S. Pulmonary biophysical effects of triiodothyronine (T3) augmentation during sepsis induced hypothyroidism. J Trauma 1993;35:104–9.

[233] Novitzsky D, Cooper DKC, Human PA, et al. Triiodothyronine therapy for heart donor and recipient. J Heart Transplant 1988;7:370–6.

[234] Dulchavsky SA, Maitra SR, Maurer J, et al. Beneficial effects of thyroid hormone administration in metabolic and hemodynamic function in hemorrhagic shock. FASEB J 1990;4:A952.

[235] Klemperer JD, Klein I, Gomez M, et al. Thyroid hormone treatment after coronary-artery bypass surgery. N Engl J Med 1995;333:1522–7.

[236] Gomberg-Maitland M. Thyroid hormone and cardiovascular disease. Am Heart J 1998;135:187–96.

[237] Dulchavsky SA, Kennedy PR, Geller ER, et al. T3 preserves respiratory function in sepsis. J Trauma 1991;31:753–9.

[238] Novitzky D, Cooper DK, Reichart B. Hemodynamic and metabolic responses to hormonal therapy in brain-dead potential organ donors. Transplantation 1987;43:852–5.

[239] Hamilton MA, Stevenson LW, Fonarow GC, et al. Safety and hemodynamic effects of intravenous triiodothyronine in advanced congestive heart failure. Am J Cardiol 1998;81:443–7.

[240] Klemperer JD, Klein IL, Ojamaa K, et al. Triiodothyronine therapy lowers the incidence of atrial fibrillation after cardiac operations. Ann Thorac Surg 1996;61:1323–9.

[241] Smidt-Ott UM, Ascheim DD. Thyroid hormone and heart failure. Curr Heart Fail Rep 2006;3:114–9.

[242] LoPresti JS, Eigen A, Kaptein E, et al. Alterations in 3,3'5'-triiodothyronine metabolism in response to propylthiouracil, dexamethasone, and thyroxine administration in man. J Clin Invest 1989;84:1650–1656.

243 Lim VS, Passo C, Murata Y, et al. Reduced triiodothyronine content in liver but not pituitary of the uremic rat model: demonstration of changes compatible with thyroid hormone deficiency in liver only. Endocrinology 1984;114(1):280–286.

244 Cremaschi GA, Gorelik G, Klecha AJ, Lysionek AE, Genaro AM. Chronic stress influences the immune system through the thyroid axis. Life Sci 2000 Nov 17;67(26):3171–9.

245 Burr WA, Ramsden DB, Griffiths RS, et al. Effect of a single dose of dexamethasone on serum concentrations of thyroid hormones. Lancet 1976;10;2(7976):58–61.

246 Saranteas T, Tachmintzis A, Katsikeris N, et al. Perioperative thyroid hormone kinetics in patients undergoing major oral and maxillofacial operations. J Oral Maxillofac Surg 2007;65:408–414.

247 Joffe RT. A perspective on the thyroid and depression. Can J Psychiatry 1990;35(9):754–8.

248 Posternak M, Novak S, Stern R, et al. A pilot effectiveness study: placebo-controlled trial of adjunctive L-triiodothyronine (T3) used to accelerate and potentiate the antidepressant response. Int J Neuropsychopharmacology 2008;11:15–25.

249 Wekking EM, Appelhof BC, Fliers E, et al. Cognitive functioning and well-being in euthyroid patients on thyroxine replacement therapy for primary hypothyroidism. Eur J Endocrinol 2005;153:747–753.

250 Escobar-Morreale HF, Escobar del Rey F, Obregon MJ, Morreale de Escobar G. Only the combined treatment with thyroxine and triiodothryoidine ensures euthyroidism in all tissue. Endocrinology 1996;137:2490–2502.

251 Duick DS, Warren DW, Nicoloff JT, Otis CL, Croxson MS. Effect of single dose dexamethasone on the concentration of serum triiodothyronine in man. J Clin Endocrinol Metab 1974;39(6):1151–4.

252 Dore C, Hesp R, Wilkins D, et al. Prediction of energy requirements of obese patients after massive weight loss. Human Nutr Clin Nutr 1982;366:41–48.

253 Drenick EJ, Dennin HF. Energy expenditure in fasting obese men. J Lab Clin Med 1973;81:421–430.

254 Tulp OL, Mckee TD. Thiiodothyronine (T3) neogenesis in lean and obese LA/N-cp rats. Biochem Biophys Res Commun 1986;140(1):134–142.

255 Silva JE, Larsen PR. Interrelationships among thyroxine, growth hormone, and the sympathetic nervous system in the regulation of 5-iodothyronine deiodinase in rat brown adipose tissue. J Clin Invest 1986;77:1214–1223.

256 Loucks AB, Heath EM. Induction of low-T3 syndrome in exercising women occurs at the threshold of energy availability. Am J Physiol Regul Integr Comp Physiol 1994;266:R817–R823.

257 Opstad PK, Falch D, Oktedalen O, Fonnum F, Wergeland R. The thyroid function in young men during prolonged exercise and the effect of energy and sleep deprivation. Clinical Endocrinology 1984;20:657–669.

258 Zhou D, Kusnecov AW, Shurin MR, DePaoli M, Rabin BS. Exposure to physical and psychological stressors elevates plasma interleukin-6: relationship to the activation of the hypothalamic–pituitary–adrenal axis. Endocrinology 1993;133:2523–30.

259 Brunner EJ, Marmot MG, Nanchahal K, et al. Social inequality in coronary risk: central obesity and the metabolic syndrome. Evidence from the Whitehall II Study. Diabetologia 1997;40:1341–9.

260 Miller GE, Blackwell E. Turning up the heat: inflammation as a mechanism linking chronic stress, depression, and heart disease. Current Directions in Psychological Science 2009;15(6):269–272.

261 Ranjit N, Diez-Roux AV, Shea S, et al. Psychosocial factors and inflammation in the multi-ethnic study of atherosclerosis. Arch Intern Med 2007;167:174–181.

262 Davis MC, Zautra AJ, Younger J, et al. Chronic stress and regulation of cellular markers of inflammation in rheumatoid arthritis: implications for fatigue. Brain Behav Immun 2008;22(1):24–32.

263 Yudkin JS, Kumari M, Humphries SE, Mohamed-Ali V. Inflammation, obesity, stress and coronary heart disease: is interleukin-6 the link? Atherosclerosis 2000;2(1):209–214.

264 Tilg H, Moschen AR. Insulin resistance, inflammation, and non-alcoholic fatty liver disease. Trends Endocrinol Metab 2008;19(10):371–9.

265 Mohamed-Ali V, Goodrick S, Rawesh A, et al. Human subcutaneous adipose tissue secretes interleukin-6 but not TNF-a in vivo. J Clin Endocrinol Metab 1997;82:4196–200.

266 Hotamisligil GS, Arner P, Caro JF, Atkinson RL, Spiegelman BM. Increased adipose tissue expression of tumor necrosis factor-a in human obesity and insulin resistance. J Clin Invest 1995;95:2409–15.

267 Fried SK, Bunkin DA, Greenberg AS. Omental and subcutaneous adipose tissues of obese subjects release interleukin-6: depot difference and regulation by glucocorticoid. J Clin Endocrinol Metab 1998;83:847–50.

268 Liu S, Tinker L, Song Y, et al. A prospective study of inflammatory cytokines and diabetes mellitus in a multiethnic cohort of postmenopausal women. Arch Intern Med 2007;167(15):1676–85.

269 Leonard BE. Inflammation, depression and dementia: are they connected? Neurochem Res 2007;32(10):1749–56.

270 Maes M. Evidence for an immune response in major depression: a review and hypothesis. Prog Neuropsychopharmacol Biol Psychiatry 1995;19(1):11–38.

271 Maes M, Scharpé S, Meltzer HY, et al. Relationships between interleukin-6 activity, acute phase proteins, and function of the hypothalamic-pituitary-adrenal axis in severe depression. Psychiatry Res 1993;49(1):11–27.

272 Maes M. Evidence for an immune response in major depression: a review and hypothesis. Prog Neuropsychopharmacol Biol Psychiatry 1995;19(1):11–38.

273 Pfeilschifter J, Koditz R, Pfohl M, Schatz H. Changes in proinflammatory cytokine activity after menopause. Endocrine Rev 2002;22(1):90–119.

274 Alexander RW. Inflammation and coronary artery disease. New Engl J Med 1994;331:468–9.

275 MRFIT Research Group, Kuller LH, Tracy RP, Shaten J, Meilahn EN. Relation of C-reactive protein and coronary heart disease in the MRFIT nested case-control study. Am J Epidemiol 1996;144:537–47.

276 Benvenuto R, Paroli M, Buttinelli C, et al. Tumor necrosis factor-alpha and interferon-alpha synthesis by cerebrospinal fluid-derived T cell clones in multiple sclerosis. Ann NY Acad Sci 1992;650:341–346.

277 Cohen MC, Cohen S. Cytokine function: a study in biologic diversity. Am J Clin Pathol 1996;105:589–598.

278 Khan G. Epstein-Barr virus, cytokines, and inflammation: a cocktail for the pathogenesis of Hodgkin's lymphoma? Exp Hematol 2006;34(4):399–406.

279 Takeshita S, Breen EC, Ivashchenko M, et al. Induction of IL-6 and IL-10 production by recombinant HIV-1 envelope glycoprotein 41 (gp41) in the THP-1 human monocytic cell line. Cell Immunol 1995;165(2):234–242.

280 Coussens LM, Raymond WW, Bergers G, et al. Inflammatory mast cells up-regulate angiogenesis during squamous epithelial carcinogenesis. Genes Dev 1999;13:1382–1397.

281 Cleeland CS, Bennett GJ, Dantzer R, et al. Are the symptoms of cancer and cancer treatment due to a shared biologic mechanism? A cytokine-immunologic model of cancer symptoms. Cancer 2003;97:2919–2925.

282   Lee BN, Dantzer R, Langley KE, et al. A cytokine-based neuroimmunologic mechanism of cancer related symptoms. Neuroimmunomodulation 2004;11:279–292.

283   Malyszko J, Malyszko JS, Pawlak K, Mysliwiec M. Thyroid function, endothelium, and inflammation in hemodialyzed patients: possible relations? J Renal Nutrition 2007;17(1):30–37.

284   Boelen A, Kwakkel J, Alkemade A, et al. Induction of type 3 deiodinase activity in inflammatory cells of mice with chronic local inflammation. Endocrinology 2005;146(12):5128–5134.

285   Pizzorno JE, Katzinger JJ. Clinical implications of persistent organic pollutants epigenetic mechanisms. J Rest Med 2013;2(1):4–13.

286   Brouwer A, Morse DC, Lans MC, et al. Interactions of persistent environmental organohalogens with the thyroid hormone system: mechanisms and possible consequences for animal and human health. Toxicol Ind Health 1998;14:59–84.

287   Hagmar L, Rylander L, Dyremark E, et al. Plasma concentrations of persistent organochlorines in relation to thyrotropin and thyroid hormone levels in women. Int Arch Occup Environ Health. 2001;74:184–8.

288 Persky V, Turyk M, Anderson HA, et al. The effects of PCB exposure and fish consumption on endogenous hormones. Environ Health Perspect. 2001;109:1275–83.

289 Chevrier J, Harley KG, Bradman A, et al. Polybrominated diphenyl ether (PBDE) flame retardants and thyroid hormone during pregnancy. Environ Health Perspect 2010;118:1444–9.

290   Lee DH, Lee IK, Song K, et al. A strong dose-response relation between serum concentrations of persistent organic pollutants and diabetes: results from the National Health and Examination Survey 1999-2002. Diabetes Care 2006;29(7):1638–44.

291   Lee DH, Steffes MW, Sjödin A, et al. Low dose organochlorine pesticides and polychlorinated biphenyls predict obesity, dyslipidemia, and insulin resistance among people free of diabetes. PLoS One 2011;6(1):e15977.

292   Lim S, Ahn SY, Song IC, et al. Chronic exposure to the herbicide, atrazine, causes mitochondrial dysfunction and insulin resistance. PLoS One 2009;4(4):e5186.

293   Lee HK. Mitochondrial dysfunction and insulin resistance: the contribution of dioxin-like substances. Diabetes Metab J 2011;35(3):207–15.

294   Takser L, Mergler D, Baldwin M, et al. Thyroid hormones in pregnancy in relation to environmental exposure to organochlorine compounds and mercury. Environmental Health Perspectives 2005;113(8):1039–1045.

295   Marsh AB, Bergman A, Bladh LG, et al. Synthesis of p-hydroxybromodiphenyl ethers and binding to the thyroid receptor. Organohalogen Compounds 1998;37:305–8.

296   Visser TJ, Leonard JL, Kaplan MM, Larsen PR. Kinetic evidence suggesting two mechanisms for iodothyronine 5'-deiodination in rat cerebral cortex. Proc Natl Acad Sci USA 1982;79:5080–5084.

297   Hesch RD, Brunner G, Soling HD. Conversion of thyroxine (T4) and triiodothyronine (T3) and the subcellular localization of the converting enzyme. Clin Chim Acta 1975;59:209–213.

298   Visser TJ, van der Does-Tobe I, Docter R, Hennemann G. Conversion of thyroxine into triiodothyronine by rat liver homogenate. Biochem J 1975;150:489–493.

299   Lakind JS, Naiman DQ. Biphenol A (BPA) daily intakes in the United States: estimates from the 2003–2004 NHANES urinary BPA data. J Exposure Environ Epidemiology 2008;18:608–615.

300   Cone M. Californians have world's highest levels of flame retardants. Environmental Health News, October 1, 2008.

301   Soldin OP, O'Mara DM, Aschner M. Thyroid hormones and methylmercury toxicity. Biol Trace Element Res 2008;126(1-3):1–12.

302   Long M, Zhao J, Wang S. Changes in trace elements contents of renal cells in cadmium poisoning. Chung Hua Yu Fang I Hsueh Tsa Chih 1998;32(2):73–5.

303   Curl CL, Fenske RA, Elgethun K. Organophosphorus pesticide exposure of urban and suburban preschool children with organic and conventional diets. Environ Health Perspect 2003;111:377–82.

304   Lu C, Barr DB, Pearson MA, et al. Dietary intake and its contribution to longitudinal organophosphorus pesticide exposure in urban/suburban children. Environ Health Perspect 2008;116(4):537–42.

305   LaSalle JM. A genomic point-of-view on environmental factors influencing the human brain methylome. Epigenetics 2011;6(7):862–9.

306   Baccarelli A, Cassano PA, Litonjua A, et al. Cardiac autonomic dysfunction: effects from particulate air pollution and protection by dietary methyl nutrients and metabolic polymorphisms. Circulation 2008;117(14):1802–9.

307   Miyashita K, Murakami M, Iriuchijima T, Takeuchi T, Mori M. Regulation of rat liver type 1 iodothyronine deiodinase mRNA levels by testosterone. Mol Cell Endocrinol 1995;115:161–167.

308   Harris AR, Vagenakis AG, Braverman LE. Sex-related differences in outer ring monodeiodination of thyroxine and 3,3',5'-triiodothyronine by rat liver homogenates. Endocrinology 1979;104:645–652.

309   Travison TG, Araujo AB, O'Donnell AB, et al. A population-level decline in serum testosterone levels in American men. J Clin Endocrinol Metab 2006;92:196–202.

310   Kupelian V, Hayes FJ, Link CL, et al. Inverse association of testosterone and the metabolic syndrome in men is consistent across race and ethnic groups. J Clin Endocrinol Metab 2008;93:3403–3410.

311   Kapoor D, Aldred H, Clark S, Channer KS, Jones TH. Clinical and biochemical assessment of hypogonadism in men with type 2 diabetes: correlations with bioavailable testosterone and visceral adiposity. Diabetes Care 2007;30(4):911–7.

312   Makhsida N, Shah J, Yan G. Hypogonadism and metabolic syndrome: implications for testosterone therapy. J Urology 2005;174:827–834.

313   Jorgensen JOL, Pedersen SA, Laurberg P, et al. Effects of growth hormone therapy on thyroid function of growth hormone-deficient adults with and without concomitant thyroxine-substituted central hypothyroidism. J Clin Endocrinol Metab 1989;69:1127–1132.

314   Darras VM, Berghman LR, Vanderpooten A, Kuhn ER. Growth hormone acutely decreases type III deiodinase in chicken liver. FEBS Lett 1992;310:5–8.

315   De Jong FJ, Peeters RP, Jeijer TD, et al. The association of pohymorphism in the type 1 and 2 deiodinase genes with circulation thyroid hormone parameters and atrophy of the medial temporal lobe. JCEM 2007;92(2):636–640.

316   Tennant F. Hormone treatments in chronic and intractable pain. Practical Pain Management 2005;57–63.

317   Bianco AC, Kim BW. Deiodinases: implications of the local control of thyroid hormone action. J Clin Invest 2006;116(10):2571–9.

318   Wu Y, Koenig RJ. Gene regulation by thyroid hormone. Trends Endocrinol Metab 2000;11(6):207–11.

319   Wondisford FE. Thyroid hormone action: insight from transgenic mouse models. J Investig Med 2003;51(4):215–20.

320   Yen PM, Ando S, Feng X, Liu Y, Maruvada P, Xia X. Thyroid hormone action at the cellular, genomic and target gene levels. Mol Cell Endocrinol 2006;246(1–2):121–7.

321 St Germain DL, Galton VA. The deiodinase family of selenoproteins. Thyroid 1997;7(4):655–68.

322 Bianco AC, Salvatore D, Gereben B, Berry MJ, Larsen PR. Biochemistry, cellular and molecular biology, and physiological roles of the iodothyronine selenodeiodinases. Endocr Rev 2002;23(1):38–89.

323 Kohrle J, Jakob F, Contempre B, Dumont JE. Selenium, the thyroid, and the endocrine system. Endocr Rev 2005;26(7):944–84.

324 Burger AG, Engler D, Sakoloff C, Staeheli V. The effects of tetraiodothyroacetic and triiodothyroacetic acid on thyroid function in euthyroid and hyperthyroid subjects. Acta Endocrinologica 1979;92(3):455–67.

325 Everts ME, Visser TJ, Moerings EP, et al. Uptake of 3,3′,5,5′-tetraiodothyroacetic acid and 3,3′,5′-triiodothyronine in cultured rat anterior pituitary cells and their effects on thyrotropin secretion. Endocrinology 1995;136:4454–61.

326 Carlin K, Carlin S. Possible etiology for euthyroid sick syndrome. Med Hypotheses 1993;40:38–43.

327 LoPresti JS, Dloll RS. Augmented conversion of T3 to triac (T3AC) is the major regulator of the low T3 state in fasting man. Thyroid 1992;2:S-94.

328 Pittman CS, Shimizu T, Burger A, Chambers JB. The nondeiodinative pathways of thyroxine metabolism: 3,5,3′,5′-tetraiodothyroacetic acid turnover in normal and fasting human subjects. J Clin Endocrinol Metab 1980;50:712–6.

329 Brenta G, Schnitiman M, Fretes O, Facco E. Comparative efficacy and side effects of the treatment of euthyroid goiter with levo-thyroxine or triiodothyroacetic acid. J Clin Endocrinol Metabol 2003;88(11):5287–92.

330 Bracco D, Morin O, Schutz Y, Liang H, Jequier E, Burger AG. Comparison of the metabolic and endocrine effects of 3,5,3′-triiodothyroacetic acid and thyroxine. J Clin Endocrinol Metab 1993;77:221–8.

331 Medeiros-Neto G, Kallas WG, Knobel M, Cavaliere H, Mattar E. Triac(3,5,3′-triiodothyroacetic acid) partially inhibits the thyrotropin response to synthetic thyrotropin releasing hormone in normal and thyroidectomized hypothyroid patients. J Clin Endocrinol Metab 1980;50:223–5.

332 Lind P, Langsteger W, Koltringer P, Eber O. 3,5,3′-triiodothyroacetic acid (TRIAC) effects on pituitary thyroid regulation and on peripheral tissue parameters. Nuklearmedizin 1989;28:217–20.

333 Everts ME, Visser TJ, Moerings EM, et al. Uptake of triiodothyroacetic acid and its effect on thyrotropin secretion in cultured anterior pituitary cells. Endocrinology 1994;135(6):2700–7.

334 Everts ME, De Jong M, Lim CF, et al. Different regulation of thyroid hormone transport in liver and pituitary: its possible role in the maintenance of low T3 production during nonthyroidal illness and fasting in man. Thyroid 1996;6(4):359–368.

335 Peeters RP, Geyten SV, Wouters PJ, et al. Tissue thyroid hormone levels in critical illness. J Clin Endocrinol Metab 2005;12:6498–507.

336 Lim C-F, Docter R, Krenning EP, et al. Transport of thyroxine into cultured hepatocytes: effects of mild nonthyroidal illness and calorie restriction in obese subjects. Clin Endocrinol (Oxf) 1994;40:79–85.

337 Sarne DH, Refetoff S. Measurement of thyroxine uptake from serum by cultured human hepatocytes as an index of thyroid status: reduced thyroxine uptake from serum of patients with nonthyroidal illness. J Clin Endocrinol Metab 1985;61:1046–52.

338 Hennemann G, Docter R, Friesema EC, et al. Plasma membrane transport of thyroid hormones and its role in thyroid hormone metabolism and bioavailability. Endocrine Reviews 2001;22(4):451–476.

339 Holm AC, Jacquemin C. Membrane transport of l-triiodothyronine by human red cell ghosts. Biochem Biophys Res Commun 1979;89:1006–1017.

340 Docter R, Krenning EP, Bos G, Fekkes DSF, Hennemann G. Evidence that the uptake of triiodo-l-thyronine by human erythrocytes is carrier-mediated but not energy-dependent. Biochem J 1982;208:27–34.

341 Holm AC, Kagedal B. Kinetics of triiodothyronine uptake by erythrocytes in hyperthyroidism, hypothyroidism, and thyroid hormone resistance. J Clin Endocrinol Metab 1989;69:364–368.

342 Osty J, Valensi P, Samson M, Francon J, Blondeau JP. Transport of thyroid hormones by human erythrocytes: kinetic characterization in adults and newborns. J Clin Endocrinol Metab 1990;71:1589–1595.

343 Moreau X, Azorin J-M, Maurel M, Jeanningros R. Increase in red blood cell triiodothyronine uptake in untreated unipolar major depressed patients compared to healthy controls. Prog Neuropsychopharmacol Biol Psychiatry 1998;22:293–310.

344 Osty J, Jego L, Francon J, Blondeau JP. Characterization of triiodothyronine transport and accumulation in rat erythrocytes. Endocrinology 1988;123:2303–2311.

345 Osty J, Zhou Y, Chantoux F, Francon J, Blondeau JP. The triiodothyronine carrier of rat erythrocytes: asymmetry and mechanism of transinhibition. Biochim Biophys Acta 1990;1051:46–51.

346 Moreau X, Lejeune PJ, Jeanningros R. Kinetics of red blood cell T3 uptake in hypothyroidism with or without hormonal replacement, in the rat. J Endocrinol Invest 1999;22:257–261.

347 McLeese JM, Eales JG. 3,5,3-Triiodo-l-thyronine and lthyroxine uptake into red blood cells of rainbow trout (*Oncorhynchus mykiss*). Gen Comp Endocrinol 1996;102:47–55.

348 McLeese JM, Eales JG. Characteristics of the uptake of 3,5,3-triiodo-l-thyronine and l-thyroxine into red blood cells of rainbow trout (*Oncorhynchus mykiss*). Gen Comp Endocrinol 1996;103:200–208.

349 Everts ME, Docter R, van Buuren JC, et al. Evidence of carrier-mediated uptake of triiodothyronine in cultured anterior pituitary cells of euthyroid rats. Endocrinology 1993;132:1278–1285.

350 Everts ME, Docter R, Moerings EP, et al. Uptake of thyroxine in cultured anterior pituitary cells of euthyroid rats. Endocrinology 1994;134:2490–2497.

351 Yan Z, Hinkle PM. Saturable, stereospecific transport of 3,5,3-triiodo-l-thyronine and l-thyroxine into GH4C1 pituitary cells. J Biol Chem 1993;268:20179–20184.

352 Goncalves E, Lakshmanan M, Pontecorvi A, Robbins J. Thyroid hormone transport in a human glioma cell line. Mol Cell Endocrinol 1990;69:157–165.

353 Francon J, Cantoux F, Blondeau JP. Carrier-mediated transport of thyroid hormones into rat glial cells in primary culture. J Neurochem 1989;53:1456–1463.

354 Beslin A, Chantoux F, Blondeau JP, Francon J. Relationship between the thyroid hormone transport system and the Na-H exchanger in cultured rat brain astrocytes. Endocrinology 1995;136:5385–5390.

355 Chantoux F, Blondeau JP, Francon J. Characterization of the thyroid hormone transport system of cerebrocortical rat neurons in primary culture. J Neurochem 1995;65:2549–2554.

356 Kastellakis A, Valcana T. Characterization of thyroid hormone transport in synaptosomes from rat brain. Mol Cell Endocrinol 1989;67:231–241.

357 Lakshmanan M, Goncalves E, Lessly G, et al. The transport of thyroxine into mouse neuroblastoma cells, NB41A3: the effect of L-system amino acids. Endocrinology 1990;126:3245–3250.

358 Pontecorvi A, Lakshmanan M, Robbins J. Intracellular transport of 3,5,3-triiodo-l-thyronine in rat skeletal myoblasts. Endocrinology 1987;121:2145–2152.

359 Everts ME, Verhoeven FA, Bezstarosti K, et al. Uptake of thyroid hormones in neonatal rat cardiac myocytes. Endocrinology 1996;137: 4235–4242.

360 Zonefrati R, Rotella CM, Toccafondi RS, Arcangeli P. Thyroid hormone receptors in human cultured fibroblasts: evidence for cellular T4 transport and nuclear binding. Horm Metab Res 1983;15:151–154.

361 Docter R, Krenning EP, Bernard HF, Hennemann G. Active transport of iodothyronines into human cultured fibroblasts. J Clin Endocrinol Metab 1987;65:624–628.

362 Cheng SY. Characterization of binding of uptake of 3,3,5-triiodo-l-thyronine in cultured mouse fibroblasts. Endocrinology 1983;112: 1754–1762.

363 Mitchell AM, Manley SW, Mortimer RH. Uptake of l-triiodothyronine by human cultured trophoblast cells. J Endocrinol 1992;133:483–486.

364 Mitchell AM, Manley SW, Mortimer RH. Membrane transport of thyroid hormone in the human choriocarcinoma cell line JAR. Mol Cell Endocrinol 1992;87:139–145.

365 Mitchell AM, Manley SW, Rowan KA, Mortimer RH. Uptake of reverse T3 in the human choriocarcinoma cell line JAR. Placenta 1999;20:65–70.

366 Bernus I, Mitchell AM, Manley SW, Mortimer RH. Uptake of l-triiodothyronine sulfate by human choriocarcinoma cell line JAR. Placenta 1999;20(2–3):161–165.

367 Mitchell AM, Manley SW, Payne EJ, Mortimer RH. Uptake of thyroxine in the human choriocarcinoma cell line JAR. J Endocrinol 1995;146:233–238.

368 Landeta LC, Gonzales-Padrones T, Rodriguez-Fernandez C. Uptake of thyroid hormones (l-T3 and l-T4) by isolated rat adipocytes. Biochem Biophys Res Commun 1987;145:105–110.

369 Kostrouch Z, Felt V, Raska J, Nedvidkova J, Holeckova E. Binding of (125I) triiodothyronine to human peripheral leukocytes and its internalization. Experientia 1987;43:1117–1118.

370 Kostrouch Z, Raka I, Felt V, Nedvidkova J, Holeckova E. Internalization of triiodothyronine-bovine serum albumin-colloidal gold complexes in human peripheral leukocytes. Experientia 1987;43:1119–1120.

371 Centanni M, Mancini G, Andreoli M. Carrier-mediated [125I]-T3 uptake by mouse thymocytes. Endocrinology 1989;124:2443–2448.

372 Centanni M, Sapone A, Taglienti A, Andreoli M. Effect of extracellular sodium on thyroid hormone uptake by mouse thymocytes. Endocrinology 1991;129:2175–2179.

373 de Jong M, Docter R, Bernard HF, et al. T4 uptake into the perfused rat liver and liver T4 uptake in humans are inhibited by fructose. Am J Physiol 1994;266:E768–E775.

374 Hennenmann G, Everts ME, de Jong M, et al. The significance of plasma membrane transport in the bioavailability of thyroid hormone. Clin Endo 1998;48:1–8.

375 Vos RA, de Jong M, Bernard BF, et al. Impaired thyroxine and 3,5,3′-triiodothyronine handling by rat hepatocytes in the presence of serum of patients with nonthyroidal illness. J Clin Endocrinol Metab 1995;80:2364–2370.

376 Hennemann G, Krenning EP. The kinetics of thyroid hormone transporters and their role in non-thyroidal illness and starvation. Best Practice & Res Clin Endo Metab 2007;21(2):323–338.

377 Hennemann G, Vos RA, de Jong M, et al. Decreased peripheral 3,5,3′-triiodothyronine (T3) production from thyroxine (T4): a syndrome of impaired thyroid hormone activation due to transport inhibition of T4- into T3-producing tissues. J Clin Endocrinol Metabol 1993;77(5):1431–1435.

378 Stump CS, Short KR, Bigelow ML, et al. Effect of insulin on human skeletal muscle mitochondrial ATP production, protein synthesis, and mRNA transcripts. Proc Natl Acad Sci 2003;100(13):7996–8001.

379 Krenning EP, Docter R, Bernard HF, et al. The essential role of albumin in the active transport of thyroid hormones into primary cultured rat hepatocytes. FEBS Lett 1979;1;107(1):227–30.

380 Krenning EP, Docter R, Bernard HF, et al. Regulation of the active transport of 3,3′,5-triiodothyronine (T$_3$) into primary cultured rat hepatocytes by ATP. FEBS Lett 1979;10(1):227–230.

381 van der Heyden JT, Docter R, van Toor H, et al. Effects of caloric deprivation on thyroid hormone tissue uptake and generation of low-T3 syndrome. Am J Physiol Endocrinol Metab 1986;251(2):E156–E163.

382 Wassen FWJS, Moerings EPCM, van Toor H, et al. Thyroid hormone uptake in cultured rat anterior pituitary cells: effects of energy status and bilirubin. J Endocrinol 2000;165:599–606.

383 Jenning AS, Ferguson DC, Utiger RD. Regulation of the conversion of thyroxine to triiodothyronine in the perfused rat liver. J Clin Invest 1979;64:1614–1623.

384 Krenning E, Docter R, Bernard B, Visser T, Hennemann G. Characteristics of active transport of thyroid hormone into rat hepatocytes. Biochim Biophys Acta 1981;676:314–320.

385 Riley WW, Eales JG. Characterization of 3,5,3-triiodo-lthyronine transport into hepatocytes isolated from juvenile rainbow trout (*Oncorhynchus mykiss*), and comparison with l-thyroxine transport. Gen Comp Endocrinol 1994;95:301–309.

386 Spencer CA, Lum SMC, Wilber JF, et al. Dynamics of serum thyrotropin and thyroid hormone changes in fasting. J Clin Endocrin Metab 1983;(5):883–888.

387 St Germain DL, Galton VA. Comparative study of pituitary-thyroid hormone economy in fasting and hypothyroid rats. J Clin Invest 1985;75(2):679–688.

388 Arem R, Wiener GJ, Kaplan SG, et al. Reduced tissue thyroid hormone levels in fatal illness. Metabolism 1993;42(9):1102–8.

389 Lim C-F, Bernard BF, De Jong M, et al. A furan fatty acid and indoxyl sulfate are the putative inhibitors of thyroxine hepatocyte transport in uremia. J Clin Endocrinol Metab 1993;76:318–324.

390 Lim C-F, Docter R, Visser TJ, et al. Inhibition of thyroxine transport into cultured rat hepatocytes by serum of non-uremic critically ill patients: effects of bilirubin and nonesterified fatty acids. J Clin Endocrinol Metab 1993;76:1165–1172.

391 Lim VS, Passo C, Murata Y, et al. Reduced triiodothyronine content in liver but not pituitary of the uremic rat model: demonstration of changes compatible with thyroid hormone deficiency in liver only. Endocrinology 1984;114:280–286.

392 Everts ME, Lim C-F, Moerings EPCM, et al. Effects of a furan fatty acid and indoxyl sulfate on thyroid hormone uptake in cultured anterior pituitary cells. Am J Physiol 1995;268:E974–E979.

393 Doyle D. Benzodiazepines inhibit temperature dependent L-[125I] triiodothyronine accumulation into human liver, human neuroblast, and rat pituitary cell lines. Endocrinology 1992;130:1211–1216.

394 Krenning EP, Docter R, Bernard HF, et al. Decreased transport of thyroxine (T4), 3,3′,5-triiodothyronine (T3) and 3,3′,5′-triiodothyronine (rT3) into rat hepatocytes in primary culture due to a decrease of cellular ATP content and various drugs. FEBS Lett 1982;140:229–233.

395 Kaptein EM, Robinson WJ, Grieb DA, et al. Peripheral serum thyroxine, triiodothyronine, and reverse triiodothyronine in the low thyroxine state of acute nonthyroidal illness. A noncompartmental analysis. J Clin Invest 1982;69:526–535.

396 Kaptein EM, Kaptein JS, Chang EI, et al. Thyroxine transfer and distribution in critical nonthyroidal illness, chronic renal failure, and chronic ethanol abuse. J Clin Endocrinol Metab 1987;65:606–616.

397 Everts ME, Visser TJ, Moerings EM, et al. Uptake of triiodothyroacetic acid and its effect on thyrotropin secretion in cultured anterior pituitary cells. Endocrinology 1994;135(6):2700–2707.

398 De Jong M, Docter R, van der Hoek HJ, Vos RA. Transport of 3,5,3′-triiodothyronine into the perfused rat liver and subsequent metabolism are inhibited by fasting. Endocrinology 1992;131(1):463–470.

399 Hennemann G, Krenning EP, Bernard B, et al. Regulation of influx and efflux of thyroid hormones in rat hepatocytes: possible physiologic significance of plasma membrane in the regulation of thyroid hormone activity. Horm Metab Res Suppl 1984;14:1–6.

400 Petersen KF, Dufour S, Shulman GI. Decreased insulin-stimulated ATP synthesis and phosphate transport in muscle of insulin-resistant offspring of type 2 diabetic parents. PLoS Med 2005;2(9):e233.

401 Szendroedi J, Schmid AI, Meyerspeer M, et al. Impaired mitochondrial function and insulin resistance of skeletal muscle in mitochondrial diabetes. Diabetes Care 2009;32(4):677–9.

402 Abdul-Ghani MA, Jani R, Chavez A, et al. Mitochondrial reactive oxygen species generation in obese non-diabetic and type 2 diabetic participants. Diabetologia 2009;52(4):574–82.

403 Verga SB, Donatelli M, Orio L, et al. A low reported energy intake is associated with metabolic syndrome. J Endocrinol Invest 2009;32: 538–541.

404 Brehm A, Krssak M, Schmid AI, et al. Increased lipid availability impairs insulin-stimulated ATP synthesis in human skeletal muscle. Diabetes 2006;55:136–140.

405 DeMarco NM, Beitz DC, Whitehurst GB. Effect of fasting on free fatty acid, glycerol and cholesterol concentrations in blood plasma and lipoprotein lipase activity in adipose tissue of cattle. J Anim Sci 1981;52:75–82.

406 Leibel RL, Jirsch J. Diminished energy requirements in reduced-obese patients. Metabolism 1984;33(2):164–170.

407 Steen SN, Opplieger RA, Brownell KD. Metabolic effects of repeated weight and regain in adolescent wrestlers. JAMA 1988;260:47–50.

408 Elliot DL, Goldberg L, Kuehl KD, Bennett WM. Sustained depression of the resting metabolic rate after massive weight loss. Am J Clin Nutr 1989;49:93–6.

409 Manore MM, Berry TE, Skinner JS, Carroll SS. Energy expenditure at rest and during exercise in nonobese female cyclical dieters and in nondieting control subjects. Am J Clin Nutr 1991;54:41–6.

410 Croxson MS, Ibbertson HK, Low serum triiodothyronine (T3) and hypothyroidism in anorexia nervosa. J Clin Endocrinol Metab 1977;44: 167–174.

411 Carlin K, Carlin S. Possible etiology for euthyroid sick syndrome. Med Hypotheses 1993;40:38–43.

412 Brownell KD, Greenwood MR, Stellar E, Shrager EE. The effects of repeated cycles of weight loss and regain in rats. Physiol Behav 1986;38(4):459–64.

413 Pieczenik SR, Neustadt J. Mitochondrial dysfunction and molecular pathways of disease. Exp Mol Pathol 2007;83(1):84–92.

414 Wallace DC. A mitochondrial paradigm of metabolic and degenerative diseases, aging, and cancer: a dawn for evolutionary medicine. Ann Rev Genetics 2005;39(1):359–407.

415 Fosslien, E. Mitochondrial medicine—molecular pathology of defective oxidative phosphorylation. Ann Clin Lab Sci 2001;31(1):25–67.

416 West IC. Radicals and oxidative stress in diabetes. Diabet Med 2000;17(3):171–180.

417 Modica-Napolitano JS, Renshaw PF. Ethanolamine and phosphoethanolamine inhibit mitochondrial function in vitro: implications for mitochondrial dysfunction hypothesis in depression and bipolar disorder. Biological Psychiatry 2004;55(3):273–277.

418 Gardner A, Boles RG. Mitochondrial energy depletion in depression with somatization. Psychother Psychosom 2008;77:127–129.

419 Burroughs S, French D. Depression and anxiety: role of mitochondria. Current Anesthesia Crit Care 2007;18:34–41.

420 Einat H, Yuan P, Manji HK. Increased anxiety-like behaviors and mitochondrial dysfunction in mice with targeted mutation of the Bcl-2 gene: further support for the involvement of mitochondrial function in anxiety disorders. Behav Brain Res 2005;165(2):172–180.

421 Stork C, Renshaw PF. Mitochondrial dysfunction in bipolar disorder: evidence from magnetic resonance spectroscopy research. Mol Psychiatry 2005;10(10):900–919.

422 Fattal O, Budur, Vaughan AJ, Franco K. Review of the literature on major mental disorders in adult patients with mitochondrial diseases. Psychosomatics 2006;47(1):1–7.

423 Hutchin T, Cortopassi G. A mitochondrial DNA clone is associated with increased risk for Alzheimer's disease. Proc Natl Acad Sci USA 1995;92:6892–95.

424 Sherer TB, Betarbet R, Greenamyre JT. Environment, mitochondria, and Parkinson's disease. Neuroscientist 2002;8(3):192–7.

425 Gomez C, Bandez MJ, Navarro A. Pesticides and impairment of mitochondrial function in relation with the Parkinsonian syndrome. Front Biosci 2007;12:1079–93.

426 Stavrovskaya IG, Kristal BS. The powerhouse takes control of the cell: is the mitochondrial permeability transition a viable therapeutic target against neuronal dysfunction and death? Free Radic Biol Med 2005;38(6):687–697.

427 Schapira AHV. Mitochondrial disease. Lancet 2006;368:70–82.

428 Richter, C. Oxidative damage to mitochondrial DNA and its relationship to aging. Int J Biochem Cell Biol 1995;27(7):647–653.

429 Papa, S. Mitochondrial oxidative phosphorylation changes in the life span. Molecular aspects and physiopathological implications. Biochimica Biophysica Acta 1996;87–105.

430 Cortopassi G, Wang A. Mitochondria in organismal aging and degeneration. Biochimica Biophysica Acta 1999;1410:183–193.

431 Harman, D. The biologic clock: the mitochondria? J Am Geriatr Soc 1972;20:145–147.

432 Miquel J, Economos AC, Fleming J, Johnson JE. Mitochondrial role in cell aging. Exp Gerontol 1980;15:575–91.

433 Miquel J. An integrated theory of aging as the result of mitochondrial DNA mutation in differentiated cells. Arch Gerontol Geriatr 1991;12: 99–117.

434 Miquel J. An update on the mitochondrial-DNA mutation hypothesis of cell aging. Mutation Research 1992;275:209–16.

435 Zs-Nagy I. A membrane hypothesis of aging. J Theor Biol 1978;75:189–195.

436 Zs-Nagy I. The role of membrane structure and function in cellular aging: a review. Mech Aging Dev 1979;9:37–246.

437 Savitha S, Sivarajan K, Haripriya D, et al. Efficacy of levo carnitine and alpha lipoic acid in ameliorating the decline in mitochondrial enzymes during aging. Clin Nutr 2005;24(5):794–800.

438 Skulachev VP, Longo VD. Aging as a mitochondria-mediated atavistic program: can aging be switched off? Ann NY Acad Sci 2005;1057:145–164.

439 Corral-Debrinski M, Shoffner JM, Lott MT, Wallace DC. Association of mitochondrial DNA damage with aging and coronary atherosclerotic heart disease. Mutat Res 1992;275(3–6):169–180.

440 Ames BN, Shigenaga MK, Hagen TM. Oxidants, antioxidants, and the degenerative diseases of aging. Proc Natl Acad Sci USA 1993;90(17): 7915–7922.

441 Fulle S, Mecocci P, Fano G, et al. Specific oxidative alterations in vastus lateralis muscle of patients with the diagnosis of chronic fatigue syndrome. Free Radic Biol Med 2000;29(12):1252–1259.

442 Buist R. Elevated xenobiotics, lactate and pyruvate in C.F.S. patients. J Orthomolec Medicine 1989;4(3):170–172.

443 Park JH, Niermann KJ, Olsen N. Evidence for metabolic abnormalities in the muscles of patients with fibromyalgia. Curr Rheumatol Rep 2000;2(2):131–140.

444 Yunus MB, Kalyan-Raman UP, Kalyan-Raman K. Primary fibromyalgia syndrome and myofascial pain syndrome: clinical features and muscle pathology. Arch Phys Med Rehabil 1988;69(6):451–454.

445 Puddu P, Puddu GM, Galletti L, Cravero E, Muscari A. Mitochondrial dysfunction as an initiating event in atherogenesis: a plausible hypothesis. Cardiology 2005;103(3):137–141.

446 Chen L, Knowlton AA. Depressed mitochondrial fusion in heart failure. Circulation 2007;116:259.

447 Kaptein EM, Feinstein EI, Nicoloff JT, Massry SG. Serum reverse triiodothyronine and thyroxine kinetics in patients with chronic renal failure. J Clin Endocrinol Metab 1983;57:181–189.

448 Kaptein EM. Thyroid hormone metabolism and thyroid disease in chronic renal failure. Endocr Rev 1996;17:45–63.

449 Kaptein EM. Clinical relevance of thyroid hormone alterations in nonthyroidal illness. Thyroid Int 1997;4:22–25.

450 Kigoshi S, Akiyama M, Ito R. Close correlation between levels of cholesterol and free fatty acids in lymphoid cells. Cell Mol Life Sci 1976;32(10):1244–1246.

451 Escobar-Morreale HF, Obregón MJ, Escobar del Rey F. Only the combined treatment with thyroxine and triiodothyronine ensures euthyroidism in all tissues of the thyroidectomized rat. Endocrinology 1996;137:2490–2502.

452 Fraser WD, Biggart EM, O'Reilly DJ, et al. Are biochemical tests of thyroid function of any value in monitoring patients receiving thyroxine replacement? BMJ 1986;293:808–810.

453 Escobar-Morreale HF, Obregón MJ, Escobar del Rey F, et al. Replacement therapy for hypothyroidism with thyroxine alone does not ensure euthyroidism in all tissues, as studied in thyroidectomized rats. J Clin Invest 1995;96(6):2828–2838.

454 Meier C, Trittibach P, Guglielmetti M, Staub JJ, Muller B. Serum TSH in assessment of severity of tissue hypothyroidism in patients with overt primary thyroid failure: cross sectional survey. BMJ 2003;326:311–312.

455 Alevizaki M, Mantzou E, Cimponeriu AT, et al. TSH may not be a good marker for adequate thyroid hormone replacement therapy. Wien Klin Wochenschr 2005;117/18:636–640.

456 Zulewski H, Muller B, Exer P, et al. Estimation of tissue hypothyroidism by a new clinical score: evaluation of patients with various grades of hypothyroidism and controls. J Clin Endocrinol Metab 1997;82(3):771–776.

457 Hackney AC, Feith S, Pozos, R, Seale J. Effects of high altitude and cold exposure on resting thyroid hormone concentrations. Aviat Space Environ Med 1995;66(4):325–9.

458 Opstad PK, Falch D, Oktedalen O, et al. The thyroid function in young men during prolonged exercise and the effect of energy and sleep deprivation. Clin Endo 1984;20:657–669.

459 Ellingsen DG, Efskind J, Haug E, et al. Effects of low mercury vapour exposure on the thyroid function in Chloralkai workers. J Appl Toxicol 2000;20:483–489.

460 den Brinker M, Joosten KFM, Visser, et al. Euthyroid sick syndrome in meningococcal sepsis: the impact of peripheral thyroid hormone metabolism and binding proteins. J Clin Endocrinol Metab 2005;90(10):5613–5620.

461 Chopra IJ, Solomon DH, Hepner GW, et al. Misleadingly low free thyroxine index and usefulness of reverse triiodothyronine measurement in nonthyroidal illnesses. Ann Intern Med 1979;90(6):905–12.

462 van den Beld AW, Visser TJ, Feelders RA, et al. Thyroid hormone concentrations, disease, physical function and mortality in elderly men. J Clin Endocrinol Metab 2005;90(12):6403–9.

463 Chopra IJ. A study of extrathyroidal conversion of thyroxine (T4) to 3,3′,5-triiodothyronine (T3) in vitro. Endocrinology 1977;101(2):453–63.

464 Sechman A, Niezgoda J, Sobocinski R. The relationship between basal metabolic rate (BMR) and concentrations of plasma thyroid hormones in fasting cockerels. Folia Biol (Krakow) 1989;37(1–2):83–90.

465 Magri F, Cravello L, Fioravanti M, et al. Thyroid function in old and very old healthy subjects. J Endocrinol Invest 2002;25(10):60–63.

466 O'Brian JI, Baybee DE, Wartofsky L, et al. Altered peripheral thyroid hormone metabolism and diminished hypothalamic pituitary responsiveness with changes in dietary composition. Clin Res 1978;26:310A.

467 Friberg L, Drvota V, Bjelak AH, Eggertsen G, Ahnve S. Association between increased levels of reverse triiodothyronine and mortality after acute myocardial infarction. Am J Med 2001;111(9):699–703.

468 McCormack PD. Cold stress, reverse T3 and lymphocyte function. Alaska Med 1998;40(3):55–62.

469 Scriba PC, Bauer M, Emmert D, et al. Effects of obesity, total fasting and re-alimentation on L-thyroxine (T4), 3,5,3-L-triiodothyronine (T3), 3,3,5-L-triiodothyronine (rT3), -thyroxine binding globulin (TBG), transferrin, 2–haptoglobin and complement C3 in serum. Acta Endocrinol 1979;91:629–43.

470 Kvetny J. Thyroxine binding and cellular metabolism of thyroxine in mononuclear blood cells from patients with anorexia nervosa. J Endocrinol 1983 Sep;98(3):343–50.

471 Germain DL. Metabolic effect of 3,3′,5′-triiodothyronine in cultured growth hormone-producing rat pituitary tumor cells. Evidence for a unique mechanism of thyroid hormone action. J Clin Invest 1985;76(2):890–893.

472 Szymanski PT. Effects of thyroid hormones and reverse T3 pretreatment on the betaadrenoreceptors in the rat heart. Acta Physiol Pol 1986;37:131–138.

473 du Pont JS. Is reverse triiodothyronine a physiological nonactive competitor for the action of triiodothyronine upon the electrical properties of GH3 cells? Neuroendocrinology 1991;54:146–150.

474 Schulte C. Low T3 syndrome and nutritional status as prognostic factors in patients undergoing bone marrow transplantation. Bone Marrow Transplant 1998;22:1171–1178.

475   Goichot B, Schlienger JL, Grunenberger F, et al. Thyroid hormone status and nutrient intake in the free-living elderly. Interest of reverse triiodothyronine assessment. Eur J Endo 1994;130:244–252.
476   Okamoto R, Leibfritz D. Adverse effects of reverse triodothyronine on cellular metabolism as assessed by 1H and 31P NMR spectroscopy. Res Exp Med 1997;197:211–217.
477   de Jong FJ, den Heijer T, Visser TJ, et al. Thyroid hormones, dementia, and atrophy of the medial temporal lobe. J Clin Endo Metab 2006;91(7):2569–2573.
478   Forestier E, Vinzio S, Sapin R, et al. Increased reverse T3 is associated with shorter survival in independently-living elderly. The Alsanut Study. Eur J Endocrinol 2009;160(2):207–14.
479   Visser TJ, Lamberts WJ, Wilson JHP, et al. Serum thyroid hormone concentrations during prolonged reduction of dietary intake. Metabolism 1978;27(4):405–409.
480   Linnoila M, Lamberg BA, Potter WZ, et al. High reverse T3 levels in manic and unipolar depressed women. Psych Res 1982;6:271–276.
481   McCormack PD, Reed HL, Thomas JR, et al. Increases in rT3 serum levels observed during extended Alaskan field operations of naval personnel. Alaska Med 1996;38(3):89–97.
482   Mariotti S, Barbesino G, Caturegli P, et al. Complex alteration of thyroid function in healthy centenarians. J Clin Endo Metab 1993;77(5):1130–1134.
483   Danforth EJ, Desilets EJ, Jorton ES, et al. Reciprocal serum triiodothryronine (T3) and reverse (rT3) induced by altering the carbohydrate content of the diet. Clin Res 1975;23:573.
484   McCormack PD, Thomas J, Malik M, Staschen CM. Cold stress, reverse T3 and lymphocyte function. Alaskan Med 1998;40(3):55–62.
485   Peeters RP, Wouters PJ, van Toor H, et al. Serum 3,3',5'-triiodothyronine (rT3) and 3,5,3'-triiodothyronine/rT3 are prognostic markers in critically ill patients and are associated with postmortem tissue deiodinase activities. J Clin Endocrinol Metab 2005;90(8):4559–65.
486   Szabolcs I, Weber M, Kovacs Z, et al. The possible reason for serum 3,3'5'-(reverse T3) triiodothyronine increase in old people. Acta Medica Acad Sci Hun Tomus 1982;39(1–2):11–17.
487   Silberman H, Eisenberg D, Ryan J, et al. The relation of thyroid indices in the critically ill patient to prognosis and nutritional factors. Surg Gynecol Obstet 1988;166(3):223–228.
488   Mitchell AM, Manley SW, Rowan KA, Mortimer RH. Uptake of reverse T3 in the human choriocarcinoma cell line Jar. Placenta 1999;20:65–70.
489   Stan M, Morris JC. Thyrotropin-axis adaptation in aging and chronic disease. Endocrinol Metab Clin N Am 2005;34:973–992.
490   LoPresti JS, Eigen A, Kaptein E, et al. Alterations in 3,3',5'-triiodothyronine metabolism in response to propylthiouracil, dexamethasone, and thyroxine administration in man. J Clin Invest 1989;84:1650–1656.
491   Palmblad J, Levi L, Burger A, et al. Effects of total energy withdrawal (fasting) on the levels of growth hormone, thyrotropin, cortisol, adrenaline, noradrenaline, T4, T3, and rT3 in healthy males. Acta Med Scand 1977;201:15–22.
492   Reinhardt W, Misch C, Jockenhovel F, et al. Triiodothyronine (T3) reflects renal graft function after renal transplantation. Clin Endo 1997;46:563–569.
493   Chopra IJ, Chopra U, Smith SR, et al. Reciprocal changes in serum concentrations of 3,3'5'-triiodothyronine (reverse T3) and 3,3'5'-triiodothyronine (T3) in systemic illnesses. J Clin Endocrinol Met 1975;41(6):1043–1049.
494   Spaulding SW, Chopra IJ, Swherwin RS, et al. Effect of caloric restriction and dietary composition on serum T3 and reverse T3 in man. J Clin Endocrinol Metab 1976;42(197):197–200.
495   Girdler SS, Pedersen CA, Light KC. Thyroid axis function during the menstrual cycle in women with premenstrual syndrome. Psychoneuroendocrinology 1995;20(4):395–403.
496   Peeters RP, Wouters PJ, Kaptein E, et al. Reduced activation and increased inactivation of thyroid hormone in tissues of critically ill patients. J Clin Endocrinol Metab 2003;88:3202–11.
497   Pittman JA, Tingley JO, Nickerson JF, Hill SR. Antimetabolic activity of 3,3',5'-triiodo-dl-thyronine in man. Metabolism 1960;9:293–5.
498   Desai M, Irani AJ, Patil K, et al. The importance of reverse triiodothyroinine in hypothyroid children on replacement treatment. Archives Dis Childhood 1984;59:30–35.
499   Chopra IJ. A radioimmunoassay for measurement of 3,3',5'-triiodothyronine (reverse T3). J Clin Invest 1974;54:583–92.
500   Kodding R, Hesch RD. L-3',5'-diiodothyronine in human serum. Lancet 1978;312(8098):1049.
501   Benua RS, Kumaoka S, Leeper RD, Rawson RW. The effect of dl-3,3',5'-triiodothyronine in Grave's disease. J Clin Endocrinol Metab 1959;19:1344–6.
502   Chopra IJ. Study of extrathyroidal conversion of T4 to T3 in vitro: evidence that reverse T3 is a potent inhibitor of T3 production. Clin Res 1976;24:142A.
503   Gavin LA, Moeller M, Shoback D, Cavalieri RR. Reverse T3 and modulators of the calcium messenger system rapidly decrease T4–5'-deiodinase II activity in cultured mouse neuroblastoma cells. Thyroidology 1988;(1):5–12.
504   Chopra IJ, Williams DE, Orgiazzi J, Solomon DH. Opposite effects of dexamethasone on serum concentrations of 3,3',5'-triiodothyronine (reverse T3) and 3,3',5-triiodothyronine (T3). JCEM 1975;41:911–920.
505   Brent GA, Hershman JM. Thyroxine therapy in patients with severe nonthyroidal illnesses and low serum thyroxine concentration. J Clin Endocrinol Metab 1986;63(1):1–8.
506   Escobar-Morreale HF, Obregon MJ, Escobar del Rey F, et al. Replacement therapy for hypothyroidism with thyroxine alone does not ensure euthyroidism in all tissues, as studied in thyroidectomized rats. J Clin Invest 1995;96(6):2828–2838.
507   Lomenick JP, El-Sayyid M, Smith WJ. Effect of levo-thyroxine treatment on weight and body mass index in children with acquired hypothyroidism. J Pediatr 2008;152(1):96–100.
508   Acker CG, Singh AR, Flick RP, et al. A trial of thyroxine in acute renal failure. Kidney Int 2000;57:293–8.
509   Samuels MH, Schuff KG, Carlson NE, Carello P, Janowsky JS. Health status, psychological symptoms, mood, and cognition in L-thyroxine-treated hypothyroid subjects. Thyroid 2007;17(3):249–58.
510   Krotkiewski M, Holm G, Shono N. Small doses of triiodothyronine can change some risk factors associated with abdominal obesity. Int J Obesity 1997;21:922–929.
511   Krotkiewski M. Thyroid hormones and treatment of obesity. Int J Obesity 2000;24(2):S116–S119.
512   Lowe JC, Garrison RL, Reichman AJ, et al. Effectiveness and safety of T3 (triiodothyronine) therapy for euthyroid fibromyalgia: a double-blind placebo-controlled response-driven crossover study. Clin Bull Myofasc Ther 1997;2(2/3):31–58.
513   Lowe JC, Reichman AJ, Yellin J. The process of change during T3 treatment for euthyroid fibromyalgia: a double-blind placebo-controlled crossover study. Clin Bull Myofasc Ther 1997;2(2/3):91–124.

514 Lowe JC, Garrison RL, Reichman AJ, et al. Triiodothyronine (T3) treatment of euthyroid fibromyalgia: a small-n replication of a double-blind placebo-controlled crossover study. Clin Bull Myofasc Ther 1997;2(4):71–88.

515 Samuels MH, Schuff KG, Carlson NE, Carello P, Janowsky JS. Health status, psychological symptoms, mood, and cognition in L-thyroxine-treated hypothyroid subjects. Thyroid 2007;17(3):249–58.

516 Cooke RG, Joffe RT, Levitt AJ. T3 augmentation of antidepressant treatment in T4-replaced thyroid patients. J Clin Psychiatry 1992;53(1):16–8.

517 Bettendorf M, Schmidt KG, Grulich-Henn J, et al. Tri-idothyronine treatment in children after cardiac surgery: a double-blind, randomized, placebo-controlled study. The Lancet 2000;356:529–534.

518 Pingitore A, Galli E, Barison A, et al. Acute effects of triiodothryronine replacement therapy in patients with chronic heart failure and low-T3 syndrome: a randomized placebo-controlled study. J Clin Endocrin Metab 2008;93(4):1351–8.

519 Meyer T, Husch M, van den Berg E, et al. Treatment of dopamine-dependent shock with triiodothyronine: preliminary results. Deutsch Med Wochenschr 1979;104:1711–14.

520 Dulchavsky SA, Hendrick SR, Dutta S. Pulmonary biophysical effects of triiodothyronine (T3) augmentation during sepsis induced hypothyroidism. J Trauma 1993;35:104–9.

521 Novitzsky D, Cooper DKC, Human PA, et al. Triiodothyronine therapy for heart donor and recipient. J Heart Transplant 1988;7:370–6.

522 Dulchavsky SA, Maitra SR, Maurer J, et al. Beneficial effects of thyroid hormone administration in metabolic and hemodynamic function in hemorrhagic shock. FASEB J 1990;4:A952.

523 Klemperer JD, Klein I, Gomez M, et al. Thyroid hormone treatment after coronary-artery bypass surgery. N Engl J Med 1995;333:1522–7.

524 Gomberg-Maitland M. Thyroid hormone and cardiovascular disease. Am Heart J 1998;135:187–96.

525 Dulchavsky SA, Kennedy PR, Geller ER, et al. T3 preserves respiratory function in sepsis. J Trauma 1991;31:753–9.

526 Novitzky D, Cooper DK, Reichart B. Hemodynamic and metabolic responses to hormonal therapy in brain-dead potential organ donors. Transplantation 1987;43:852–5.

527 Hamilton MA, Stevenson LW, Fonarow GC, et al. Safety and hemodynamic effects of intravenous triiodothyronine in advanced congestive heart failure. Am J Cardiol 1998;81:443–7.

528 Klemperer JD, Klein IL, Ojamaa K, et al. Triidothyronine therapy lowers the incidence of atrial fibrillation after cardiac operations. Ann Thorac Surg 1996;61:1323–9.

429 Smidt-Ott UM, Ascheim DD. Thyroid hormone and heart failure. Curr Heart Fail Rep 2006;3:114–9.

530 Englebienne P, Verhas M, Herst CV, et al. Type I interferons induce proteins susceptible to act as thyroid receptor (TR) corepressors and to signal the TR for destruction by the proteasome: possible etiology for unexplained chronic fatigue. Med Hypotheses 2003;60(2):175–80.

531 Garrison RL, Breeding PC. A metabolic basis for fibromyalgia and its related disorders: the possible role of resistance to thyroid hormone. Med Hypotheses 2003;61(2):182–89.

532 Primary Care Provider Education Project. Chronic Fatigue Syndrome: A Diagnostic and Management Challenge. Center for Disease Control and Prevention; 2003:3.

533 Refetoff S, Weiss RE, Usala SJ. The syndromes of resistance to thyroid hormone. Endocr Rev 1993;14(3):348–99.

534 Braverman LE, Utiger RD. Introduction to hypothyroidism. In: Werner and Ingbar's The Thyroid: A Fundamental and Clinical Text. Baltimore, MD: Lippincott; 1991, p.919–920.

535 Iranmanesh A, Lizarralde G, Johnson M, et al. Dynamics of 24-hour endogenous cortisol secretion and clearance in primary hypothyroidism assessed before and after partial thyroid hormone replacement. J Clin Endocrinol Metab 1990;70:155.

536 Scott LV, Svec F, Dinan T. A preliminary study of dehydroepiandrosterone response to low-dose ACTH in chronic fatigue syndrome and in healthy subjects. Psychiatry Res 2000;97(1):21–8.

537 Ciloglu F, Peker I, Pehlivan A, et al. Exercise intensity and its effects on thyroid hormones. Neuro Endocrinol Lett. 2005;26(6):830-4.

2

Hyperthyroidism

T

he three main types of hyperthyroidism are Graves' disease, thyroid multinodular goiter, and toxic adenoma.

Graves' Disease

The most common cause of hyperthyroidism is Graves' disease, which is an autoimmune disorder that directs antibodies against thyroid-stimulating hormone (TSH) receptors, destroying them in the process. The autoimmune activity associated with Graves' disease involves both B and T lymphocytes and is directed at four specific thyroid antigens. These antigens include the sodium/iodide symporter (NIS), thyroglobulin (Tg), thyroid peroxidase (TPO), and the thyrotropin receptor (TSH-R). Each of these antigens serves a specific role, and each is key to normal thyroid function.[1] NIS transports iodine from blood into the thyroid follicular cells. TPO organifies iodine by attaching it to tyrosine moieties on the Tg molecule as a step in the formation of thyroxine (T4). T4 is converted to triiodothyronine (T3) in the peripheral tissues by iodothyronine deiodinase.

Thyroglobulin antibody (TgAb) is directed against Tg, and thyroid peroxidase antibody (TPOAb) is directed against TPO. The formation of TgAb and TPOAb is associated with all types of autoimmune thyroid diseases, so their presence in the blood can be used to diagnose underlying autoimmunity without the presence of clinical symptoms.[2] For instance, an elevation of these autoimmune antibodies may precede diagnosis of autoimmune disease diagnosis by 2–7 years.[3]

Thyroid stimulating immunoglobulins (TSIs) are considered diagnostic for Graves' disease even though only about 80% of Graves' patients (both treated and untreated) have them. In addition, TSIs are elevated in 5–10% of patients with Hashimoto's thyroiditis (one reason Hashimoto's patients can go hyperthyroid sometimes). TPO antibodies are a sign of thyroid tissue destruction and are found in about 90% of Hashimoto's patients and about 75% of Graves' patients.[4-6]

The sensitive TSH (or thyrotropin) assay has become the single best screening test for hyperthyroidism and is the most sensitive test for detecting mild thyroid hormone excess.[7] There is no complete agreement on the TSH levels diagnostic of hyperthyroidism. Whereas the low end of the reference range for TSH listed by many laboratories is 0.5 µIU/ml, the American Association of Clinical Endocrinologists recommends that hyperthyroidism be diagnosed with TSH less than 0.3 µIU/ml.[7,8]

Although Hashimoto's (autoimmune) thyroiditis is accompanied by elevated TgAb in more than 90% of cases, the presence of TgAb alone does not necessarily suggest thyroid disease.[9] Elevation of TgAb is also indicative of other autoimmune disorders (e.g., systemic lupus erythematosus). Diseases linked to an elevation of both TgAb and TPOAb include autoimmune thyroiditis, rheumatoid arthritis, pernicious anemia, and type I diabetes.[6] The presence of TgAb, but not TPOAb, is an independent risk factor for thyroid cancer.[10]

Ophthalmopathy and pre-tibial myxedema are common symptoms of Graves' disease, and are caused by thyroid antibodies that cross-react with antigens in fibroblasts and adipocytes behind the eye. All hyperthyroid patients can develop eyelid retraction and a distinctive stare/bulging eyes (exophthalmos). Patients with high TSI antibodies and absent TPO antibodies are particularly susceptible to exophthalmos.

Graves' ophthalmopathy

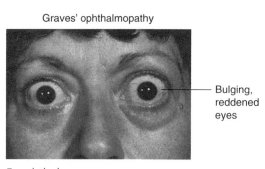

Bulging, reddened eyes

Exophthalmos

Toxic Multinodular Goiter and Toxic Adenoma

Goiter is swelling of the thyroid gland that can occur whether the gland is functioning properly or not. In toxic multinodular goiter, rogue thyroid cells form nodules that autonomously produce excess thyroid hormone. Toxic multinodular goiter is the second most common cause of hyperthyroidism (after Graves' disease).[11] A toxic thyroid adenoma is distinguished from a toxic multinodular goiter of the thyroid in that an adenoma is a benign neoplasm that is typically solitary, but both require treatment. Twenty to 80 percent of toxic adenomas and some nodules of multinodular goiters have somatic mutations of the TSH receptor gene, causing the follicular cells to escape from the normal control exerted by the pituitary gland.[12,13] These autonomous follicular cells then begin to produce and secrete thyroid hormone in an uncontrolled manner (i.e., unregulated by TSH).[14]

The prevalence of toxic nodular goiter increases with age and tends to be more common in areas where iodine intake is relatively low (i.e., places where iodine deficiency is common).[15] Toxic thyroid adenoma (unlike toxic nodular goiter) is not related to iodine intake, but rather results from a genetic abnormality in a single precursor cell.[16]

By definition, both of these types of thyroid nodule disorders are benign. Therefore, there is a very low risk that the follicular cells will spread/invade other parts of the neck or the body. However, careful pathological examination may be necessary to distinguish a thyroid adenoma from a minimally invasive follicular thyroid carcinoma.[13]

Conventional Medical Treatment

Conventional treatment of hyperthyroidism includes propylthiouracil (PTU), radioiodine (RAI), and surgery. PTU works in two ways: 1) inhibiting the enzyme thyroperoxidase, which normally acts in thyroid hormone synthesis by oxidizing the anion iodide (I⁻) to iodine (I⁰), and 2) blocking conversion of T4 to T3 in the peripheral tissues. RAI is the conventional treatment of choice for Graves' disease because it eliminates the hyperthyroid condition. However, patients treated with RAI will usually be hypothyroid for life. In rare cases of Graves' disease, patients may require surgery to partially or fully remove the thyroid gland.

Complementary and Alternative Medicine

Due to potential side effects associated with many conventional hyperthyroid medications, complementary and alternative therapies should almost always be tried first. Obviously, this is not advised in a hyperthyroid emergency. Table 2.1 summarizes some herbs and nutrients commonly used to provide support in autoimmune hyperthyroidism.

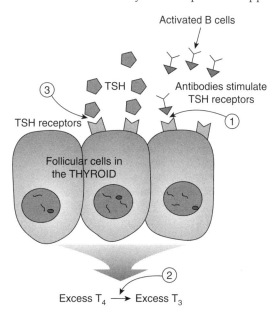

① Inhibition of thyroid activation by immunoglobulins

② Inhibition of $T_4 \rightarrow T_3$ conversion

③ Inhibition of TSH binding

④ (+) ionotrophic, (−) chronotrophic, antioxidant, antimicrobial, antispasmodic

Thyroid Stimulating Immunoglobulins stimulate TSH receptors. Four mechanisms of action of herbal constituents rosmarinic acid, lithospermic acid, and caffeic acid in Graves' disease.

Table 2.1. Key herbs and nutrients that provide thyroid support in autoimmune hyperthyroidism

Herb/Nutrient*	Action	Dose
Rosmarinic Acid[17–22]	• Helpful in lowering antithyroid antibodies in both hyper- and hypothyroidism • Induces T cell apoptosis of only actively proliferating T cells • Directs T cell activity • Inhibits T cell activation and proliferation • Modulates T cell promotion of pro-inflammatory cytokine release • Believed to prevent TSH effects on receptor sites, block immunoglobulin effects on TSH receptors, and inhibit peripheral conversion of T4 to T3	335 mg twice per day
Bugleweed *(Lycopus virginacus)*[23]	• Vascular sedative (e.g., decreases blood pressure) • Good for rapid pulse with a weak heart • Targets the pituitary thyroidal and gonadal system • Decreases T4, T3, and TSH levels within 24 hours • Inhibits iodine metabolism and T4	
Iris Versicolor (Blue flag)**[24]	• Stimulates glandular secretion and removal of wastes through the lymphatic system • Anti-inflammatory actions reduces thyroid enlargement	750 mg per day
Motherwort *(Leonurus cardiaca)*[25]	• Central nervous depressant • Hypotensive effects • Adjuvant therapy for hyperthyroidism • Action due to the alkaloid leonurine	
Commiphora mukul (Guggul)*[21–30]	• Naturally increases T3 levels; also effective in decreasing T3 levels in hyperthyroid patients	750 mg per day
Selenium[31]	• Decreases TPO antibodies • Increases glutathione peroxidase (GPX), decreasing hydrogen peroxide which damages the thyroid	400 µg per day
Potassium Iodide[32–34]	• Critical component for thyroid hormone metabolism • Extra iodine with hidden hot nodule can lead to thyroid storm; stop iodine if thyrotoxic symptoms appear or worsen	6 mg per day
Vitamin D3[35–41]	• Modulates T cell response and inhibits Th1 cytokines	50,000 IU twice per week

* These supplements should be used under supervision and physicians need to be cognizant of potential side effects and contraindications with medications. Mild and transient gastrointestinal side effects may occur when first using some of these supplements and include nausea, bloating, and loose stools/diarrhea. These side effects have generally been reported with higher dosages of these supplements.

** The overuse or abuse of blue iris can increase the risk of adverse effects from cardiac glycoside drugs such as digoxin (Lanoxin®) and therefore should not be taken concomitantly.

*** Large amounts of guggulsterones might increase the adverse effects of hormone replacement therapy through estrogen-alpha receptor agonist activity and should not be taken with estrogens.

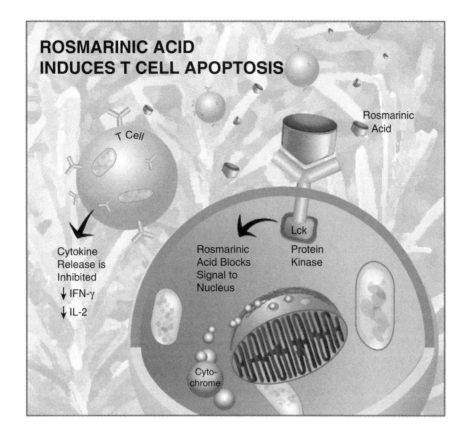

ROSMARINIC ACID INDUCES T CELL APOPTOSIS

In addition to natural supplementation, there are certain dietary modifications that may be beneficial for managing hyperthyroidism; this would include ensuring healthy digestion and absorption. The single most important lifestyle factor for maintaining and improving thyroid function is exercise because it reduces stress and stimulates the peripheral production of T3 by inducing 5′-deiodinase.

1   Spitzweg C, Joba W, Heufelder AE. Expression of thyroid-related genes in human thymus. Thyroid 1999;9:133–41.
2   McLeod DS, Cooper DS. The incidence and prevalence of thyroid autoimmunity. Endocrine 2012;42:252–65.
3   Hutfless S, Matos P, Talor MV, Caturegli P, Rose NR. Significance of prediagnostic thyroid antibodies in women with autoimmune thyroid disease. J Clin Endocrinol Metab 2011;96:E1466–E1471.
4   Chardes T, Chapal N, Bresson D, et al. The human anti-thyroid peroxidase autoantibody repertoire in Graves' and Hashimoto's autoimmune thyroid diseases. Immunogenetics 2002;54(3):141–57.
5   Werner SC, Ingbar SH, Braverman LE, Utiger RD, editors. Werner & Ingbar's the thyroid: a fundamental and clinical text. 9th ed. Philadelphia: Lippincott Williams & Wilkins; 2005.
6   Saravanan P, Dayan CM. Thyroid autoantibodies. Endocrinol Metab Clin North Am 2001;30(2):315–37.
7   Baskin HJ, Cobin RH, Duick DS, et al. American Association of Clinical Endocrinologists medical guidelines for clinical practice for the evaluation and treatment of hyperthyroidism and hypothyroidism. Endocr Pract 2006;8:457–69; Erratum in: Endocr Pract 2008;14(6):802–3.
8   Walsh JP, Brenner AP, Feddema P, Leedman PJ, Brown SJ, O'Leary P. Thyrotropin and thyroid antibodies as predictors of hypothyroidism: a 13-year, longitudinal study of a community-based cohort using current immunoassay techniques. J Clin Endocrinol Metab 2010;95:1095–104.
9   Gallagher CM, Meliker JR. Mercury and thyroid autoantibodies in U.S. women, NHANES 2007–2008. Environ Int 2012;40:39–43.
10   Kim ES, Lim DJ, Baek KH, et al. Thyroglobulin antibody is associated with increased cancer risk in thyroid nodules. Thyroid 2010;20(8):885–91.
11   de Rooij A, Vandenbroucke JP, Smit JW, Stokkel MP, Dekkers OM. Clinical outcomes after estimated versus calculated activity of radioiodine for the treatment of hyperthyroidism: systematic review and meta-analysis. Eur J Endocrinol 2009;161(5):771–7.
12   Russo D, Arturi F, Suarez HG, et al. Thyrotropin receptor gene alterations in thyroid hyperfunctioning adenomas. J Clin Endocrinol Metab 1996;81(4):1548–51.
13   Tonacchera M, Chiovato L, Pinchera A, et al. Hyperfunctioning thyroid nodules in toxic multinodular goiter share activating thyrotropin receptor mutations with solitary toxic adenoma. J Clin Endocrinol Metab 1998;83(2):492–8.
14   Reid JR, Wheeler SF. Hyperthyroidism: diagnosis and treatment. Am Fam Physician 2005;72(4):623–30.
15   Laurberg P, Pedersen KM, Vestergaard H, Sigurdsson G. High incidence of multinodular toxic goitre in the elderly population in a low iodine intake area vs. high incidence of Graves' disease in the young in a high iodine intake area: comparative surveys of thyrotoxicosis epidemiology in East-Jutland Denmark and Iceland. J Intern Med 1991;229(5):415–20.
16   Cotran RS, Kumar V, Collins T, editors. Robbins Pathological Basis of Disease. Philadelphia: WB Saunders Co.; 1999.
17   Sourgens H, Winterhoff H, Gumbinger HG, Kemper FH. Effects of *Lithospermum officinale* and related plants on hypophyseal and thyroid hormones in the rat. Pharmaceutical Biology 1986;24:55–63.

18 Hur YG, Yun Y, Won J. Rosmarinic acid induces p56lck-dependent apoptosis in Jurkat and peripheral T cells via mitochondrial pathway independent from Fas/Fas ligand interaction. J Immunol 2004;172:79–87.

19 Hur YG, Suh CH, Kim S, Won J. Rosmarinic acid induces apoptosis of activated T cells from rheumatoid arthritis patients via mitochondrial pathway. J Clin Immunol 2007;27:36–45.

20 Park SH, Oh HS, Kang MA, et al. The structure-activity relationship of the series of non-peptide small antagonists for p56lck SH2 domain. Bioorg Med Chem 2007;15:3938–50.

21 Won J, Hur YG, Hur EM, et al. Rosmarinic acid inhibits TCR-induced T cell activation and proliferation in an Lck-dependent manner. Eur J Immunol 2003;33:870–9.

22 Kang MA, Yun SY, Won J. Rosmarinic acid inhibits Ca^{2+}-dependent pathways of T-cell antigen receptor-mediated signaling by inhibiting the PLC-gamma 1 and Itk activity. Blood 2003;101:3534–42.

23 Winterhoff H, Gumbinger HG, Vahlensieck U, Kemper FH, Schmitz H, Behnke B. Endocrine effects of *Lycopus europaeus* L. following oral application. Arzneimittelforschung 1994;44(1):41–45.

24 Frances D. Botanical approaches to hypothyroidism: avoiding supplemental thyroid hormone. Medical Herbalism 2002;12:1–5.

25 Kelly GS. Peripheral metabolism of thyroid hormones: a review. Altern Med Rev 2000;5(4):306–33.

26 Singh AK, Tripathi SN, Prasad GC. Response of commiphora mukul (guggulu) on melatonin induced hypothyroidism. Anc Sci Life 1983; 3:85–90.

27 Tripathi YB, Malhotra OP, Tripathi SN. Thyroid stimulating action of Z-guggulsterone obtained from Commiphora mukul. Planta Med 1984;50:78–80.

28 Tripathi YB, Tripathi P, Malhotra OP, Tripathi SN. Thyroid stimulatory action of (Z)-guggulsterone: mechanism of action. Planta Med 1988;54:271–7.

29 Antonio J, Colker CM, Torina GC, Shi Q, Brink W, Kaiman D. Effects of a standardized guggulsterone phosphate supplement on body composition in overweight adults: a pilot study. Current Therapeutic Research 1999;60:220–7.

30 Panda S, Kar A. Gugulu (Commiphora mukul) induces triiodothyronine production: possible involvement of lipid peroxidation. Life Sci 1999;65:L137–L141.

31 Zagrodzki P, Ratajczak R. Selenium supplementation in autoimmune thyroiditis female patient–effects on thyroid and ovarian functions (case study). Biol Trace Elem Res 2008;126:76–82.

32 Grineva EN, Malakhova TV, Tsoi UA, Smirnov BI. [Efficacy of thyroxine and potassium iodide treatment of benign nodular thyroid lesions]. Ter Arkh 2003;75:72–5.

33 Vanderpump MP. The epidemiology of thyroid disease. Br Med Bull 2011;99:39–51.

34 Kahaly GJ, Dienes HP, Beyer J, Hommel G. Iodide induces thyroid autoimmunity in patients with endemic goitre: a randomised, double-blind, placebo-controlled trial. Eur J Endocrinol 1998;139:290–7.

35 Tamer G, Arik S, Tamer I, Coksert D. Relative vitamin D insufficiency in Hashimoto's thyroiditis. Thyroid 2011;21:891–6.

36 Cantorna MT, Mahon BD. Mounting evidence for vitamin D as an environmental factor affecting autoimmune disease prevalence. Exp Biol Med (Maywood) 2004;229:1136–42.

37 Ginanjar E, Sumariyono, Setiati S, Setiyohadi B. Vitamin D and autoimmune disease. Acta Med Indones 2007;39:133–41.

38 Chen W, Lin H, Wang M. Immune intervention effects on the induction of experimental autoimmune thyroiditis. J Huazhong Univ Sci Technolog Med Sci 2002;22:343–5, 354.

39 Fournier C, Gepner P, Sadouk M, Charreire J. *In vivo* beneficial effects of cyclosporin A and 1,25-dihydroxyvitamin D3 on the induction of experimental autoimmune thyroiditis. Clin Immunol Immunopathol 1990;54:53–63.

40 Lemire JM, Archer DC, Beck L, Spiegelberg HL. Immunosuppressive actions of 1,25-dihydroxyvitamin D3: preferential inhibition of Th1 functions. J Nutr 1995;125:1704S–8S.

41 Kivity S, Agmon-Levin N, Zisappl M, et al. Vitamin D and autoimmune thyroid diseases. Cell Mol Immunol 2011;8:243–7.

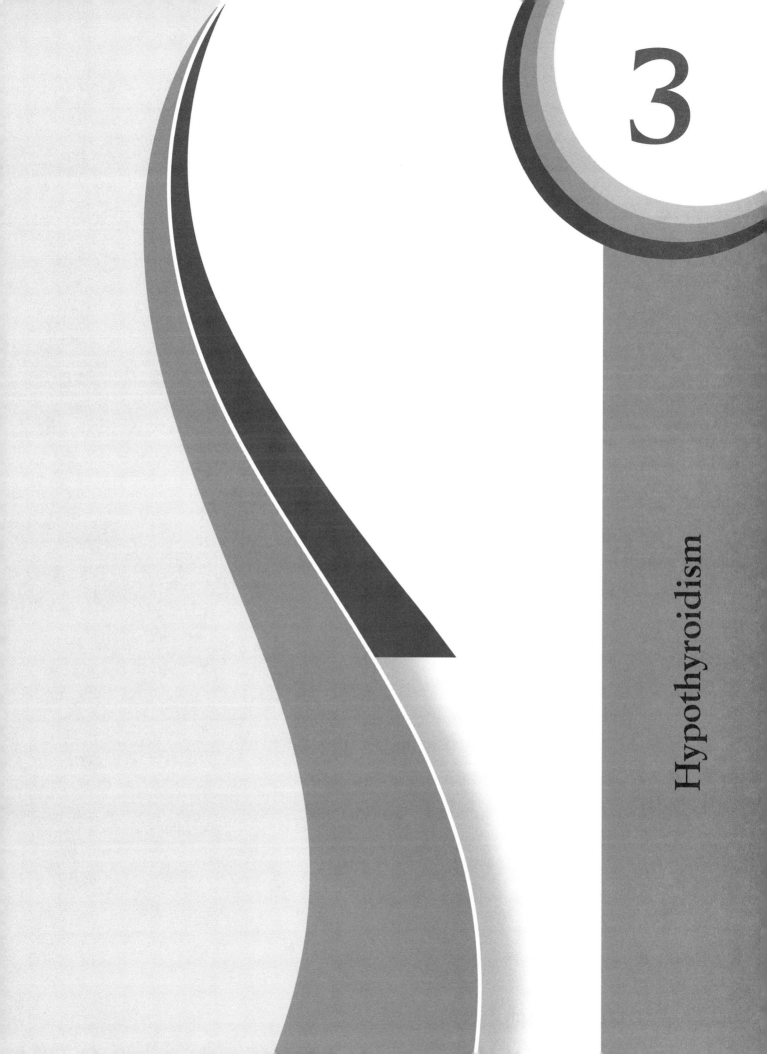

3

Hypothyroidism

Central Tertiary Hypothyroidism (Hypothalamic Dysfunction)

Just as the pituitary gland releases thyroid-stimulating hormone (TSH) to tell the thyroid gland to produce thyroid hormone, the hypothalamus also releases a hormone called thyrotropin-releasing hormone (TRH) that tells the pituitary gland to release TSH. Although it is rare, there is sometimes a problem with the hypothalamus, which inhibits the release of TRH. This can be caused by radiation to the brain, trauma to the head, or other conditions that affect the hypothalamus.[1]

Central Secondary Hypothyroidism (Pituitary Dysfunction)

Pituitary disease can be caused by tumors, surgery, radiation therapy, or Sheehan's syndrome. Each of these disorders can reduce the size and function of the pituitary gland. When the pituitary gland gets smaller, it cannot produce enough TSH. Sheehan's syndrome occurs when there is necrosis (cell death) of the pituitary gland, typically related to childbirth in women.[1]

Primary Hypothyroidism

Primary hypothyroidism, which accounts for over 95% of hypothyroidism cases, is characterized by a failure of the thyroid gland to produce a sufficient supply of thyroid hormones. Primary hypothyroidism can be caused by a variety of underlying conditions.

Thyroid Gland

Iodine Deficiency

The trace mineral iodine is an integral component of the thyroid hormones [thyroxine (T4) and triiodothyronine (T3)]. Therefore, it should come as no surprise that iodine deficiency is the most common cause of hypothyroidism (and goiter) worldwide,[2] and is associated with an increased risk of high cholesterol, atherosclerosis, autoimmune disease (e.g., Hashimoto's), and thyrotoxicosis resulting from Grave's disease.[3–5] Iodine deficiency can be devastating to the developing brain, causing a mental retardation (i.e., cretinism). Approximately 30% of the world's population lives in areas of iodine deficiency; these areas see a prevalence of goiter as high as 80%.[3,5]

Median Population Urinary Iodine Values and Iodine Nutrition		
Median Urinary Iodine Concentration (μg/l)	Corresponding Iodine Intake (μg/day)	Iodine Nutrition
<20	<30	Severe deficiency
20–49	30–74	Moderate deficiency
50–99	75–149	Mild deficiency
100–199	150–299	Optimal
200–299	300–449	More than adequate
>299	>499	Possible excess

Iodine urinary output, iodine intake, and iodine nutritional status.

When defined as an iodine intake less than 100 mcg/day, iodine deficiency affects approximately two billion people, many of whom live in mountainous areas.[6] According to the World Health Organization, iodine deficiency is defined by the following urine levels: mild = 149–100 mcg/l, moderate = 99–50 mcg/l, and severe = <49 mcg/l. Today, iodine deficiency is less common in North America than in other parts of the world because of the ubiquity of iodized salt (beginning in 1924 by the state of Michigan). Dietary intake of iodine decreased dramatically in the 1970s. The National Health and Nutrition Examination Surveys (NHANESs) of 2001–2002, 2005–2006, and 2007–2008 have shown that US dietary iodine intake has stabilized near this low level.[7,8] Now, 16–50% of pregnant women may be iodine deficient (some recent studies show it might be as high as 60%).[9] Babies of iodine-deficient women can be born with neonatal goiter, hypothyroidism and impaired mental development. By the same token, there have been case reports of babies born with high TSH and low T4 (T3 levels were not mentioned) to mothers who consumed iodine in excess of 13 mg/day during pregnancy.[10]

Iodine can primarily be found in sea life. Therefore, dietary iodine can be obtained through the consumption of sea vegetables and seafood (e.g., fish and shellfish). Other foods such as beans, nuts, seeds, and vegetables (e.g., peppers, spinach, chard, summer squash, turnip, onion, garlic) are also good sources of iodine provided that the soil in which they were grown contains sufficient quantities of iodine. Dairy and eggs also contain appreciable quantities of iodine depending on the dietary sources provided to the animals in question. The recommended daily allowance (RDA) of iodine is 150 µg for an adult male. For comparison, the consumption of 1 g of iodized salt provides 76 µg of iodine, while sea salt also contains iodine but in lesser amounts.

Iodine is absorbed quickly through the skin or intestinal tract. On average (and depending on need), 30% is absorbed by the thyroid gland, where it is incorporated into thyroid hormones (T4 and T3). Iodine is also found in the salivary glands, breasts, choroid plexus, and gastric mucosa. Ingested iodide can be prematurely oxidized in the follicular cells by hydrogen peroxide, which is kept in check by glutathione peroxidase (GPX). Low levels of GPX in the thyroid tissue can lead to oxidative damage of the iodine transporter sodium/iodide symporter (NIS). High doses of iodide can lead to increased TSH and decreased T4 but, at the same time, T3 levels can go up.

Iodine Therapy

Anecdotal experience from many practitioners demonstrates that the use of replenishing iodine therapy can be helpful for symptoms of low body temperature and hypothyroidism (including Hashimoto's) as well as Graves' disease (not hot nodule). For these indications iodine supplementation is usually very well tolerated, and helps many patients feel more energetic. Some practitioners report that supplementing their patients with iodine sometimes obviates the need for them to use thyroid hormones like T3 or dessicated thyroid, or reduces the dose needed. When used to treat autoimmune thyroid disease (AIT) in one study, iodine improved autoimmunity at lower doses, but made it worse with high doses. However, the best improvement in autoimmunity was evident when selenium was added to those higher doses of iodine.[11] Potassium iodide and T4 therapy are often used for treating thyroid disorders because they have been shown to inhibit and prevent the growth of benign thyroid nodules in 66% of patients.[12] Additionally, iodine supplementation has been reported to reduce thyroid volume with sustained effects seen up to 12 months post-therapy in patients with goiter.[13] Iodine supplementation is a better solution for iodine deficiency than T4 supplementation is because goiter quickly returns when T4 is discontinued in untreated iodine deficiency.

Iodine also plays a major role in female breast physiology. For example, women with fibrocystic breast disease experience a 70% improvement with appropriate iodine supplementation. Furthermore, breast cancer is linked with increased TPO antibodies as well as goiter, and subsequent iodine supplementation can inhibit breast tumor development. This is evidenced by the low rate of breast cancer found in Japanese women who some have asserted consume iodine-rich seaweed regularly (13.8 mg/day).[14–16] However, other research has shown Japanese consumption at only 10% this level. The typical study shows that 1.2 mg/day of iodine is due to the ingestion of seaweed in Japan[17] while one study found 1.5 mg/day of iodine due to the ingestion of seaweed in one city.

Because iodine is water soluble, excess iodine is excreted in the urine or the sweat, tears, and bile (feces). This explains why there have been no reported cases of iodine toxicity from naturally occurring sources in food or water. However, when a large amount of highly concentrated iodine is taken orally, it can cause side effects such as metallic taste, burning mouth, increased salivation, headache, edema, acne, and gastric upset. However, replenishing iodine in iodine-deficient populations results in hyperthyroidism in a small but significant percentage. The American Academy of Allergy, Asthma, and Immunology states that reactions to iodine-containing sources should not be considered an iodine allergy (i.e., involving IgE).[18] Moreover, these iodine-related side effects can often be alleviated via concomitant supplementation with adequate selenium therapy.[19,20]

Replenishing iodine supplementation for a few months can be very beneficial for a large percentage, and less than 10% of people respond adversely to excess iodine.[21] Nevertheless, there have been reports that some people that take more than 6 mg/day can develop hypothyroidism or hyperthyroidism. When giving a therapeutic trial of iodine to improve symptoms of slow metabolism, practitioners should monitor the treatment to make sure the patient's condition is improving. Prolonged use of high-dose iodine supplementation can sometimes cause thyroid gland hyperplasia, thyroid adenoma, and hypothyroidism, therefore, we recommend higher replenishing doses of iodine (up to about 48 mg/day as potassium iodide) for only a few months before reducing it back to maintenance levels of 1–12 mg/day (and the dose can be reduced to 150 mcg/day if indicated or preferred).[22] Some people can have flu-like symptoms (tired, malaise, headache, loss of appetite, not feeling well) about 1 week after starting iodine. Because this is mainly due to the competitive inhibition of Br and Cl, patients should consider reducing the dose for 2 weeks and trying again.

Topically, iodine may stain skin, irritate tissues, and cause iodine burns in concentrations of 7% or more. Although iodine therapy can cause side effects in some people, experts believe that its benefits far outweigh its risks, which can be minimized through proper monitoring.[23]

Prior to establishing a maintenance dose of iodine, baseline measures of TSH, T4, free T3, thyroid stimulating immunoglobulin (TSI), TPO antibody, 24-hour urinary iodine and body temperatures should be documented when appropriate, especially if a nodule is observed. These levels should be checked after 1 month and then every 3–6 months during the first year. It is normal for TSH to rise upon the initiation of iodine supplementation. If the free T3 is not going down, then this is not hypothyroidism. TSH usually normalizes after 6–9 months. Remember, no baseline tests are going to guarantee that a patient will respond well to iodine, therefore judicious clinical follow-up is always necessary. These follow-up assessments should include not only blood testing, but also involve a thorough physical examination (e.g., body temperatures) as well as an extensive assessment of possible hypo- or hyperthyroid symptoms. In the unusual case that iodine appears to be making a person's autoimmunity or hypo- or hyperthyroid symptoms worse, then the iodine supplementation can be discontinued.

Baseline iodine levels can be checked via 24-hour urine testing or load urine testing. Variation in urinary excretion of iodine throughout the day is variable, which makes spot testing inaccurate. If the patient is only willing to do spot testing, 10 consecutive days are necessary to achieve an accurate assessment. Iodine load testing involves a 50 mg bolus dose of oral iodine, followed by a 24-hour urine iodine measurement. Proponents of load testing feel that 90% excretion is iodine replete and that many patients feel better if they can just get it up to 70% excretion. Some practitioners also find blood iodine testing to be convenient.

With respect to dosing, the rule is "start low and go slow." Because some people may have a hidden hot nodule that will quickly generate excess thyroid hormone when supplied iodine, it is good to start with 6 mg/day (as potassium iodide) for a few days to check for any adverse reactions. Then, the dose can be gradually built up to about 48 mg/day for a few months. Concomitant use of selenium 200–800 mcg/day is also strongly advised to counter autoimmunity in susceptible individuals. Elemental iodine in the form of potassium iodide has been prescribed in very high doses such as 50 mg/day, decreasing the need for T4 in hypothyroid patients, and decreasing hypothyroid symptoms.[24] However, such high doses can potentially cause side effects such as skin outbreaks, palpitations, and aggravations of thyroid (hot/hidden) nodules (TSI antibodies normal). Hyperthyroidism may be a particularly problematic side effect for iodine-deficient patients who are replenished with high doses of iodine too quickly.[25] For some, even 25 mg/day of iodine or less may cause problems.[22] Once an appropriate dose has been found, therapy should be continued for up to 3 months, then slowly reduced back to physiologic levels (i.e., 1–12 mg/day, selenium 100–200 mcg/day).

Hashimoto's Thyroiditis

Hashimoto's disease (i.e., chronic lymphocytic thyroiditis) is an autoimmune disorder. The thyroid gland is the organ most commonly affected by autoimmune disease.[26] Hashimoto's is considered the most common cause of thyroid problems in the United States, and studies suggest that the incidence of thyroid disease throughout the world is increasing.[26] This disorder commonly begins between the ages of 30 and 50 years, affects women more often than men (8:1), and often causes a goiter. The reason for the difference between genders is not clear.[27] Approximately 20% of patients have symptoms of hypothyroidism when first diagnosed, while for the majority, hypothyroid symptoms will follow later, after a goiter. Thyroglobulin (Tg) antibodies are elevated in more than 90% of these patients.[28] Other forms of autoimmune disease may exist concomitantly with Hashimoto's thyroiditis, such as Addison's disease, rheumatoid arthritis, systemic lupus erythematosus, Sjögren's syndrome, and pernicious anemia. TPO antibodies and Tg antibodies are usually elevated in Hashimoto's. Interestingly, patients with elevated TPO and Tg antibodies may be asymptomatic and these elevations may precede diagnosis of autoimmune disease by 2–7 years.[29] The production of antibodies is stimulated by the iodination of Tg. Although it is reported that there is a genetic predisposition for autoimmune thyroiditis, onset of the disease can be triggered by environmental factors such as iodine intake, toxins, halogens, pesticides, heavy metals, nutrient deficiencies, and proliferation of lymphocytes.

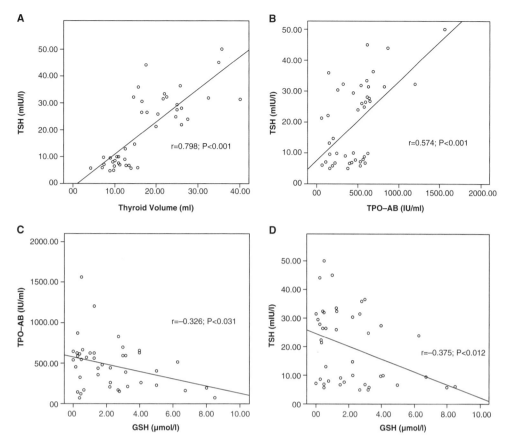

Associations between markers of thyroid malfunction and/or oxidative stress in individuals with Hashimoto's thyroiditis (n=44). A: Thyroid Volume (Tvol) and thyroid stimulating hormone (TSH) levels; B: TSH levels and anti-thyroperoxidase antibody (TPO-AB) titers; C: Glutathione (GSH) levels and TPO-AB titers; D: GSH contents and TSH levels.[30]

Iatrogenic (Treatment-Induced) Hypothyroidism

Treatments for hyperthyroidism, such as thyroidectomy, iodine-131 therapy, and antithyroid drugs, are common causes of hypothyroidism. Other prescribed agents that may block thyroid hormone synthesis include lithium carbonate, oral hypoglycemic agents, 6-mercaptopurine, P-aminosalicylic acid (PAS), antiarrhythmic drugs (e.g., amiodarone), anti-anginal drugs, tricyclic antidepressants, and interferon. Drugs associated with altered peripheral conversion of T4 to T3 include corticosteroid (e.g., dexamethasone), propylthiouracil (PTU), radiographic contrast agents (e.g., lopanic acid), amiodarone, and beta blockers (e.g., propanolol).[31]

Post-Partum Thyroiditis

Fluctuating thyroid function after childbirth (first described in the 1970s) occurs in 5–10% of new mothers. Thyroid inflammation may occur several months after childbirth, resulting in the development of clinical hyperthyroidism. In some patients, the hyperthyroid phase will be associated with significant inflammatory damage to the thyroid, which leads to the development of hypothyroidism.

Depression

For many patients, undiagnosed thyroid dysfunction maybe the underlying cause or major contributor to their depression or bipolar disorder.[32–46] The dysfunction present with these conditions includes the down-regulation of D1 (reduced T4 to T3 conversion) and reduced uptake of T4 into the cell, resulting in increased serum T4 levels with low intracellular T3 levels.[32–34,38,39,43,47–53] These conditions may also involve the upregulation of D3, resulting in elevated reverse T3,[32,38,39] which blocks the thyroid effect[54,55–65] and is an indicator of reduced transport of T4 into the cell.[64,66] Additionally, studies show that depressed patients have reduced T4 transport across the blood brain barrier due to a defective transport protein (i.e., transthyretin), resulting in significantly reduced thyroid levels in the brain; all of this, despite "normal" serum levels and standard thyroid tests[32,47,48] as well as a reduced TSH response to TRH.[36–39,51–53,67–71]

It is not surprising that T4 and T4/T3 combinations may have some benefit in depression; but due to the suppressed T4 to T3 conversion from suppressed D1[32–34,38] and reduced uptake of T4 into the cell and brain,[33,39,47,48] time-release T3 is significantly more beneficial than T4 or T4/T3 combination supplementation.[33,49,72–76]

In the *International Journal of Neuropsychopharmacology*, Posternak et al. published a double-blind placebo-controlled trial of 50 patients with normal thyroid function as defined by a normal TSH (1.5 ± 0.8). The patients were randomized to receive 25 mcg of T3 or placebo in addition to antidepressant therapy.[77] The study found that T3 therapy was associated with almost a 2-fold increase in response rate and a 4.5 times greater likelihood of experiencing a positive response at any point over the 6-week period. Side effects were higher in the placebo group on 10/11 criteria, including a significant increase in nervousness.

Kelly and Lieberman investigated the effectiveness of T3 for the treatment of bipolar disorder in patients who had failed to adequately respond to an average of 14 medications used to treat their bipolar disorder. The average dose of T3 used was 90.4 mcg (range 13–188 mcg). The medication was found to be well tolerated and 84% experienced significant improvement. Furthermore, 33% of T3 patients experienced full remission. Again, this is in patients who had not previously responded to numerous medications. One patient who was switched to T4 for cost reasons experienced a return of symptoms, which resolved upon the reintroduction of T3. The authors concluded, "Augmentation with supraphysiologic doses of T3 should be considered in cases of treatment resistant bipolar depression...."[76] The authors thanked several doctors who encouraged them to go beyond the traditional 50 mcg of T3 because it has helped so many of their patients.

With over 4000 patients, The STAR*D Report is the largest trial comparing antidepressant effectiveness for depression. It found that 66% of patients fail to respond to antidepressants or have side effects severe enough to discontinue their use. Of those who do respond, over half will relapse within 1 year.[78] The trial found that T3 was effective even when cognitive therapy or medications such as citalopram (Celexa®), bupropion (Wellbutrin®), sertraline (Zolft®), and venlafaxine (Effexor®) were not. T3 was shown to be 50% more effective than commonly used therapeutic approaches with standard antidepressants, even with the less than optimal dose of 50 mcg. T3 therapy was also associated with significantly less side effects. The authors included a case study to exemplify the effectiveness of T3, especially when other medications are not effective:

> "Ms. "B," a 44-year-old divorced white woman, became depressed after losing her job as a secretary in a law firm. She initially sought treatment from her primary care physician and then entered the STAR*D study. Ms. B met criteria for major depressive disorder and generalized anxiety disorder. Her baseline QIDS-SR [Quick Inventory of Depressive Symptomatology – Self Report] score was 16. After 12 weeks on citalopram, her QIDS-SR score was 10 [minimal response]. She was then randomly assigned to augmentation with buspirone; she soon experienced gastrointestinal distress, and she stopped taking buspirone after 6 weeks. She elected to try one more augmentation agent and was randomly assigned to T3 augmentation. When she started T3 augmentation, her QIDS-SR score was 12. After 4 weeks, she felt that her mood and energy had lifted substantially. She felt better able to make decisions, organize, and prioritize and felt that she was able and ready to look for another job. "I felt as if my brain suddenly had oxygen," she said, "and everything became clearer." After 12 weeks, Ms. B felt back to normal, and her QIDS-SR score was 0 [complete resolution of symptoms]."[78]

Given the accumulating data implicating thyroid dysfunction in depressed and bipolar patients, it is clear that time-release T3 supplementation should be considered in this patient population despite "normal" serum thyroid levels. Additionally, straight T4 should be considered inappropriate and suboptimal therapy for replacement in such patients.

Environmental Factors

Heavy Metals

Heavy metals (cadmium, lead, and mercury) have been linked to alterations in thyroid function.[79–82] The association of mercury with Tg antibody positivity, but not TPO antibody positivity, indicates a relationship between mercury and autoimmunity. Laboratory evidence suggests that TPO enzyme is inhibited by inorganic mercury but not mercury.[83] Both organic and inorganic mercury inhibit the iodination of Tg.[84] Further, it has been hypothesized that mercury induces protein alterations that result in cell-specific antigenicity as well as a theory that formation of polyclonal B lymphocytes and autoantibodies result from mercury-induced T lymphocyte stimulation.[85,86] Mercury exposure typically reflects consumption of fish in the general population.[87] Cadmium exposure leads to lipid peroxidation in the thyroid, which can be protected against by ascorbic acid supplementation.[79] Alterations in antioxidant enzyme systems and lipid peroxidation in response to heavy metals are hypothesized to lead to membrane integrity dysfunction and suboptimal 5'-deiodinase activity.[88–90] In order for the body to remove cadmium, selenium becomes bound to the cadmium and is expelled from the body via the bile system. Therefore, cadmium toxicity can deplete selenium, which is an essential component of deiodinase enzymes responsible for conversion of T4 to T3, and reduced selenium can also lead to an increase in rT3, which in turn can result in hypothyroidism.[91] Selenium is also an essential component of the antioxidant, GPX. Reduction in selenium reduces the formation of GPX, resulting in increased levels of reactive oxygen species and hydrogen peroxide, which can damage the thyroid.

Halogens

Iodination of Tg and the NIS are affected by halogens including perchlorate, chlorine, fluorine, and bromine. These chemicals have differing effects on the thyroid and vary in their mechanisms of action. Perchlorate (ClO_4) competitively inhibits iodide uptake by the NIS and displaces T4 from serum.[92] Chlorine inhibits iodide trapping and decreases serum T4.[93] Fluoride decreases T3 and T4 and increases TSH in the blood; however, the mechanism by which this occurs remains unclear.[94] Bromine displaces iodine, increases plasma TSH, and has an inhibitory effect on thyroid activity.[95] These individual chemicals are found in our environment and often in household products including beverages, drinking water, toothpastes, and cleaning agents; however, adverse effects on the thyroid are generally seen only with exposure to high amounts of these compounds. Usually the thyroid hormone concentration change occurs in response to a mixture of chemicals, but not to individual chemicals.[96]

Pesticides

Organochlorine pesticides, which contain the chlorine molecule, have also been associated with increased incidence of euthyroid goiter or hypothyroidism.[97] Organophosphate pesticide levels correlate well with endocrine pathologies, and have been shown to decrease TSH levels, free T4, and free T3. They also increase adrenocorticotropic hormone and cortisol levels. Hexachlorobenzene (HCB), a commonly used pesticide, is highly lipophilic and accumulates in fat tissue. A study performed at the Environmental and Respiratory Unit in Spain found that there was a negative association between serum HCB concentrations and total T4 levels (a decrease of 0.32 mcg/dl of T4 for every 1 ng/ml increase in HCB). These results suggest some type of thyroid function involvement. HCB may also impair peripheral metabolism of thyroid hormones. Given the negative impact that organophosphate pesticide can have on endocrine health, the importance of eating organic foods cannot be overemphasized.[31]

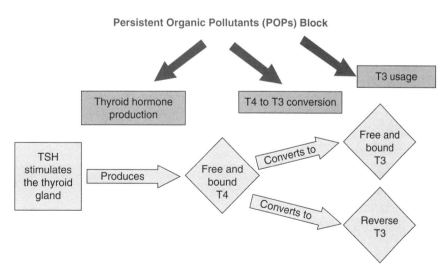

Persistent Organic Pollutants (POPs) can block thyroid hormone production, conversion, and expression.

When organic foods are not available because of expense or location, it is advisable that people use the following list (see Table 3.1) from the Environmental Working Group (www.ewg.org) indicating which foods in US supermarkets are more likely to have toxins ("dirty") or not ("clean").

Table 3.1. Environmental Working Group's Dirty Dozen Plus and Clean 15

Dirty Dozen Plus (avoid)	Clean 15 (eat)
Apples	Asparagus
Celery	Avocados
Cherry tomatoes	Cabbage
Cucumbers	Cantaloupe
Grapes	Sweet corn
Hot peppers	Eggplant
Nectarines (imported)	Grapefruit
Peaches	Kiwi
Potatoes	Mangos
Spinach	Mushrooms
Strawberries	Onions
Sweet bell peppers	Papayas
Kale, collard greens	Pineapples
Summer squash	Sweet peas (frozen)
	Sweet potatoes

Factors that influence thyroid antigens and Hashimoto's disease:

- Polychlorinated biphenyls (PCBs)
- Iodine (in excess or when intake increases significantly)
- Perchlorate
- Radiation
- Fluoride
- Bromine
- Lithium
- Mercury
- Bisphenol A
- Teflon

T3 and T4

3,3',5–Triiodothyronine (T3)

3,3',5,5'–Tetraiodothyronine (T4)

PCBs

4–Hydroxy–3,3',4',5–tetrachlorobiphenol
(4–OH–tetraCB)

4–Hydroxy–2,3,3',4,5–pentachlorobiphenol
(4–OH–PentaCB)

BPAs

Bisphenol A (BPA)

Tetrachlorobisphenol A (TCBPA)

Tetramethylbisphenol A (TMBPA)

Persistent Organic Pollutants (POPs) can be disruptive to thyroid physiology because they are so similar in structure to T3 and T4.[98]

Toxic Metal Exposure

Exposure to toxic metals, such as cadmium, mercury, and lead, can result in altered thyroid hormone metabolism. Researchers have concluded that heavy metal toxicity directly poison the enzymes involved in the production/conversion of thyroid hormones and damage the antioxidant enzyme systems that protect cell membranes from lipid peroxidation. This heavy metal-induced increase in lipid peroxidation can affect thyroid gland function and peripheral conversion of thyroid hormones.[31] High levels of lead in the body can be detrimental to thyroid function. The use of oral DMSA (2,3-dimercaptosuccinic acid) at a dose of 30 mg/kg over 5 days has been shown to lower blood lead by 72.5%.[99] A lower dosage of 10 mg/kg will lower blood lead by 35.5% and may be safer for some patients.

Radiation and Pollution

Radiation, heavy industry pollutants, coal pollution, motor vehicle emissions, and agricultural fungicides have also been suggested to play a role in autoimmune thyroid disease.[100–102]

Environmental Goitrogens

Environmental goitrogens include perchlorate, fluoride, and mercury. In some cases, iodine in excess of 1000 mcg/day can lead to hypothyroidism, or hyperthyroidism.

Medications

Medications that induce goiters and suppress thyroid function include amiodarone, carbamazepine, lithium, potassium iodine, phenobarbitone, phenytoin, and rifampin. Medications that have reported effects on thyroid antigens include beta blockers, theophyline, amiodarone, phenytoin, PTU, and chemotherapy.

Stress

Trauma and/or grief often triggers low thyroid function as a physiological coping mechanism for dealing with stressful circumstances. The stress response is mediated in the central nervous system as well as peripheral organs.[103] The typical response to stress is an increase in production of cortisol, decrease in production of TSH, decrease in T3, and increase in rT3. Altered peripheral metabolism of T4 to T3 and rT3 may be due to increased cortisol. Even changes in serum cortisol within normal range can cause significant alterations in thyroid hormone levels.[31]

Nutrition

Fasting or a deficiency of vitamins (e.g., A, E, B12, riboflavin, niacin), minerals (e.g., Se, I, Fe, Zn, K), or amino acids (e.g., cysteine, tyrosine) can lead to hypothyroidism.[104–106] For example, vitamin B12 deficiency results in decreased levels of 5'-deiodinase, which is utilized in the metabolism of T4 to T3 in peripheral tissues.[107] Conversely, excess consumption of certain foods, such as goitrogens, can also induce hypothyroidism. These include uncooked brassicas (e.g., cabbage, kale, Brussels sprouts, mustard, cauliflower), rutabagas, peanuts, turnips, peaches, pears, spinach, and soy.[31] Vegans are at risk for developing iodine deficiency especially if their diets are high in raw foods, which can contain goitrogens.

Lifestyle

Aerobic exercise and stress management seem to support proper thyroid function and peripheral conversion, whereas sleep deprivation and excess alcohol intake appear to have the opposite effect.[31]

Hypothyroidism on the Rise

In the mid-to-late 1960s, diseases of the thyroid were not common in medical practice. Almost 30 years later (in 1995), 11.7% of the population had abnormal TSH, and 13 million may have been living with undiagnosed thyroid dysfunction.[108] The Colorado Prevalence Study (published in 2000) found that approximately 10% of subjects who were not taking any thyroid medications had some form of thyroid dysfunction; extrapolated to the United States adult population, this represents a possible 13 million cases of undetected thyroid gland abnormalities.[109] A 2008 recent systematic review revealed that hypothyroidism had an estimated incidence between 80:100,000 per year in males and

350:100,000 per year in females.[108] Research by McLeod and Cooper, published in 2012, concluded that the incidence and prevalence of autoimmune thyroid disease is on the rise.[110] The incidence of congenital hypothyroidism has also significantly increased, doubling in the last two decades (1987–2005).

Although no scientific consensus exists regarding the exact cause of this increase in hypothyroidism, some experts have pointed to contamination as a possible contributor. After all, pesticide use in the US has increased 10-fold in the last 40 years.[111] In addition, factors promoting iodine insufficiency include the reduced use of iodized salt in home food preparation as a result of recommendations to lessen salt consumption, lack of homogeneity in the actual amount of iodine found in containers of iodized salt, no use of iodized salt in restaurant meals or processed foods, the dairy industry no longer using iodine-based disinfectants and reducing use of iodine in feed supplements, and replacement of iodate-based bread conditioners with potassium bromate (an iodide inhibitor) in breads and baked goods.[112] Regardless of what factors are driving this increase, data suggest that physicians should consider monitoring TSH levels of all patients, especially in those who present with symptoms related to thyroid dysfunction.

Evaluation and Management

Therapeutic Approach

Natural treatment strategies for normalizing thyroid function vary depending on whether there is an autoimmune hypothyroid condition, Wilson's Temperature Syndrome (WTS), or subclinical or clinical hypothyroidism.

Hypothyroidism may be caused by a number of factors including a reduction in hormone synthesis by the thyroid gland, thyroid gland ablation (surgery/radiation), deficient TSH, and other peripheral causes. Hormone synthesis is also reduced with iodine deficiency, Hashimoto's disease, high intake of dietary goitrogens, pharmaceutical inhibitors of the thyroid, sub-acute thyroiditis, infiltrative thyroid disease, and congenital thyroid disease. Peripheral causes include deficient T4 to T3 conversion, excess RT3, and thyroid hormone resistance.

Thyroid Replacement Hormones

- Thyroid hormones are useful in hypothyroidism and WTS. They can also decrease thyroid nodule sizes.
- Thyroid hormone replacement should be used cautiously because it can exacerbate a variety of common conditions including: adrenal cortical insufficiency (i.e., Addison's or subclinical Addison's syndrome), coronary artery disease (e.g., angina pectoris), cardiac arrhythmias, tachycardia, cardiomyopathy, anxiety disorders, diabetes mellitus type II, syndrome X, diabetes insipidus, osteoporosis, and thyrotoxicosis.
- Thyroid hormone replacement should be used cautiously with stimulant herbs and pharmaceuticals such as steroid hormones, anticoagulants, hypoglycemic agents, antidepressants, and cardiac medications. When given in high doses, thyroid hormone preparations can be very cardio-active, and therefore increase the risk of tachycardia and atrial fibrillation, even in individuals with no history of cardiac symptoms. Thus, patients taking thyroid hormone replacement must be encouraged to report adverse events as well as be educated in the symptoms of thyrotoxicosis.

Thyroid Hormone Replacement Options

- T3 (Liothyronine) sustained release: 7.5–90 mcg BID in incremental dosages (see WT3 protocol) to establish a normal body temperature. Among both euthyroid and hypothyroid patients, the object of T3 therapy is to return the body's temperature back to normal (98.6°F), which in turn resets the body's metabolism. For euthyroid patients, T3 therapy can be restorative, with the patient not needing any exogenous thyroid hormones after the treatment to continue feeling well. The WT3 (Wilson's T3) protocol, designed by Denis Wilson, MD and described in Chapter 5 of this book requires patient education and good compliance. Patients should also be educated about potential side effects so that they do not worry unnecessarily. If side effects appear, they should be addressed early.
- T3 Pure (Cytomel): 7.5–100 mcg daily. The research of John C. Lowe, DC showed very good results for fatigue and fibromyalgia in euthyroid patients using a once-a-day Cytomel regimen of about 75 mcg/day. Although it is easy to use, Cytomel can be prone to side effects because it is not sustained release, and the symptoms tend to return once the T3 is discontinued if the treatment is not directed toward and does not succeed at normalizing the body temperature.
- Desiccated Natural Thyroid: prepared from domesticated animals, one grain (60 mg desiccated thyroid) contains approximately 38 mcg T4 and 9 mcg T3. One-grain increments of desiccated thyroid can be increased once a week, but be vigilant for possible cardiac side effects. Although this is a simple treatment option, it almost never resets

the metabolism back to normal. Consequently, patients are not able to wean off the medicine without having symptoms return.

- T3 and T4 mixed: 50 mcg T3, 100 mcg T4.
- Levothyroxine: 25–200 mcg. This is the most popular thyroid hormone replacement, and provides a standard dose of T4, but does not include T3, and thus adequate T3 is maintained only if T4 to T3 conversion is adequate.
- Natural Progesterone: oral micronized progesterone 200 mg/day potentiates thyroid hormone and is indicated in patients with an estrogen-to-progesterone imbalance (estrogen dominance).

Thyroid Support

Thyroid botanical and nutritional support (e.g., Iris Versicolor, Guggul, potassium iodide) is beneficial for the treatment of WTS, low body temperature, fatigue, arthritis, mild hypercholesterolemia, and Hashimoto's disease (see Table 3.2). Thyroid support can be beneficial for almost any hypothyroid patient regardless of its etiology. For patients with mild to moderate WTS, thyroid support may also be used as an alternative to WT3 therapy.

- **Diet:** As in any autoimmune disease, natural therapies that focus on immune system regulation are particularly helpful. Hair mineral analysis can be a great tool for identifying low levels of selenium, zinc, and iron, which contribute to thyroid hormone dysfunction. Consider testing for antigens, as well as avoiding dietary antigens when appropriate. Gluten sensitivity may also be a concern because it is linked with most autoimmune conditions (e.g., Hashimoto's disease). Hypothyroid patients are deficient in heat and energy and should thus eat warming foods when possible. A diet high in goitrogens should also be avoided.
- **Digestion:** For thyroid support, it is critical to ensure a healthy digestive tract in order to maintain proper absorption. Supplements such as HCl, bitter herbs, and digestive enzymes with meals can support healthy digestion. If leaky gut is identified, a medium- to long-term gut repair protocol is indicated, including the treatment of dysbiosis. Treating dysbiosis can reduce the production of endotoxins in the gut and reduce intestinal hyperpermeability, in turn helping to modulate an overactive immunity.
- **Exercise:** The single most important lifestyle factor one can do in improving thyroid function is exercise. Aerobic exercise stimulates the peripheral production of T3 by inducing 5'-deiodinase (type I monoiodinase), an enzyme outside the thyroid gland that converts T4 into the more active T3. Aerobic exercise of a minimum of three times a week should therefore be prescribed.
- **Stress Reduction:** Thyroid malfunction is epidemic in this century, possibly due to pesticides and chemicals ubiquitously found in our environment. Chronic emotional stress can be a causative factor as well. Thus, stress management techniques and the consumption of chemical-free whole foods should be encouraged.
  - **Adaptogenic (Stress-Reducing) Herbs:** Adding dietary adaptogenic herbs is often beneficial in the treatment of Hashimoto's disease because they act as endocrine tonics that help mitigate autoimmune diseases. This is especially true if chronic stress or adrenal insufficiency is a factor. Adrenal supportive herbs include: Eleuthero, Sarsaparilla, Rhodiola, and Ashwagandha.
- **DHEA:** Dehydroepiandrosterone (DHEA), a major adrenal hormone, has been found to benefit a variety of autoimmune diseases in dosages of 100–200 mg/day. However, many clinicians prefer lower physiological doses, such as 10–50 mg/day in men and 5–15 mg/day in women. Lab work should be done to confirm physiological ranges with DHEA supplementation.
- **Detoxification:** The traditional use of detoxification has a place in the treatment of autoimmune disease. Therapies that support the liver to process endogenous and exogenous toxins have demonstrated benefits in managing autoimmune disease including thyroiditis.
  - General detoxification ideas
    - Some fasting
    - Clean protein, like fish low in mercury
    - Lots of water, soup broths
    - Avoid sugar (when possible)
    - Fresh organic fruit
    - Plenty of detoxifying herbs
    - Enemas, colonics, emesis
    - Sweating (through exercise or sauna)
- **WT3:** Wilson's T3 therapy (discussed in Chapter 5) can lower thyroid antibodies and ensure a better chance of controlling Hashimoto's disease. There are some patients who need thyroid hormone supplementation for life, due to either permanent glandular hypothyroidism or thyroidectomy. Even so, it is not uncommon for such patients to do better on less T4 after WT3 therapy than they did on more T4 before WT3 therapy. For example, patients may have low temperatures and debilitating symptoms on 200 mcg/day of Synthroid®. They can be switched to WT3

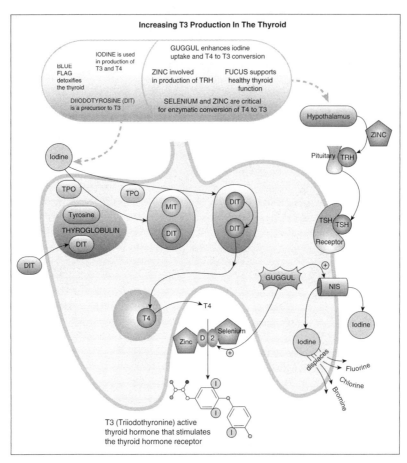

Increasing T3 Production In The Thyroid

BLUE FLAG detoxifies the thyroid

IODINE is used in production of T3 and T4

GUGGUL enhances iodine uptake and T4 to T3 conversion

ZINC involved in production of TRH

FUCUS supports healthy thyroid function

DIIODOTYROSINE (DIT) is a precursor to T3

SELENIUM and ZINC are critical for enzymatic conversion of T4 to T3

Hypothalamus

ZINC

Pituitary

TRH

Iodine

TPO

TPO

MIT

DIT

DIT

DIT

TSH

TSH

Receptor

Tyrosine

THYROGLOBULIN

DIT

DIT

GUGGUL

NIS

Iodine

T4

T4

Zinc

D 2

Selenium

Iodine

displaces

Fluorine

Chlorine

Bromine

T3 (Triiodothyronine) active thyroid hormone that stimulates the thyroid hormone receptor

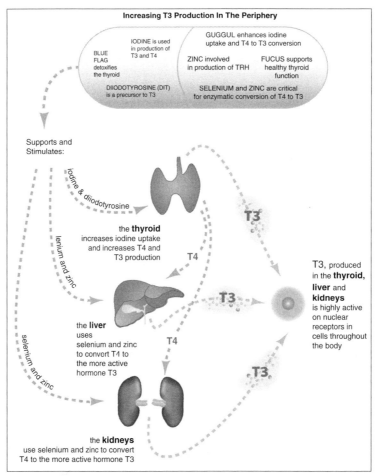

Increasing T3 Production In The Periphery

BLUE FLAG detoxifies the thyroid

IODINE is used in production of T3 and T4

GUGGUL enhances iodine uptake and T4 to T3 conversion

ZINC involved in production of TRH

FUCUS supports healthy thyroid function

DIIODOTYROSINE (DIT) is a precursor to T3

SELENIUM and ZINC are critical for enzymatic conversion of T4 to T3

Supports and Stimulates:

iodine & diiodotyrosine

selenium and zinc

selenium and zinc

the **thyroid** increases iodine uptake and increases T4 and T3 production

the **liver** uses selenium and zinc to convert T4 to the more active hormone T3

the **kidneys** use selenium and zinc to convert T4 to the more active hormone T3

T3

T4

T3

T4

T3

T3, produced in the **thyroid, liver** and **kidneys** is highly active on nuclear receptors in cells throughout the body therapy for a time, and then when they are switched back to Synthroid®, they may have normal temperatures and no symptoms on a much lower dose of Synthroid® (e.g., 50 mcg/day).

WT3 therapy (as opposed to Synthroid® or Armour®) not only resets but also tends to clear out the thyroid system pathways by reducing T4 and RT3 levels. Lowering T4 and RT3 may reduce proteoytic destruction of 5'-deiodinase and thereby help restore outer ring deiodination (ORD; conversion of T4 to T3). Patients with WTS who are not permanently hypothyroid can often be restored to normal temperatures, subsequently experiencing a resolution of related symptoms. Although this can sometimes be accomplished without the need for thyroid medicine, the combination of WT3 therapy and herbal thyroid support provides a better chance of complete recovery.

Table 3.2. Botanicals and nutraceuticals for thyroid support

Herb/Nutrient*	Action	Dose
Fucus vesiculosis (Bladderwrack or Kelp)	• Provides the organ with the nutrition and substrates it requires • Can increase metabolic rate and stimulate weight loss	5 g/day
Iris Versicolor (Blue flag)**[113]	• Anti-inflammatory • Stimulates glandular secretion and removal of wastes through the lymphatic system	750 mg/day
Commiphora mukul (Guggul)***[25,28,31,99,108–111,113–118]	• Naturally increases T3 levels • Effective in decreasing T3 levels in hyperthyroid patients • Improved conversion • Anti-inflammatory	750 mg/day
Selenium	• Decreases TPO antibodies	500 mcg BID week 1, then 500 mcg QD week 2, then 200 mcg QD thereafter
Potassium Iodide[119–121]	• Element necessary for thyroid hormone metabolism	100 mcg–50 mg QD
Rosmarinic Acid	• Helpful in reducing antithyroid antibodies in hyper- and hypothyroidism	335 mg twice per day
Tyrosine	• Amino acid required for the synthesis of thyroid hormones	Max 2 grams QD in divided doses between meals
Vitamin D3[122–125]	• Helpful in preventing autoimmune thyroiditis • Modulates T cell responses, inhibits Th1 cell cytokines	Up to 50,000 IU two times per week (blood levels should be monitored)
3,5 Diiodotyrosine	• Immediate precursor to thyroid hormone	800 mcg/day

* These supplements should be used under supervision, and physicians need to be cognizant of potential side effects and contraindications with medications. Mild and transient gastrointestinal side effects may occur when first using some of these supplements and include nausea, bloating and loose stools/diarrhea. These side effects have generally been reported with higher dosages of these supplements.
** The overuse or abuse of blue iris can increase the risk of adverse effects from cardiac glycoside drugs such as digoxin (Lanoxin®) and therefore should not be taken concomitantly.
*** Large amounts of guggulsterones might increase the adverse effects of hormone replacement therapy through estrogen-alpha receptor agonist activity and should not be taken with estrogens.

Suggested Thyroid Support Formula

- 225 mg Iris versicolor
- 225 mg Guggul
- 200 mg Fucus
- 80 mcg Selenomethionine (1 cap 3x/day)
- Topical (massage over thyroid once a day)
  ○ Myrrh essential oil:olive oil (diluted 1:3–4 parts)

This optional formula provides nutritional support and stimulation to the thyroid gland, improving the peripheral conversion of T4 to T3, and increasing body temperature. It can not only decrease thyroid antibodies in Hashimoto's thyroiditis, but with long-term use, often increases thyroid hormone production in hypothyroid patients. This thyroid support formula, especially with high doses of selenomethionine, can bring thyroid antibodies down. Patients with mild to moderate cases of WTS can often recover with the use of this herbal formula, or WT3, or a combination of both.[10,21]

1   Lania A, Persani L, Beck-Peccoz P. Central hypothyroidism. Pituitary 2008;11(2):181–6.

2   Andersson M, Takkouche B, Egli I, Allen HE, de Benoist B. Current global iodine status and progress over the last decade towards the elimination of iodine deficiency. Bull World Health Org 2005;83(7):518–25.

3   Aghini-Lombardi F, Antonangeli L. The spectrum of thyroid disorders in an iodine-deficient community: the Pescopagano survey. J Clin Endocrinol Metab 1999 Feb;84(2):561–6.

4   Human Vitamin and Mineral Requirements. Report of a joint FAO/WHO expert consultation, Bangkok, Thailand. Chapter 12, Iodine.

5   Vanderpump MP. The epidemiology of thyroid disease. Br Med Bull 2011;99:39–51.

6   Caldwell KL, Makhmudov A, Ely E, Jones RL, Wang RY. Iodine status of the U.S. population, National Health and Nutrition Examination Survey, 2005–2006 and 2007–2008. Thyroid 2011;21(4):419–27.

7   Caldwell KL, Jones R, Hollowell JG. Urinary iodine concentration: United States National Health And Nutrition Examination Survey 2001–2002. Thyroid 2005;15(7):692–9.

8   Caldwell KL, Miller GA, Wang RY, Jain RB, Jones RL. Iodine status of the U.S. population, National Health and Nutrition Examination Survey 2003–2004. Thyroid 2008;18(11):1207–14.

9   Pessah-Pollack R, Eschler DC, Pozharny Z, Davies T. Apparent insufficiency of iodine supplementation in pregnancy. J Womens Health (Larchmt) 2013, Oct 12. [Epub ahead of print]

10   Crawford BA, Cowell CT. Iodine toxicity from soy milk and seaweed ingestion is associated with serious thyroid dysfunction. Med J Aust 2010;193(7):413–5.

11   Chen X, Liu L, Yao P, et al. Effect of excessive iodine on immune function of lymphocytes and intervention with selenium. J Huazhong Univ Sci Technolog Med Sci 2007;27(4):422–5.

12   Grineva EN, Malakhova TV, et al. Efficacy of thyroxine and potassium iodide treatment of benign nodular thyroid lesions. Ter Arkh 2003;75(8):72–75.

13   Kahaly GJ, Dienes HP, Beyer J, Hommel G. Iodide induces thyroid autoimmunity in patients with endemic goitre: a randomised, double-blind, placebo-controlled trial. Eur J Endocrinol 1998;139:290–7.

14   Ghent WR, Eskin BA, Low DA. Iodine replacement in fibrocystic disease of the breast. Canadian J Surg 1993;36(5):453–60.

15   Smyth PPA. The thyroid, iodine and breast cancer. Breast Cancer Res 2003;5:235–8.

16   Kawamura T, Sobue T. Comparison of Breast Cancer Mortality in Five Countries: France, Italy, Japan, the UK and the USA from the WHO Mortality Database (1960–2000). Japanese J Clin Oncol 2005;35(12):758(59).

17   Nagataki S. The average of dietary iodine intake due to the ingestion of seaweeds is 1.2 mg/day in Japan. Thyroid. 2008 Jun;18(6):667–8.

18   Sicherer S. Risk of severe allergic reactions from the use of potassium iodide for radiation emergencies. J Allergy Clin Immunol 2004 Dec;114(6): 1395–7.

19   Xu J, Liu XL, Yang XF, et al. Supplemental selenium alleviates the toxic effects of excessive iodine on thyroid. Biol Trace Elem Res 2011; 141(1–3):110–8.

20   Xue H et al. Selenium upregulates CD4(+)CD25(+) regulatory T cells in iodine-induced autoimmune thyroiditis model of NOD.H-2(h4) mice. Endocr J 2010;57(7):595–601.

21   International Programme on Chemical Safety (IPCS), http://www.inchem.org/documents/jecfa/jecmono/v024je11.htm.

22   Crawford BA, Cowell CT. Iodine toxicity from soy milk and seaweed ingestion is associated with serious thyroid dysfunction. Med J Aust 2010;193(7):413–5.

23   Delange F, Lecomte P. Iodine supplementation: benefits outweigh risks. Drug Safety 2000;22(2):89–95.

24   Abraham GE, Flechas JD, Hakala JC. Orthoiodosupplementation: iodine sufficiency of the whole human body. The Original Internist, 2002 – optimox.com. http://www.optimox.com/pics/Iodine/IOD-02/IOD_02.htm

25   Roti E, Uberti ED. Iodine excess and hyperthyroidism. Thyroid 2001;11(5):493–500.

26   McLeod DS, Cooper DS. The incidence and prevalence of thyroid autoimmunity. Endocrine. 2012;42:252–65.

27   McGrogan A, Seaman HE, Wright JW, de Vries CS. The incidence of autoimmune thyroid disease: a systematic review of the literature. Clin Endocrinol (Oxf). 2008;69:687–96.

28   Gallagher CM, Meliker JR. Mercury and thyroid autoantibodies in U.S. women, NHANES 2007–2008. Environ Int 2012;40:39–43.

29   Baskin HJ, Cobin RH, Duick DS, et al. American Association of Clinical Endocrinologists medical guidelines for clinical practice for the evaluation and treatment of hyperthyroidism and hypothyroidism. Endocr Pract. 2002;8:457–69.

30   Rostami R, Aghasi MR, Mohammadi A, Nourooz-Zadeh J. Enhanced oxidative stress in Hashimoto's thyroiditis: Inter-relationships to biomarkers of thyroid function. Clinical Biochemistry. 2013;46(4–5):308–12.

31   Kelly GS. Peripheral metabolism of thyroid hormones: a review. Altern Med Rev 2000;5(4):306–33.

32   Linnoila M, Lamberg BA, Potter WZ, Gold PW, Goodwin FK. High reverse T3 levels in manic and unipolar depressed women. Psychiatry Research 1982;6:271–276.

33   Jackson I. The thyroid axis and depression. Thyroid 1998;8(10):951–956.

34   Gitlin M, Altshuler LL, Frye MA, et al. Peripheral thyroid hormones and response to selective serotonin reuptake inhibitors. J Psychiatry Neurosci 2004;29(5):383–386.

35   Clausen P, Mersebach H, Nielsen B, et al. Hypothyroidism is associated with signs of endothelial dysfunction despite 1-year replacement therapy with levothyroxine. Clinical Endocrinology 2009;70:932–937.

36   Duval F, Mokrani MC, Bailey P, et al. Thyroid axis activity and serotonin function major depressive episode. Psychoneuroendocrinology 1999;24:695–712.

37   Unden F, Ljunggren JG, Kjellman BF, Beck-Friis J, Wetterberg L. Twenty-four-hour serum levels of T4 and T3 in relation to decreased TSH serum levels and decreased TSH response to TRH in affective disorders. Acta Psychiatr Scand 1986;73:358–365.

38   Linnoila M, Lamberg BA, Rosberg G, Karonen SL, Welin MG. Thyroid hormones and TSH, prolactin and LH responses to repeated TRH and LRH injections in depressed patients. Acta Psychiat Scand 1979;59:536–544.

39   Kirkegaard C, Faber J. Altered serum levels of thyroxine, triiodothyronines and diiodothyronines in endogenous depression. Acta Endocrinologica 1981;96:199–207.

40   Sintzel F, Mallaret M, Bougerol T. Potentializing of tricyclics and serotoninergics by thyroid hormones in resistant depressive disorders. Encephale 2004;30(3):267–75.

41   Panicker V, Evans J, Bjoro T, Asvold BO. A paradoxical difference in relationship between anxiety, depression and thyroid function in subjects on and not on T4: findings from the Hunt study. Clinical Endocrinology 2009;71:574–580.

42   Thompson FK. Is there a thyroid-cortisol-depression axis? Thyroid Science 2007;2(10):1.

43   Forman-Hoffman V, Philibert RA. Lower TSH and higher T4 levels are associated with current depressive syndrome in young adults. Acta Psychiatry Scand 2006;114:132–139.

44   Cole DP, Thase ME, Mallinger AG, et al. Slower treatment response in biolar depression predicted by lower pretreatment thyroid function. Am J Psychiatry 2002;159:116–121.

45   Premachandra1 BN, Kabir MA, Williams IK. Low T3 syndrome in psychiatric depression. J Endocrinol Invest 2006;29:568–572.

46   Isogawa K, Haruo Nagayama H, Tsutsumi T, et al. Simultaneous use of thyrotropin-releasing hormone test and combined dexamethasone/-corticotropine-releasing hormone test for severity evaluation and outcome prediction in patients with major depressive disorder. J Psych Res 2005;39:467–473.

47   Sullivan GM, Hatterer JA, Herbert J, Chen X, Rosse SP. Low levels of transthyretin in CSF of depressed patients. Am J Psych 1999;156:710–715.

48   Hatterer JA, Herbert J, Jidaka C, Roose SP, Gorman JM. CSF transthyretin in patients with depression. Am J Psychiatry 1993;150:813–815.

49   Whybrow PC, Coppen A, Prange AJ, Noguera R, Bailey JE. Thyroid function and the response to liothyronine in depression. Arch Gen Psychiatry 1972;26:242–245.

50   Kirkegaard C, Faber J. Free thyroxine and 3,3',5'-triiodothyronine levels in cerebrospinal fluid in patients with endogenous depression. Acta Endocrinol 1991;124:166–172.

51   Kirkegaard C. The thyrotropin response to thyrotropin-releasing hormone in endogenous depression. Psychoneuroendocrinology 1981;6:189–212.

52   Baumgartner A, Graf KJ, Kurten I, Meinhold H. The hypothalamic-pituitary-thyroid axis in psychiatric patients and healthy subjects. Psychiatry Research 12988;24:271–332.

53   Stipcevic T, Pivac N, Kozaric-Kovacic D, Muck-Seler D. Thyroid activity in patients with major depression. Coll Antropol 2008;32(3):973–976.

54   Silva JE, Gordon MB, Crantz FR, Leonard JL, Larsen PR. Qualitative and quantitative differences in pathways of extrathyroidial triiodothyronine generation between euthyroid and hypothyroid rats. J Clin Invest 1984;73:898–907.

55   Okamoto R, Leibfritz D. Adverse effects of reverse triiodothyronine on cellular metabolism as assessed by 1H and 31P NMR spectroscopy. Res Exp Med (Berl) 1997;197(4):211–7.

56   Tien ES, Matsui K, Moore R, Negishi M. The nuclear receptor constitutively active/androstane receptor regulates type 1 deiodinase and thyroid hormone activity in the regenerating mouse liver. J Pharmacol Exp Ther 2007;320(1):307–13.

57   Benvenga S, Cahnmann HJ, Robbins J. Characterization of thyroid hormone binding to apolipoprotein-E: localization of the binding site in the exon 3-coded domain. Endocrinology 1993;133:1300–1305.

58   Sechman A, Niezgoda J, Sobocinski R. The relationship between basal metabolic rate (BMR) and concentrations of plasma thyroid hormones in fasting cockerels. Follu Biol 1989;37(1–2):83–90.

59   Pittman JA, Tingley JO, Nickerson JF, Hill SR. Antimetabolic activity of 3,3',5'-triiodo-dl-thyronine in man. Metabolism 1960;9:293–5.

60   Santini F, Chopra IJ, Hurd RE, Solomon DH, Teco GN. A study of the characteristics of the rat placental iodothyronine 5-monodeiodinase: evidence that is distinct from the rat hepatic iodothyronine 5-monodeiodinase. Endocrinology 1992;130:2325–2332.

61   Silva JE, Leonard JL. Regulation of rat cerebrocortical and adenophypophyseal type II 5'-deiodinase by thyroxinem triiodothyronine, and reverse triiodothyronine. Endocrinology 1985;116(4):1627–1635.

62   Obregon MJ, Larsen PR, Silva JE. The role of 3,3',5'-triiodothyroinine in the regulation of type II iodothyronin 5'-deiodinase in the rat cerebral cortex. Endocrinology 1986;119(5):2186–2192.

63   Chopra IJ. A study of extrathyroidal conversion of thyroxine (T4) to 3,3',5-triiodothyronine (T3) in vitro. Endocrinology 1977;101(2):453–63.

64   Mitchell AM, Manley SW, Rowan KA, Mortimer RH. Uptake of reverse T3 in the human choriocarcinoma cell line Jar. Placenta 1999;20:65–70.

65   Van der Geyten S, Buys N, Sanders JP, et al. Acute pretranslational regulation of type III iodothyronine deiodinase by growth hormone and dexamethasone in chicken embryos. Mol Cell Endocrinol 1999;147:49–56.

66   Visser TJ, Lamberts WJ, Wilson JHP, Docter WR, Hennemann G. Serum thyroid hormone concentrations during prolonged reduction of dietary intake. Metabolism 1978;27(4):405–409.

67   Cheron RG, Kaplan MM, Larsen PR. Physiological and pharmacological influences on thyroxine to 3,5,3'-triiodothyronine conversion and nuclear 3,5,3'-triiodothyronine binding in rat anterior pituitary. J Clin Invest 1979;64:1402–1414.

68   Araujo RL, Andrade BM, da Silva ML, et al. Tissue-specific deiodinase regulation during food restriction and low replacement dose of leptin in rats. Am J Physiol Endocinol Metab 2009;296:E1157–E1163.

69   Leibel RL, Jirsch J. Diminished energy requirements in reduced-obese patients. Metabolism 1984;33(2):164–170.

70   Fontana L, Klein S, Holloszy JO, Premachandra BN. Effect of long-term calorie restriction with adequate protein and micronutrients on thyroid hormones. J Clin Endocrinol Metab 2006;91(8):3232–3235.

71   Croxson MS, Ibbertson HK. Low serum triiodothyronine (T3) and hypothyroidism. J Clin Endocrinol Metab 1977;44:167–174.

72   Cooke RG, Joffe RT, Levitt AJ. T3 augmentation of antidepressant treatment in T4-replaced thyroid patients. J Clin Psychiatry 1992;53(1):16–8.

73   Joffe RT. A perspective on the thyroid and depression. Can J Psychiatry 1990;35(9):754–8.

74   Sawka AM, Gerstein HC, Marriott MJ, MacQueen GM, Joffe RT. Does a combination regimen of thyroxine (T4) and 3,5,3'-triiodothyronine improved depressive symptoms better than T4 alone in patients with hypothyroidism? Results of a double-blind, randomized, controlled trial. J Clin Endocrinol Metab 2003;88(10):4551–4555.

75   Cooper-Kazaz R, Apter JT, Cohen R, et al. Combined treatment with sertraline and liothyronine in major depression. Arch Gen Psych 2007;64:679–688.

76   Kelly T, Lieberman DZ. The use of triiodothyronine as an augmentation agent in treatment resistant bipolar II and bipolar disorder NOS. J Affect Disord 2009;116:222–226.

77   Posternak M, Novak S, Stern R, et al. A pilot effectiveness study: placebo-controlled trial of adjunctive L-triiodothyronine (T3) used to accelerate and potentiate the antidepressant response. Int J Neuropsychopharmacology 2008;11:15–25.

78   Nierenberg AA, Fava M, Trivedi MH, et al. A comparison of lithium and T3 augmentation following two failed medication treatments for depression: A STAR*D Report. Am J Psychiatry 2006;163:1519–1530.

79   Gupta P, Kar A. Role of ascorbic acid in cadmium-induced thyroid dysfunction and lipid peroxidation. J Appl Toxicol. 1998;18:317–20.

80   Swarup D, Naresh R, Varshney VP, et al. Changes in plasma hormones profile and liver function in cows naturally exposed to lead and cadmium around different industrial areas. Res Vet Sci. 2007;82:16–21.

81   Wade MG, Parent S, Finnson KW, et al. Thyroid toxicity due to subchronic exposure to a complex mixture of 16 organochlorines, lead, and cadmium. Toxicol Sci. 2002;67:207–18.

82   Yoshizuka M, Mori N, Hamasaki K, et al. Cadmium toxicity in the thyroid gland of pregnant rats. Exp Mol Pathol. 1991;55:97–104.

83   Nishida M, Sato K, Kawada J. Differential effects of methylmercuric chloride and mercuric chloride on oxidation and iodination reactions catalyzed by thyroid peroxidase. Biochem Int. 1990;22:369–78.

84   Kawada J, Nishida M, Yoshimura Y, Mitani K. Effects of organic and inorganic mercurials on thyroidal functions. J Pharmacobiodyn. 1980;3:149–59.

85   Pusey CD, Bowman C, Morgan A, Weetman AP, Hartley B, Lockwood CM. Kinetics and pathogenicity of autoantibodies induced by mercuric chloride in the brown Norway rat. Clin Exp Immunol. 1990;81:76–82.

86   Powell JJ, Van de Water J, Gershwin ME. Evidence for the role of environmental agents in the initiation or progression of autoimmune conditions. Environ Health Perspect. 1999;107 (Suppl 5):667–72.

87   Agency for Toxic Substances and Disease Registry (ASTDR). Toxicological Profile for Mercury. 1999 Atlanta, GA: U.S. Department of Health and Human Services, Public Health Service.

88   Chaurasia SS, Kar A. Influence of lead on type-I iodothyronine 5′-monodeiodinase activity in male mouse. Horm Metab Res. 1997;29:532–3.

89   Chaurasia SS, Kar A. Protective effects of vitamin E against lead-induced deterioration of membrane associated type-I iodothyronine 5′-monodeiodinase (5′D-I) activity in male mice. Toxicology. 1997;124:203–9.

90   Gupta P, Kar A. Cadmium induced thyroid dysfunction in chicken: hepatic type I iodothyronine 5′-monodeiodinase activity and role of lipid peroxidation. Comp Biochem Physiol C Pharmacol Toxicol Endocrinol. 1999;123:39–44.

91   Yoshida K, Sugihira N, Suzuki M, et al. Effect of cadmium on T4 outer ring monodeiodination by rat liver. Environ Res. 1987;42:400–5.

92   Merrill EA, Clewell RA, Gearhart JM, et al. PBPK predictions of perchlorate distribution and its effect on thyroid uptake of radioiodide in the male rat. Toxicol Sci. 2003;73:256–69.

93   Harrington RM, Shertzer HG, Bercz JP. Effects of chlorine dioxide on thyroid function in the African green monkey and the rat. J Toxicol Environ Health. 1986;19:235–42.

94   Wang H, Yang Z, Zhou B, Gao H, Yan X, Wang J. Fluoride-induced thyroid dysfunction in rats: roles of dietary protein and calcium level. Toxicol Ind Health. 2009;25:49–57.

95   Allain P, Berre S, Krari N, et al. Bromine and thyroid hormone activity. J Clin Pathol. 1993;46:456–8.

96   Porter WP, Jaeger JW, Carlson IH. Endocrine, immune, and behavioral effects of aldicarb (carbamate), atrazine (triazine) and nitrate (fertilizer) mixtures at groundwater concentrations. Toxicol Ind Health. 1999;15:133–50.

97   Howdeshell KL. A model of the development of the brain as a construct of the thyroid system. Environ Health Perspect. 2002;110 (Suppl 3):337–48.

98   Kashiwagi K, Furuno N, Kitamura S, Ohta S, Sugihara K, Utsumi K, Hanada H, Taniguchi K, Suzuki K, Kashiwagi A. Disruption of thyroid hormone function by environmental chemicals. J Health Sci. 2009;55:147–160.

99   Graziano JH, Siris ES, Lolacono N, et al. 2,3-dimercaptosuccinic acid as an antidote for lead intoxication. Clin Pharmacol Ther 1985;37:432–8.

100   Mangano JJ. A post-Chernobyl rise in thyroid cancer in Connecticut, USA. Eur J Cancer Prev 1996;5:75–81.

101   Duntas LH. Environmental factors and autoimmune thyroiditis. Nat Clin Pract Endocrinol Metab 2008;4:454–60.

102   Safran M, Paul TL, Roti E, Braverman LE. Environmental factors affecting autoimmune thyroid disease. Endocrinol Metab Clin North Am 1987;16:327–42.

103   Chrousos GP. Stress and disorders of the stress system. Nat Rev Endocrinol. 2009;5:374–81.

104   Delange F. The disorders induced by iodine deficiency. Thyroid 1994;4:107–28.

105   Pizzulli A, Ranjbar A. Selenium deficiency and hypothyroidism: a new etiology in the differential diagnosis of hypothyroidism in children. Biol Trace Elem Res 2000;77:199–208.

106   Watts DL. The nutritional relationships of the thyroid. J Orthomol Med. 1989;4:165–9.

107   Stangl GI, Schwarz FJ, Kirchgessner M. Cobalt deficiency effects on trace elements, hormones and enzymes involved in energy metabolism of cattle. Int J Vitam Nutr Res 1999;69:120–6.

108   McGrogan A, Seaman HE, Wright JW, de Vries CS. The incidence of autoimmune thyroid disease: a systematic review of the literature. Clin Endocrinol (Oxf) 2008;69:687–96.

109   Canaris GJ, Manowitz NR, Mayor G, Ridgway EC. The Colorado thyroid disease prevalence study. Arch Intern Med 2000;160:526–34.

110   McLeod DS, Cooper DS. The incidence and prevalence of thyroid autoimmunity. Endocrine 2012 Oct;42(2):252–65.

111   Crinnion W. Clean, green, & lean. Hoboken, New Jersey: John Wiley & Sons; 2010.

112   Pizzorno L. Iodine: the next vitamin D? Part I: Americans at high risk for iodine insufficiency. Longevity Medicine Review, May 2009, http://www.lmreview.com/articles/view/iodine-the-next-vitamin-d-part-I/.

113   Frances D. Botanical approaches to hypothyroidism: avoiding supplemental thyroid hormone. Medical Herbalism 2002;12:1–5.

114   Singh AK, Tripathi SN, Prasad GC. Response of commiphora mukul (guggulu) on melatonin induced hypothyroidism. Anc Sci Life 1983;3:85–90.

115   Tripathi YB, Malhotra OP, Tripathi SN. Thyroid stimulating action of Z-guggulsterone obtained from Commiphora mukul. Planta Med 1984;50:78–80.

116   Tripathi YB, Tripathi P, Malhotra OP, Tripathi SN. Thyroid stimulatory action of (Z)-guggulsterone: mechanism of action. Planta Med 1988;54:271–7.

117   Antonio J, Colker CM, Torina GC, Shi Q, Brink W, Kaiman D. Effects of a standardized guggulsterone phosphate supplement on body composition in overweight adults: a pilot study. Curr Ther Res 1999;60:220–7.

[118] Panda S, Kar A. Gugulu (Commiphora mukul) induces triiodothyronine production: possible involvement of lipid peroxidation. Life Sci 1999;65:L137–L141.

[119] Grineva EN, Malakhova TV, Tsoi UA, Smirnov BI. Efficacy of thyroxine and potassium iodide treatment of benign nodular thyroid lesions. Ter Arkh 2003;75:72–5.

[120] Vanderpump MP. The epidemiology of thyroid disease. Br Med Bull 2011;99:39–51.

[121] Kahaly GJ, Dienes HP, Beyer J, Hommel G. Iodide induces thyroid autoimmunity in patients with endemic goitre: a randomised, double-blind, placebo-controlled trial. Eur J Endocrinol 1998;139:290–7.

[122] Tamer G, Arik S, Tamer I, Coksert D. Relative vitamin D insufficiency in Hashimoto's thyroiditis. Thyroid 2011;21:891–6.

[123] Ginanjar E, Sumariyono, Setiati S, Setiyohadi B. Vitamin D and autoimmune disease. Acta Med Indones 2007;39:133–41.

[124] Chen W, Lin H, Wang M. Immune intervention effects on the induction of experimental autoimmune thyroiditis. J Huazhong Univ Sci Technol Med Sci 2002;22:343–5, 354.

[125] Fournier C, Gepner P, Sadouk M, Charreire J. *In vivo* beneficial effects of cyclosporin A and 1,25-dihydroxyvitamin D3 on the induction of experimental autoimmune thyroiditis. Clin Immunol Immunopathol 1990;54:53–63.

4

Diagnosing Tissue Thyroid Status

Why Conventional Blood Tests are Not Accurate

The thyroid-stimulating hormone (TSH) test is generally considered the most sensitive marker of thyroid hormone levels in the peripheral tissue. This view, however, is incorrect. Most endocrinologists and other physicians mistakenly assume that, except for unique situations, a normal TSH is a clear indication that the person's tissue thyroid levels are adequate (thus concluding that symptoms are not due to low thyroid). But a more thorough understanding of the hypothalamic–pituitary–thyroid (HPT) axis and thyroid hormone regulation casts doubt on this common misconception. As discussed in depth in Chapter 1, the pituitary conversion of thyroxine (T4) to triiodothyronine (T3) is not susceptible to the same inhibiting factors as cellular conversion resulting in a faulty feedback mechanism.

The pituitary is both anatomically and physiologically unique, reacting differently to inflammation, chronic calorie reduction (dieting), environmental toxins, nutritional deficiencies, and physiologic stress than every other tissue in the body.[1–25] During physiologic stress or dieting, there is a reduced conversion of T4 to T3 and an increase in the formation of the anti-thyroid reverse T3 (rT3) in tissues throughout the body, except for in the pituitary, where local mechanisms increase T3 levels.[1–63]

Serum Levels of Thyroid Hormones

Due to the differences in the pituitary's response to physiological stress, depression, dieting, aging, and inflammation (as discussed previously), most individuals with diminished tissue levels of thyroid will have a normal TSH.[1–63] Doctors are taught that if active thyroid (T3) levels drop, the TSH will increase. Thus, endocrinologists and other doctors tell patients that an elevated TSH is the most useful marker for diminished T3 levels, and that a normal TSH indicates that their thyroid status is "fine." The TSH, however, is primarily a marker of pituitary levels of T3 and not of T3 levels in any other part of the body. Only under ideal conditions of total health do pituitary T3 levels correlate with T3 levels in the rest of the body.

The relationship between TSH and tissue T3 is lost in the presence of:

- Physiologic or emotional stress[1–20,26–37]
- Depression[38–43]
- Insulin resistance and diabetes[33,44,65–66]
- Aging[35,45–54]
- Calorie deprivation (dieting)[21–23,55–59]
- Inflammation[5–8,27,67–70]
- Premenstrual syndrome (PMS)[60,61]
- Chronic fatigue syndrome (CFS) and fibromyalgia[62,63]
- Obesity[71–73]
- Numerous other conditions[1–63]

In the presence of these conditions, the TSH is a poor marker of active thyroid levels and thyroid status. Thus, a normal TSH cannot be used as a reliable indicator that a person is euthyroid (normal thyroid) on the level of the tissues.

Accumulating data suggest that using TSH as a measure of thyroid function will miss 20–95% of patients with low thyroid in the tissues (depending on comorbid conditions).[1–63] One study exemplifying the failure of TSH to detect low thyroid in the tissues was published in the *Journal of Rheumatology* and evaluated thyroid system function in patients with fibromyalgia.[62] Using thyrotropin releasing hormone (TRH) testing, which is a more accurate measure of thyroid function, they found that all of the patients with fibromyalgia were low thyroid despite the fact that their standard thyroid function tests, including TSH, T4, and T3, were in the normal range. These patients also tended to have low normal TSH levels that averaged 0.86 vs. 1.42 in controls, with high normal free T4 and low normal T3 levels. Therefore, doctors erroneously feel these patients are on the high side of normal because of the low normal TSH and high normal T4.

A study published in the *New England Journal of Medicine* investigated the incidence of low thyroid in women with PMS via TRH testing and iodine uptake scans as well as measuring of TSH, T4, T3, T3U (T3 uptake), and thyroid antibodies. The study found that 94% of patients with PMS had thyroid dysfunction (low thyroid in the tissues) compared to 0% of the asymptomatic patients. Sixty-five percent of the low thyroid patients had thyroid tests in "normal" range and could only be diagnosed by TRH testing (which is not included in the usual thyroid function tests). They also found that all PMS patients had complete resolution of symptoms with thyroid treatment even though the standard blood tests were "normal".[60]

A study published in the *American Journal of Psychiatry* also investigated thyroid function in women with PMS with the use of TRH testing. The study found 70% of women with PMS had abnormal TRH testing, showing thyroid dysfunction despite having normal TSH levels.[74]

A study in the *Journal of Clinical Endocrinology and Metabolism* examined the accuracy of using TSH to identify thyroid dysfunction in obese individuals.[72] The study found that although TSH levels were not significantly different between normal weight and obese individuals, 36% of obese patients had severe thyroid dysfunction that was detected by TRH, but not standard TSH testing. Similarly, a study published in the journal *Psychoneuroendocrinology* also evaluated the accuracy of TSH to detect thyroid dysfunction in obese patients by testing the TSH as well as performing TRH testing.[75] It was found that in obese individuals, the TSH failed to detect low thyroid patients 40% of the time.

A large study published in the journal *BMC Endocrine Disorders* evaluated the accuracy of TSH testing in 2,570 women attending a reproductive endocrine clinic for menstrual irregularities or infertility.[76] The study found that TSH was a very poor indicator of abnormal thyroid function as over half the women with a TSH between 2 and 4 mIU/l, which would be interpreted as normal thyroid function, were shown to be low thyroid when the more accurate and sensitive TRH testing was done.

A study published in *The Lancet* performed thyroid biopsies in patients with CFS and found that 40% of these patients had lymphocytic thyroiditis (Hashimoto's thyroiditis), with only 40% of these being positive for thyroid peroxidase (TPO), antithyroglobulin antibodies, or an abnormal TSH. Therefore, thyroid dysfunction among these patients would have gone undetected if the biopsy had not been done.[77,78] This study also demonstrated that because the TSH is a poor indicator of thyroid function, it also does not predict whose symptoms will respond to thyroid replacement. The authors state, "After treatment with thyroxine, clinical response was favorable, irrespective of baseline TSH concentration."[77]

This research demonstrates that many fatigued patients have Hashimoto's thyroiditis that is undetectable by standard auto-antibody and TSH testing. Many of these patients fit the diagnostic criteria of CFS. Further, the test demonstrates that many such patients will likely respond to thyroid replacement regardless of their baseline thyroid function tests. The authors suggest that the TSH not be relied upon to accurately detect thyroid dysfunction in chronically fatigued patients.[77,78]

A study published in the *British Medical Journal* examined the accuracy of using the TSH as a marker for adequate thyroid replacement.[79] This study also found that TSH was a very poor indicator of optimal thyroid replaced and that a suppressed TSH was not an accurate indicator of over-replacement. The authors showed that a suppressed TSH was not an indication of hyperthyroidism or over-replacement in 80% of cases, thus they discourage reliance on the TSH for optimal dosing.

Many other studies have confirmed the fact that standard thyroid function tests (TSH, T4, and T3) cannot be used to rule out central hypothyroidism (such as secondary hypothyroidism that is due to hypo-function of the pituitary gland, or tertiary hypothyroidism that is due to hypo-function of the hypothalamus) as occurs with numerous conditions discussed above. One such study clearly demonstrating this fact was published in the *Journal of Clinical Endocrinology and Metabolism*; this study determined how often central hypothyroidism was confirmed with TRH testing, but yet went undetected by standard thyroid function tests.[80] The authors found that 92% of patients with central hypothyroidism would have remained undiagnosed using baseline thyroid function tests. The authors conclude, "… most prior studies have failed to accurately identify many cases of central or mixed hypothyroidism because of diagnostic criteria that require a T4 or FT4 value below the normal range in addition to a low TSH value. However, patients with central hypothyroidism most often have normal TSH values and T4 or FT4 levels at least within the low normal range."[80]

Value of Serum T4

Given that physiologic and emotional stress tend to suppress TSH, you might expect that serum T4 levels would also be lower.[1,2,9,81–85] In the presence of such conditions, however, there are competing effects that result in an increase in serum T4 while further reducing tissue levels of T3, making serum T4 (or free T4) a poor marker of tissue thyroid level. Such effects include a suppression of tissue T4 to T3 conversion (misleadingly increasing serum T4 levels),[1–63,81–86] an increased conversion of T4 to rT3,[2,14,18,40,41,46,61,87–94] an induced thyroid resistance, and reduced uptake of T4 into the cells (misleadingly increasing serum T4 levels);[16,19,86,95–102] this is true in all tissues except for the pituitary.[102]

Although all such effects reduced intracellular T3 concentrations in all tissues except for the pituitary, the serum T4 level can be increased, decreased, or unchanged. Consequently, serum T4 levels frequently do not correlate with tissue T3 levels and, as with the TSH, the serum T4 level is often misleading and unreliable for measuring the body's overall thyroid status.

Current Best Method to Diagnosis

With growing knowledge of the complexities of thyroid function at the cellular level, it is becoming increasingly clear that TSH and T4 levels are not reliable markers of tissue thyroid levels as once thought, especially with chronic physiologic or emotional stress, illness, inflammation, depression, and aging. The TRH test is a reliable method but such testing is expensive, burdensome, requires trained personnel, and entails multiple blood draws. Thus, TRH testing is not practical to use in a clinical setting. Although there are limitations to all testing and there is no perfect test, research shows that signs (like body temperature) and symptoms are still the most reliable indicators of thyroid status in the tissues. Also, obtaining free T3, rT3, and T3/rT3 ratios can be helpful to determine tissue thyroid status; they may also be useful for predicting who may respond favorably to thyroid supplementation.[1,11,12,14,40,41,46,61,88–94] However, remember that signs, symptoms, and body temperature are the best measures of cellular thyroid deficiency. Many symptomatic patients with low tissue levels of active thyroid hormone but normal TSH and T4 levels will significantly benefit from T3 replacement, often experiencing an improvement in fatigue, depression, diabetes, weight gain, PMS, fibromyalgia, and numerous other chronic conditions.[103–116]

Test	Lower limit	Upper limit	Unit
TSH	0.3	2.0–3.0	mIU/l
Total T4/serum T4	4.5	12.3	µg/dl
	60	140	nmol/l
Free T4	0.7	1.8	ng/dl
	9	18	pmol/l
Total T3/serum T3	80	220	ng/dl
	0.9	3	nmol/l
Free T3	3.0	7.0	pg/ml
Reverse T3	11	32	ng/dl

Normal thyroid lab values.

A deeper understanding of thyroid physiology reveals that a large percentage of patients treated with T4-only preparations continue to be symptomatic. Therefore, T4-only preparations are not effective, and should not be considered the treatment of choice in conditions associated with reduced T4 to T3 conversion, reduced uptake of T4, or increased T4 to rT3 conversion. As discussed above, with any physiologic stress (emotional or physical), inflammation, depression, inflammation, aging, or dieting, the conversion of T4 to T3 is reduced and T4 will be preferentially converted to rT3,[12,14,18,40,41,46,55,88–94] which acts as a competitive inhibitor of T3 (blocks T3 at the receptor),[117–121] reduces metabolism,[117,120,121] suppresses T4 to T3 conversion,[118,120] blocks T4 and T3 uptake into the cell, and decreases the half-life of the deiodinase enzyme.[122] T4 can also reduce the half-life of the deiodinase enzyme.[9]

While a normal TSH cannot be used as a reliable indicator of global tissue thyroid effect, even a minimally elevated TSH (above 2) demonstrates that there is a diminished intra-pituitary T3 level. It is also a clear indication (except in unique situations such as a TSH-secreting tumor) that the rest of the body is suffering from inadequate thyroid activity. This is because the pituitary T3 level is usually significantly higher than the rest of the body and the most rigorously screened individuals for absence of thyroid disease have a TSH below 2 to 2.5.[76,124] Thus, treatment should likely be initiated in any symptomatic person with a TSH greater than 2.

Due to a lack of correlation between TSH and tissue thyroid levels, a normal TSH should not be used as the sole reason to withhold treatment in a symptomatic patient. A symptomatic patient with a low body temperature can be considered for T3 therapy. High rT3, low free T3, and a free T3/reverse T3 ratio less than 2 can further support the indication.[13,14,18,86,88–94,103–121,124–126,] A relatively low sex hormone binding globulin (SHBG) and slow reflex time can also be useful markers for low tissue thyroid levels and can aid in the diagnosis of tissue hypothyroidism.[110,127]

A study published in the *Journal of Clinical Endocrinology and Metabolism* assessed the functional thyroid status of 332 female patients based on a clinical score of 14 common signs and symptoms of hypothyroidism and assessments of peripheral thyroid action (tissue thyroid effect). The study found that the clinical score and ankle reflex time correlated well with tissue thyroid effect but the TSH had no correlation with the tissue effect of thyroid hormones.[128]

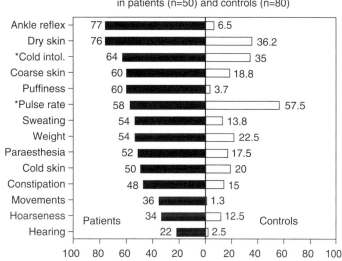

Frequency of hypothyroid symptoms and signs (in %)
in patients (n=50) and controls (n=80)

The ankle reflex itself had a specificity of 93% (93% of those with slow relaxation phase of the reflexes had tissue hypothyroidism) and a sensitivity of 77% (77% of those with tissue hypothyroidism had a slow relaxation phase of the reflexes), making both reflex speed and clinical assessment a more accurate measurement of tissue thyroid effect than the TSH.

Croxson et al. in *Journal of Endocrinology and Metabolism* found that the Achilles reflex relaxation time (ARRT) was a better marker of tissue peripheral T3 levels than TSH and T4 levels. The ARRT correlated with T3 levels and was able to correctly detect low tissue T3 levels in chronically dieting individuals, while the TSH and T4 failed to detect dramatically low tissue and serum T3 levels. The inadequacy of standard TSH and T4 testing was demonstrated in that they both failed to detect the dramatic reduction in T3 tissue levels among all of the patients.[80]

In addition to history and clinical assessment, a combination of the serum levels of TSH, free T3, free T4, rT3, anti-TPO antibody, antithyroglobulin antibody, SHBG, and measurement of reflex speed and basal metabolic rate can add to the assessment of the overall thyroid status in a patient. Forgoing treatment based on a normal TSH without further assessment will result in the misdiagnosis or mismanagement of a large number of low thyroid patients who may greatly benefit from treatment. Simply relying on a TSH to determine the thyroid status of a patient does not demonstrate current understanding of thyroid physiology and is not evidence-based medicine. In symptomatic patients with low body temperatures and normal TSH tests (especially with elevated or high normal reverse T3 levels), T4-only preparations should not be considered adequate and T3-containing preparations, in particular sustained-released T3, should be considered the treatment of choice.

Why Don't All Endocrinologists Know This?

Historically, the sole reliance on consensus statements to treat or not to treat a particular patient has been shown to result in poor care. As such, society consensus statements and practice guidelines are considered to be the worst level of evidence in support of a particular therapy or treatment. A number of organizations, including the World Health Organization, have ranked the strength and accuracy of various types of evidence used in the medical decision process. In all scoring systems, the highest strength of evidence is applied to randomized control trials and meta-analyses, with lower scores given to other forms of evidence. All grading systems place consensus statements and expert opinion by respected authorities (societies) as the poorest level of evidence, because historically they have failed to adopt new concepts and treatments based on new knowledge or new-found understanding demonstrated in the medical literature.[129–134] For instance, a recent study published in the 2009 *Journal of American Medical Association* studied the evidence supporting the claims of practice guidelines and consensus statements published by the American College of Cardiology and the American Heart Association. It was found that only 11% of the recommendations, practice guidelines, and consensus statements were based on quality evidence, and over half were based on poor quality evidence that was little more than the panel's opinion. The review also found that even the strongest (Class 1) recommendations, which are considered medical dogma, cited as a legal standard, and often go unquestioned as medical fact, were only supported by high quality evidence 19% of the time, and not revised based on new evidence.[134]

Guidelines are often out-of-date even before they are published. Additionally, once a guideline is published, there is major resistance to making needed changes or revisions as new information becomes available. They are often inappropriately used to define "gold standard" treatment for decades to come.[135–138] Groups such as the Endocrine Society, the American Association of Clinical Endocrinologists, and the American Thyroid Association have a long history of publishing guidelines and recommendations that are not supported by the weight of medical evidence. They have also failed to adjust or abandon recommendations when new understanding and knowledge contradicts their previous statements. This includes the mistaken notion that a normal TSH adequately rules out thyroid dysfunction, or that T4-only replacement is adequate for most patients. These mistaken hypotheses continue to be perpetuated despite massive amounts of research calling them into doubt (see Why conventional blood tests are not accurate).

A doctor who simply follows outdated society treatment guidelines that rely on a simple laboratory test and ignores the clinical aspects of a patient is not practicing evidence-based medicine.[129–135,139] Doctors and clinicians can do more than just practice "laboratory medicine".[129–134,139] This method of practice is consistently identified as inappropriate and poor medicine, but has become the standard used by a large percentage of endocrinologists and physicians who reduce medicine to simply reading "normal" or "abnormal" in a laboratory column.

While discussing the lack of scientific basis of most medical society's consensus statements and treatment guidelines, Dr. Diana Petritti states (*Internal Medicine News*),

> "Expert opinion and consensus statements can be quite misleading when used as the basis for a practice. Expert opinions imply that there is something that the experts know that the clinician doesn't know. I don't think it's always appreciated that it's only opinion. There is a tendency to make guidelines and recommendations seem authoritative. I believe that physicians think that there is a great deal more behind authoritative recommendations than there might be when you lift the lid off the box and see what's underneath."[140]

There has been significant concern by health care organizations and medical experts that physicians are placing too much reliance on consensus statements that over-generalize and may not apply to large groups of patients. Physicians are also being criticized for failing to learn new information presented in medical journals.[129–131,134,139–154] Thus, physicians are not only unable to translate new information into treatments for their patients, but they are also resistant to changing treatment philosophies based on accumulating evidence. This appears to be especially true of endocrinologists, at least with respect to assessing and treating thyroid dysfunction.

This concern is particularly clear in an article published in the *New England Journal of Medicine* entitled "Clinical research to clinical practice: lost in translation".[141] The article was written by Claude Lenfant MD, Director of National Heart, Lung, and Blood Institute. He states that there is great concern that doctors continue to rely on what they learned 20 years before and are uninformed about recent/current scientific findings. According to Dr. Lenfant, medical researchers, along with public officials and political leaders, are increasingly concerned about physicians' inability to translate research findings into their medical practice to benefit their patients. He says that very few physicians learn about new discoveries from reading medical journals or by attending scientific conferences; thus, they lack the ability to translate new knowledge into the field where it has the potential to enhance treatments for their patients. He states that a review of past medical discoveries reveals how excruciatingly slow the medical establishment is to adopt novel concepts; noting that even simple methods to improve medical quality are often met with fierce resistance.

"Given the ever-growing sophistication of our scientific knowledge and the additional new discoveries that are likely in the future, many of us harbor an uneasy, but quite realistic suspicion that this gap between what we know about diseases and what we do to prevent and treat them will become even wider. And it is not just recent research results that are not finding their way into clinical practice; there is plenty of evidence showing that 'old' research outcomes have been lost in translation as well."[141]

Dr. Lenfant discusses the fact that the proper practice of medicine involves the combination of medical knowledge, intuition, and judgment, and that physicians' knowledge is lacking because they don't keep up with the medical literature. He states that there is often a difference of opinion among physicians and reviewing entities, but that judgment and knowledge of the research pertaining to the patient's condition is central to the responsible practice of medicine.

"Enormous amounts of new knowledge are barreling down the information highway, but they are not arriving at the doorsteps of our patients."[141]

These thoughts are echoed by physicians who have researched this issue as well, such as William Shankle MD, Professor, University of California, Irvine. He states,

"Most doctors are practicing 10 to 20 years behind the available medical literature and continue to practice what they learned in medical school. ... There is a breakdown in the transfer of information from the research to the overwhelming majority of practicing physicians. Doctors do not seek to implement new treatments that are supported in the literature or change treatments that are not."[142]

This view is reiterated by Dr. Philip A. Pizzo, Dean of Stanford University School of Medicine, who states that in the absence of translational medicine, the delivery of medical care would remain stagnant and uninformed by the tremendous progress taking place in science and medicine.[143]

This concern has also received significant publicity in the mainstream media. This is illustrated by an article quoting Sidney Smith MD, former president of the American Heart Association, published in 2003 in the *Wall Street Journal* entitled "Too Many Patients Never Reap the Benefits of Great Research." Dr. Smith is very critical of physicians for not seeking out available information and applying that information for their patients. He argues that doctors feel the best medicine is what they've been doing and thinking for years. They discount new research, because it is not what they have been taught or practiced, and they refuse to admit that what they have been doing or thinking for many years is not the best medicine. He states,

"A large part of the problem is the real resistance of physicians ...; many of these independent-minded souls don't like being told that science knows best, and the way they've always done things is second-rate."[144]

The National Center for Policy Analysis also expresses concern for the lack of ability of physicians to translate medical therapies into practice.[145] A review published in *The Annals of Internal Medicine* found that there is clearly a problem with physicians not seeking to advance their knowledge by reviewing the current literature, believing proper care is what they learned in medical school or residency, and not basing their treatments on the most current research. The review found that the longer a physician is in practice, the more inappropriate and substandard was their care.[146] Thus, it is not a surprise that the scientific evidence as expressed in the literature is often opposite to what is continually repeated as dogma by most physicians and those considered to be "experts."

Another example is a study published in the *Journal of the American Medical Informatics Association*.[147] In reviewing the study, the National Institute of Medicine reports that there is an unacceptable lag between the discovery of new treatment modalities and their acceptance into routine care:

"The lag between the discovery of more effective forms of treatment and their incorporation into routine patient care averages 17 years."[148]

In response to this unacceptable lag, the Business and Professions Code passed an amendment relating to the healing arts. This amendment – CA Assembly Bill 592; An Act to Amend Section 2234.1 of the Business and Professions Code – states:

"Since the National Institute of Medicine has reported that it can take up to 17 years for a new best practice to reach the average physician and surgeon, it is prudent to give attention to new developments not only in general medical care but in the actual treatment of specific diseases, particularly those that are not yet broadly recognized [such as the concept of low thyroid in the tissues, chronic fatigue syndrome, and fibromyalgia]."[149]

The Principals of Medical Ethics adopted by the American Medical Association in 1980 states that a physician shall continue to study, apply, and advance scientific knowledge, as well as make relevant information available to patients, colleagues, and the public.[150] In the case of thyroid function assessment, this principal has unfortunately fallen to the wayside, in favor of being able to make rapid decisions on a patient's thyroid status based almost exclusively on the "normal or abnormal" column on the lab results for a single test; this despite the fact that hundreds of studies document the inaccuracy of the TSH (see Why conventional blood tests are not accurate).

In many cases, evidence for thyroid dysfunction that is based on signs and symptoms, medical history, and/or a physical exam is considered irrelevant if the TSH test is normal. Although completely incorrect, this method is vehemently defended. Fostering this bad practice is the United States insurance reimbursement system, which rewards physicians for seeing too many patients per day, and penalizes doctors who are methodically assessing and treating each and every patient that comes into their care. While it is true that the best physicians are continually fighting to provide cutting edge treatments and superior care that the insurance companies deem not medically necessary, even these physicians eventually get worn down and are forced to surrender to the current system that promotes substandard care.

This concept was clearly demonstrated in a study published in the March 2006 edition of *The New England Journal of Medicine* entitled "Who is at greater risk for receiving poor-quality health care." The study found that the majority of individuals received substandard, poor-quality care, and that there was no significant disparity between different income levels or whether or not the individual was covered by insurance. It used to be the case that only those in low socioeconomic classes and/or those without insurance received poor-quality care, but insurance company restrictions on treatments and diagnostic procedures have made the same poor care afforded to those of low socioeconomic status the new standard-of-care for society at large.[151] An example of this is a physician's failing to spend the time to adequately assess a potential low thyroid patient and instead simply ordering a TSH test.

Although medical societies profess to operate for the public good, there is significant concern that the medical societies not only use guidelines and recommendations to further their own economic interests, but they also use the opportunity to "sit in judgment of their competitors." They are essentially putting their interests above those of patients.[135,152–155] Potential resolutions of this problem have been discussed in a number of medical journals, including *Journal of the American Medical Association*.[135,155] It states that practice guidelines, such as those published by the Endocrine Society and the American Thyroid Association stating that the TSH should be the sole means to diagnosed low thyroid, have evolved into marketing and opinion pieces that have less to do with the proper treatment and more about expanding the societies' influence in a competitive marketplace.[135,155]

A review article published in the 2009 *American Family Physician* recommends that family physicians should avoid using such "opinion" or "consensus-based" guidelines all together and argues that good guidelines offer flexibility, incorporate patient's wishes, and emphasize patient-oriented outcomes (i.e., quality of life) over laboratory results and other surrogate markers.[156]

Evidence-based medicine involves the synthesis of all available data when comparing therapeutic options for patients. Evidence-based medicine does not mean that data should be ignored until a randomized control trial of a particular size and duration is completed. The best doctors who truly practice evidence-based medicine will not be overly reliant on consensus statements. In a review article of evidence-based medicine by Toriello and Goldenberg, the authors emphasize that,

> "Evidence-based medicine is the integration of research evidence with both clinical expertise and patients' specific values and circumstances."[157]

Instead of relying on old dogma, the best physicians will seek out and translate both basic science results and clinical outcomes to decide on the safest, most efficacious treatment for their patients. Furthermore, the best physicians will continually assess the current available data to decide which therapies are likely to carry the greatest benefits for patients and involve the lowest risks.

Additionally, an essential component of informed consent requires that in the absence of medical certainty, patients have the opportunity to choose among the available medically indicated treatments.[152] Thomas May from the Medical

College of Wisconsin's Center for the Study of Bioethics addressed the question of patient choice when there is medical controversy regarding the treatment. May concluded that it is vital to preserve choice and allow the individual whose life is most affected by that choice (i.e., the patient) to exercise autonomy of management decisions.[158] This is in total agreement with the American Medical Association's code of ethics, which states:

> "The principle of patient autonomy holds that an individual's physical, emotional, and psychological integrity should be respected and upheld. This principle also recognizes the human capacity to self-govern and choose a course of action from among different alternative options."[157]

Choice can only be preserved by understanding and acknowledging divergent viewpoints on the treatment options available, and translating that data into lay terms so that the patients can make an informed decision for themselves.[59,158,159]

---

1   Peeters RP, Geyten SV, Wouters PJ, et al. Tissue thyroid hormone levels in critical illness. J Clin Endocrinol Metab 2005;12:6498–507.
2   Docter R, Krenning EP, de Jong M, et al. The sick euthyroid syndrome: changes in thyroid hormone serum parameters and hormone metabolism. Clin Endocrinol (Oxf) 1993;39:499–518.
3   Fliers E, Alkemade A, Wiersinga WM. The hypothalamic-pituitary-thyroid axis in critical illness. Best Practice & Research Clinical Endocrinology & Metabolism 2001;15(4):453–64.
4   Chopra IJ. Euthyroid sick syndrome: is it a misnomer? J Clin Endocrinol Metab 1997;82(2):329–34.
5   Van der Poll T, Romijn JA, Wiersinga WM, et al. Tumor necrosis factor: a putative mediator of the sick euthyroid syndrome in man. J Clin Endocrinol Metab 1990;71(6):1567–72.
6   Stouthard JM, van der Poll T, Endert E, et al. Effects of acute and chronic interleukin-6 administration on thyroid hormone metabolism in humans. J Clin Endocrinol Metab 1994;79(5):1342–6.
7   Corssmit EP, Heyligenberg R, Endert E, et al. Acute effects of interferon-alpha administration on thyroid hormone metabolism in healthy men. Clin Endocrinol Metab 1995;80(11):3140–4.
8   Nagaya T, Fujieda M, Otsuka G, et al. A potential role of activated NF-Kappa B in the pathogenesis of euthyroid sick syndrome. J Clin Invest 2000;106(3):393–402.
9   Bianco AC, Salvatore D, Gereben B, et al. Biochemistry, cellular and molecular biology, and physiological roles of the iodothyronine selenodieidinases. Endocr Rev 2002;23:38–89.
10 Chopra IJ, Huang TS, Beredo A, et al. Evidence for an inhibitor of extrathyroidal conversion of thyroxine to 3,5,3′-triiodothyronine in sera of patients with nonthyroidal illnesses. J Clin Endocrinol Metab 1985;60:666–72.
11 Peeters RP, Wouters PJ, Kaptein E, et al. Reduced activation and increased inactivation of thyroid hormone in tissues of critically ill patients. J Clin Endocrinol Metab 2003;88:3202–11.
12 Chopra IJ, Chopra U, Smith SR, et al. Reciprocal changes in serum concentrations of 3,3′,5-triiodothyronine (T3) in systemic illnesses. J Clin Endocrinol Metab 1975;41:1043–9.
13 Iervasi G, Pinitore A, Landi P, et al. Low-T3 syndrome a strong prognostic predictor of death in patients with heart disease. Circulation 2003;107(5):708–13.
14 Peeters RP, Wouters PJ, van Toor H, et al. Serum 3,3′,5′-triiodothyronine (rT3) and 3,5,3′-triiodothyronine/rT3 are prognostic markers in critically ill patients and are associated with postmortem tissue deiodinase activities. J Clin Endocrinol Metab 2005;90(8):4559–65.
15 Wartofsky L, Burman K. Alterations in thyroid function in patients with systemic illness: the "euthyroid sick syndrome." Endocr Rev 1982;3(2):164–217.
16 Hennemann G, Everts ME, de Jong M, et al. The significance of plasma membrane transport in the bioavailability of thyroid hormone. Clin Endocrinol 1998;48:1–8.
17 Vos RA, de Jong M, Bernard HF, et al. Impaired thyroxine and 3,5,3′-triodothyronine handling by rat hepatocytes in the presence of serum of patients with nonthyroidal illness. J Clin Endocrinol Metab 1995;80:2364–70.
18 Chopra IJ, Solomon DH, Hepner GW, et al. Misleadingly low free thyroxine index and usefulness of reverse triiodothyronine measurement in nonthyroidal illnesses. Ann Intern Med 1979;90(6):905–12. Usefulness of rT3 in NTI.
19 De Jong M, Docter R, Van Der Hoek HJ, et al. Transport of 3,5,3′-triiodothyronine into the perfused rat liver and subsequent metabolism are inhibited by fasting. Endocrinology 1992;131:463–70.
20 Mooradian AD, Reed RL, Osterweil D, et al. Decreased serum triiodothyronine is associated with increased concentrations of tumor necrosis factor. J Clin Endocrinol Metab 1990;71(5):1239–42.
21 Cheron RG, Kaplan MM, Larsen PR. Physiological and pharmacological influences on thyroxine to 3,5,3′-triiodothyronine conversion and nuclear 3,5,3′-triiodothyronine binding in rat anterior pituitary. J Clin Invest 1979;64:1402–14.
22 Kaplan MM, Utiger RD. Iodothyronine metabolism in rate liver homogenates. J Clin Invest 1978;61:459–71.
23 Kaplan MM. Subcellular alterations causing reduced hepatic thyroxine 5′-monodeiodinase activity in fasted rats. Endocrinology 1979;104:58–64.
24 Chopra IJ. A study of extrathyroidal conversion of thyroxine (T4) to 3,3′,5-triiodothyronine (T3) in vitro. Endocrinology 1977;101:453–463. Blocks T4 to T3 conversion.
25 Kaplan MM. Thyroxine 5′-monodeiodination in rat anterior pituitary homogenates. Endocrinology 1980;106(2):567–76.
26 Carrero JJ, Qureshi AR, Axelsson J, et al. Clinical and biochemical implications of low thyroid hormone levels (total and free forms) in euthyroid patients with chronic kidney disease. J Intern Med 2007;262:690–701.
27 Zoccali C, Tripepi G, Cutrupi S, et al. Low triiodothyronine: a new facet of inflammation in end-stage renal disease. J Am Soc Nephrol 2005;16:2789–95.
28 Zoccali C, Mallamaci F, Tripepi G, et al. Low triiodothyronine and survival in endstage renal disease. Kidney Int 2006;70:523–8.
29 Pingitore A, Landi P, Taddei MC, et al. Triiodothyronine levels for risk stratification of patients with chronic heart failure. Am J Med 2005;118(2):132–6.

30   Kozdag G, Ural D, Vural A, et al. Relation between free triiodothyronine/free thyroxine ratio, echocardiographic parameters and mortality in dilated cardiomyopathy. Eur J Heart Fail 2005;7(1):113–8.

31   Karadag F, Ozcan H, Karul AB, et al. Correlates of non-thyroidal illness syndrome in chronic obstructive pulmonary disease. Respir Med 2007;101:1439–46.

32   Kok P, Roelfsema F, Langendonk JG, et al. High circulating thyrotropin levels in obese women are reduced after body weight loss induced by caloric restriction. J Clin Endocrinol Metab 2005;90:4659–63.

33   Parr JH. The effect of long-term metabolic control on free thyroid hormone levels in diabetics during insulin treatment. Ann Clin Biochem 1987;24(5):466–9.

34   Dimopoulou I, Ilias I, Mastorakos G, et al. Effects of severity of chronic obstructive pulmonary disease on thyroid function. Metabolism 2001;50(12):1397–401.

35   Mariotti S, Barbesino G, Caturegli P, et al. Complex alterations of thyroid function in healthy centenarians. J Clin Endocrinol Metab 1993;77(5):1130–4.

36   Nomura S, Pittman CS, Chambers JB, et al. Reduced peripheral conversion of thyroxine to triiodothyronine in patients with hepatic cirrhosis. J Clin Invest 1975;56:643–8.

37   Pingitore A, Galli E, Barison A, et al. Acute effects of triiodothyronine replacement therapy in patients with chronic heart failure and low T3 syndrome: a randomized placebo-controlled study. J Clin Endocrinol Metab 2008;93:1351–8.

38   Premachandra BN, Kabir MA, Williams IK. Low T3 syndrome in psychiatric depression. J Endocrinol Invest 2006;29:568–72.

39   Jackson I. The thyroid axis and depression. Thyroid 1998;8(10):952–6.

40   Linnoila M, Lamberg BA, Potter WZ, Gold PW, Goodwin FK. High reverse T3 levels in manic and unipolar depressed women. Psychiatry Research 1982;6:271–6.

41   Kjellman BF, Ljunggren JG, Beck-Friis J, Wetterberg L. Reverse T3 levels in affective disorders. Psychiatry Research 1983;10:1–9.

42   Stipcevic T, Pivax N, Kozaric-Kovacic D, Muck-Seler D. Thyroid activity in patients with major depression. Coll Antropol 2008;32(3):973–6.

43   Gold MS, Pottash LC, Extein I. Hypothyroidism and depression. JAMA 1981;245(19):1919–22.

44   Islam S, Yesmine S, Khan SA, Alam NH, Islam S. A comparative study of thyroid hormone levels in diabetic and non-diabetic patients. SE Asian J Trop Med Public Health 2008;39(5):913–916. 50% reduction in free t3 in diabetics.

45   Carle A, Laurberg P, Pedersen IB, et al. Thyrotropin secretion decreases with age in patients with hypothyroidism. Clinical Thyroidology 2007;17:139–44.

46   Annewieke W, van den Beld AW, Visser TJ, et al. Thyroid hormone concentrations, disease, physical function and mortality in elderly men. J Clin Endocrinol Metab 2005;90(12):6403–9.

47   Van Coevorden A, Laurent E, Decoster C, et al. Decreased basal and stimulated thyrotropin secretion in healthy elderly men. J Clin Endocrinol Metab 1989;69:177–85.

48   Rubenstein HA, Butler VPJ, Werner SC. Progressive decrease in serum triiodothyronine concentrations with human aging: radioimmunoassay following extraction of serum. J Clin Endocrinol Metab 1973;37:247–53.

49   Chakraborti S, Chakraborti T, Mandal M, et al. Hypothalamic–pituitary–thyroid axis status of humans during development of ageing process. Clin Chim Acta 1999;288(1–2):137–45.

50   Piers LS, Soars MJ, McCormack LM, et al. Is there evidence for an age-related reduction in metabolic rate? J Appl Phys 1998;85:2196–204.

51   Poehlman ET, Berke EM, Joseph JR, et al. Influence of aerobic capacity, body composition, and thyroid hormones on the age-related decline in resting metabolic rate. Metabolism 1992;41:915–21.

52   Magri F, Fioravanti CM, Vignati G, et al. Thyroid function in old and very old healthy subjects. J Endocrinol Invest 2002;25(10):60–3.

53   Goichot B, Schlienger JL, Grunenberger F, et al. Thyroid hormone status and nutrient intake in the free-living elderly. Interest of reverse triiodothyronine assessment. Eur J Endocrinol 1994;130:244–52.

54   Cizza G, Brady LS, Calogero AE, et al. Central hypothyroidism is associated with advanced age in male Fischer 344/n rats: in vivo and in vitro studies. Endocrinology 1992;131:2672–80.

55   Portnay GI, O'Brien JT, Bush J, et al. The effect of starvation on the concentration and binding of thyroxine and triiodothyronine in serum and on the response to TRH. J Clin Endocrinol Metab 1974;39:191–4.

56   Croxson MS, Hall TD, Kletzky OA, et al. Decreased serum thyrotropin induced by fasting. J Clin Endocrinol Metab 1977;45:560–8.

57   Carlson HE, Drenick EJ, Chopra IJ, Hershman JM. Alterations in basal and TRH-stimulated serum levels of thyrotropin, prolactin and thyroid hormones in starved obese men. J Clin Endocrinol Metab 1977;45:707–13.

58   Vinik AI, Kalk W, McLaren JH, Paul M. Fasting blunts the TSH response to synthetic thyrotropin releasing hormone (TRH). J Clin Endocrinol Metab 1975;40:509–11.

59   Azizi F. Effect of dietary composition of fasting induced changes in serum thyroid hormones and thyrotropin. Metab Clin Exp 1978;27:935–42.

60   Brayshaw ND, Brayshaw DD. Thyroid hypofunction in premenstrual syndrome. NEJM 1986;315(23):1486–7.

61   Girdler SS, Pedersen CA, Light CK. Thyroid axis function during the menstrual cycle in women with premenstrual syndrome. Psychoneuroendocrinology 1995;20(4):395–403.

62   Neeck G, Riedel W. Thyroid function in patients with fibromyalgia syndrome. J Rheum 1992;19(7):1120–2.

63   Wikland B, Lowhagen T, Sandberg PO. Fine needle aspiration cytology of the thyroid in chronic fatigue. Lancet 2001;357:956–7.

64   Meier C, Trittibach P, Guglielmetti M, et al. Serum thyroid stimulating hormone in assessment of severity of tissue hypothyroidism in patients with overt primary thyroid failure: cross sectional survey. BMJ 2003;326(8):311–2.

65   Pittman CS, Suda AK, Chambers JB, McDaniel HG, Ray GY. Abnormalities of thyroid hormone turnover in patients with diabetes mellitus before and after insulin therapy. JCEM 1979;48(5):854–60.

66   Saunders J, Hall SHE, Sonksen PH. Thyroid hormones in insulin requiring diabetes before and after treatment. Diabetologia 1978;15:29–32.

67   Chopra IJ, Sakane S, Teco GNC. A study of the serum concentration of tumor necrosis factor in thyroidal and nonthyroidal illnesses. J Clin Endocrinol Metab 1991;72:1113–6.

68   Boelen A, Platvoet-Ter Schiphorst MC, Wiersinga WM. Association between serum interleukin-6 and serum 3,5,3'-triiodothyronine in nonthyroidal illness. J Clin Endocrinol Metab 1993;77:1695–9.

69   Hashimoto H, Igarashi N, Yachie A, et al. The relationship between serum levels of interleukin-6 and thyroid hormone in children with acute respiratory infection. J Clin Endocrinol Metab 1994;78:288–91.

[70] van der Poll T, Romijn JA, Wiersinga WM. Tumor necrosis factor: a putative mediator of the sick euthyroid syndrome in man. J Clin Endo Metab;71:1567–72.

[71] Coiro V, Passeri M, Capretti L. Serotonergic control of TSH and PRL secretion in obese men. Psychoneuroendocrinology 1990;15(4):261–8.

[72] Donders SH, Pieters GF, Heevel JG, et al. Disparity of thyrotropin (TSH) and prolactin responses to TSH-releasing hormone in obesity. JCEM 1985;61(1):56–9.

[73] Ford M, Cameron E, Ratcliffe W, et al. TSH response to TRH in substantial obesity. Int J Obes 1980;4:121–5.

[74] Roy-Byrne PP, Rubinow DR, Hoban C, et al. TSH and prolactin responses to TRH in patients with premenstrual syndrome. Am J Psychiatry 1987;144(4):480–4.

[75] Coiro V, Passeri M, Capretti L, et al. Serotonergic control of TSH and PRL secretion in obese men. Psychoneuroendocrinology 1991;15(4):261–8.

[76] Moncay H, Dapunt O, Moncayo R. Diagnostic accuracy of basal TSH determinations based on the intravenous TRH stimulation tests: an evaluation of 2570 tests and comparison with the literature. BMC Endocrine Disorders 2007;7(5):1–5.

[77] Wikland B, Lowhagen T, Sandberg PO. Fine needle aspiration cytology of the thyroid in chronic fatigue. Lancet 2001;357:956–7.

[78] Wikland B, Sanberg PO, Wallinder H. Subchemical hypothyroidism. Lancet 2003;361:1305.

[79] Fraser WD, Biggart EM, O'Reilly DJ, et al. Are biochemical tests of thyroid function of any value in monitoring patients receiving thyroxine replacement? British Medical Journal 1986;293(27):808–10.

[80] Croxson MS, Ibbertson HK. Low serum triiodothyronine (T3) and hypothyroidism. J Clin Endocrinol Metab 1977;44:167–74.

[81] Wartofsky L, Burman KD. Alterations in thyroid function in patients with systemic illness: the "euthyroid sick syndrome." Endocr Rev 1982;3:164–217.

[82] Rothwell PM, Lawler PG. Prediction of outcome in intensive care patients using endocrine parameters. Crit Care Med 1995;23:78–83.

[83] De Groot LJ. Non-thyroidal illness syndrome is a manifestation of hypothalamic-pituitary dysfunction, and in view of the current evidence, should be treated with appropriate replacement therapies. Crit Care Clin 2006;22:57–86.

[84] Schilling JU, Zimmermann T, Albrecht S, et al. Low T3 syndrome in multiple trauma patients – a phenomenon or important pathogenetic factor? Medizinische Klinik 1999;3:66–9.

[85] Girvent M, Maestro S, Hernandez R, et al. Euthyroid sick syndrome, associated endocrine abnormalities, and outcome in elderly patients undergoing emergency operation. Surgery 1998;123:560–7.

[86] Hennemann G, Krenning EP, Bernard B, et al. Regulation of influx and efflux of thyroid hormones in rat hepatocytes: possible physiologic significance of the plasma membrane in the regulation of thyroid hormone activity. Horm Metab Res Suppl 1984;14:1–6.

[87] Lam KS, Lechan RM, Minamitani N, et al. Vasoactive intestinal peptide in the anterior pituitary is increased in hypothyroidism. Endocrinology 1989;124(2):1077–84.

[88] Chopra IJ, Williams DE, Orgiazzi J, Solomon DH. Opposite effects of dexamethasone on serum concentrations of 3,3′,5′-triiodothyronine (reverse T3) and 3,3′-5-triiodothyronine (T3). JCEM 1975;41:911–920. Increased rt3 decrease t3 with steroids.

[89] Danforth EJ, Desilets EJ, Jorton ES, et al. Reciprocal serum triiodothyronine (T3) and reverse (rT3) induced by altering the carbohydrate content of the diet. Clin Res 1975;23:573. Increased reverse T3 with carbohydrate diet.

[90] Palmbald J, Levi J, Burger AG, et al. Effects of total energy withdrawal (fasting) on the levels of growth hormone, thryrotropin, cortisol, noradrenaline, T4, T3 and rT3 in healthy males. Acta Med Scand 1977;201:150.

[91] Islam S, Yesmine S, Khan SA, et al. A comparative study of thyroid hormone levels in diabetic and non-diabetic patients. SE Asian J Trop Med Public Health 2008;39(5):913–6. 50% reduction in free t3 in diabetics.

[92] De Jong F, den Heijer T, Visser TJ, et al. Thyroid hormones, dementia, and atrophy of the medical temporal lobe. J Clin Endocrinol Met 2006;91(7):2569–73. High reverse t3 with brain atrophy.

[93] Goichot B, Schlienger JL, Grunenberger F, et al. Thyroid hormone status and nutrient intake in the free-living elderly. Interest of reverse triiodothyronine assessment. Eur J Endocrinol 1994;130:244–52.

[94] Visser TJ, Lamberts WJ, Wilson JHP, Docter WR, Hennemann G. Serum thyroid hormone concentrations during prolonged reduction of dietary intake. Metabolism 1978;27(4):405–9.

[95] Wassen FW, Moerings EP, van Toor H, Hennemann G, Everts ME. Thyroid hormone uptake in cultured rat anterior pituitary cells: effects of energy status and bilirubin. J Endocrinology 2000;165:599–606. Pituitary: different transport not suppressed with decreased energy.

[96] Hennemann G, Vos RA, de Jong M, Krenning EP, Docter R. Decreased peripheral 3,5,3′-triiodothyronine (T3) production from thyroxine (T4): a syndrome of impaired thyroid hormone activation due to transport inhibition of T4- into T3-producing tissues. JCEM 1993;77(5):1431–5.

[97] De Jong M, Docter R, Bernard BF, van der Heijden JT, van Toor H. T4 uptake into the perfused rat liver and liver T4 uptake in humans are inhibited by fructose. Am J Physiol Endocrinol Metab 1994;266:E768–E775.

[98] De Jong M, Docter R, Van Der Hoek HJ, et al. Transport of 3,5,3′-triiodothyronine into the perfused rat liver and subsequent metabolism are inhibited by fasting. Endocrinology 1992;131:463–70.

[99] Hennemann G, Krenning EP. The kinetics of thyroid hormone transporters and their role in non-thyroidal illness and starvation. Best Practice & Research Clinical Endo & Metab 2007;21(2):323–38.

[100] Krenning EP, Docter R, Bernard B, Visser T, Hennemann G. Decreased transport of thyroxine (T4), 3,3′,5-triiodothyronine (T3) and 3,3′,5′-triiodothyronine (rT3) into rat hepatocytes in primary culture due to a decrease of cellular ATP content and various drugs. FEBS Lett 1982;140(2):229–33.

[101] Hennemann G, Krenning EP, Bernard B, et al. Regulation of influx and efflux of thyroid hormones in rat hepatocytes: possible physiologic significance of the plasma membrane in the regulation of thyroid hormone activity. Horm Metab Res Suppl 1984;14:1–6.

[102] Wassen FW, Moerings EP, van Toor H, Hennemann G, Everts ME. Thyroid hormone uptake in cultured rat anterior pituitary cells: effects of energy status and bilirubin. J Endocrinology 2000;165:599–606. Pituitary: different transport not suppressed with decreased energy.

[103] Lowe JC, Garrison RL, Reichman AJ, Yellin J, Thompson M, Kaufman D. Effectiveness and safety of T3 (triiodothyronine) therapy for euthyroid fibromyalgia: a double-blind placebo-controlled response-driven crossover study. Clin Bulletin Myofascial Therapy 1997;2(2/3):31–57.

[104] Lowe JC, Reichman AJ, Yellin J. The process of change during T3 treatment for euthyroid fibromyalgia: a double-blind placebo-controlled crossover study. Clin Bulletin of Myofascial Therapy 1997;2(2/3):91–124.

[105] Lowe JC, Reichman AJ, Garrison R, Yellin J. Triiodothyronine (T3) treatment of euthyroid fibromyalgia: a small-n replication of a double-blind placebo-controlled crossover study. Clin Bulletin of Myofascial Therapy 1997;2(4):71–88.

[106] Yellin BA, Reichman AJ, Lowe JC. The process of change during T3 treatment for euthyroid fibromyalgia: a double-blind placebo-controlled crossover study. Clin Bull Myofascial Ther 1996;2(2–3):91–124.

107 Wikland B, Lowhagen T, Sandberg PO. Fine needle aspiration cytology of the thyroid in chronic fatigue. Lancet 2001;357:956–7.

108 Teitelbaum JE, Bird B, Greenfield RM, Weiss A, Muenz L, Gould L. Effective treatment of chronic fatigue syndrome (CFIDS) and fibromyalgia (FMS) – a randomized, double-blind, placebo-controlled, intent to treat study. J Chronic Fatigue Syndrome 2000;8(2):3–28.

109 Gitlin M, Altshuler LL, Frye MA, et al. Peripheral thyroid hormones and response to selective serotonin reuptake inhibitors. J Psychiatry Neurosci 2004;29(5):383–6.

110 Krotkiewski M, Holm G, Shono N. Small doses of triiodothyronine can change some risk factors associated with abdominal obesity. Int J Obesity 1997;21:922–9.

111 Nierenberg AA, Fava M, Trivedi MH, Wisniewski SR. A comparison of lithium and T3 augmentation following two failed medication treatments for depression: a STAR*D report. Am J Psychiatry 2006;163:1519–30.

112 Brayshaw ND, Brayshaw DD. Thyroid hypofunction in premenstrual syndrome NEJM 1986;315(23):1486–7.

113 Abraham G, Milev R, Lawson JS. T3 augmentation of SSRI resistant depression. J Affective Disorders 2006;91:211–215.

114 Posternak M, Novak S, Stern R, et al. A pilot effectiveness study: placebo-controlled trial of adjunctive L-triiodothyronine (T3) used to accelerate and potentiate the antidepressant response. Int J Neuropsychopharmacol 2008;11:15–25.

115 Klein I, Danzi S. Thyroid hormone treatment to mend a broken heart. J Clin Endocrinol Metab 2008;93(4):1172–4.

116 Pingitore A, Galli E, Barison A, et al. Acute effects of triiodothyronine replacement therapy in patients with chronic heart failure and low-T3 syndrome: a randomized, placebo-controlled study. J Clin Endocrinol Metab 2008;93(4):1351–8.

117 Okamoto R, Leibfritz D. Adverse effects of reverse triiodothyronine on cellular metabolism as assessed by 1H and 31P NMR spectroscopy. Res Exp Med (Berl) 1997;197(4):211–7. Blocks T3 lower metabolism.

118 Tien ES, Matsui K, Moore R, Negishi M. The nuclear receptor constitutively active/androstane receptor regulates type 1 deiodinase and thyroid hormone activity in the regenerating mouse liver. J Pharmacol Exp Ther 2007;320(1):307–13. Blocks thyroid receptor and suppresses D1.

119 Benvenga S, Cahnmann HJ, Robbins J. Characterization of thyroid hormone binding to apolipoprotein-E: localization of the binding site in the exon 3-coded domain. Endocrinology 1993;133:1300–5. Reduced thyroid binding and activity.

120 Sechman A, Niezgoda J, Sobocinski R. The relationship between basal metabolic rate (BMR) and concentrations of plasma thyroid hormones in fasting cockerels. Follu Biol 1989;37(1–2):83–90. Decreased BMR with fasting and increased rT3 (decreased T4 to T3 conversion and metabolism).

121 Pittman JA, Tingley JO, Nickerson JF, Hill SR. Antimetabolic activity of 3,3′,5′-triiodo-dl-thyronine in man. Metabolism 1960;9:293–5. Reduced metabolism.

122 Steinsapir J. Type 2 iodothyronine deiodinase in rat pituitary tumor cells is inactivated in proteasomes. J Clin Invest 1998;102:11.

123 Shekelle PG, Ortiz E, Rhodes S, et al. Validity of the Agency for Healthcare Research and Quality clinical practice guidelines: how quickly do guidelines become outdated? JAMA 2001;286(12):1461–7.

124 Demers LM, Spencer CA. NACB: Laboratory support for the diagnosis and monitoring of thyroid disease–thyrotropin/thyroid stimulating hormone (TSH). Academy of the American Association for Clinical Chemistry, Washington, DC; 2003.

125 Peeters RP, Wouters PJ, van Toor H, Kaptein E, Visser TJ, Van den Berghe G. Serum 3,3′,5′-triiodothyronine (rT3) and 3,5,3′-triiodothyronine/rT3 are prognostic markers in critically ill patients and are associated with postmortem tissue deiodinase activities. J Clin Endocrinol Metab 2005;90(8):4559–65.

126 Mitchell AM, Manley SW, Rowan KA, Mortimer RH. Uptake of reverse T3 in the human choriocarcinoma cell line, J Ar. Placenta 1999;20:65–70. Inhibits uptake of T3 and T4 into the cell.

127 Lecomte P, Lecureuil N, Lecureuil M, Salazar CO, Valat C. Age modulates effects of thyroid dysfunction on sex hormone binding globulin (SHBG) levels. Exp Clin Endocrinol 1995;103:339–42.

128 Zulewski H, Muller B, Exer P, Miserez AR Staub JJ. Estimation of tissue hypothyroid by a new clinical score: evaluation of patients with various grades of hypothyroidism and controls. JCEM 1997;82:771–6.

129 Amerling R, Winchester JF, Ronco C. Guidelines have done more harm than good. Blood Purification 2008;26:73–6.

130 Guirguis-Blake J, Calonge N, Miller T, et al. Current processes of the U.S. Preventive Services Task Force: refining evidence-based recommendation development. Ann Intern Med 2007;147(2):117–22.

131 Barton MB, Miller T, Wolff T, et al. How to read the new recommendation statement: methods update from the U.S. Preventive Services Task Force. Ann Intern Med 2007;147(2):123–7.

132 Oxford Centre for Evidence-based Medicine (EBM) > EBM Tools > Finding the Evidence > Levels of Evidence. http://www.cebm.net/index.aspx?o=5653.

133 Atkins D, Best D, Briss PA, et al. Grading quality of evidence and strength of recommendations. BMJ 2004;328(7454):1490.

134 Tricoci P, Allen JM, Kramer KM, et al. Scientific evidence underlying the ACC/AHA clinical practice guidelines. JAMA 2009;301(8):831–41.

135 Shaneyfelt TM, Centor RM. Reassessment of clinical practice guidelines: go gently into that good night. JAMA 2009;301:868–9.

136 Tricoci P, Allen JM, Kramer JM, et al. Scientific evidence underlying the ACC/AHA clinical practice guidelines. JAMA 2009;301(8):831–841.

137 Shekelle PG, Ortiz E, Rhodes S, et al. Validity of the Agency for Healthcare Research and Quality clinical practice guidelines: how quickly do guidelines become outdated? JAMA 2001;286(12):1461–7.

138 Burgers JS, Grol R, Klazinga NS, et al. AGREE Collaboration. Towards evidence-based clinical practice: an international survey of 18 clinical guideline programs. Int J Qual Health Care 2003;15(1):31–45.

139 Sackett DL, Rosenberg WM, Gray JA, et al. Evidence based medicine: what it is and what it isn't. BMJ 1996;312(7023):71–2.

140 Zoler ML. Half of cardiac guidelines are not evidence based: expert opinion under scrutiny. Internal Medicine News 2009;42(7):1, 8.

141 Lenfant C. Clinical research to clinical practice: lost in translation. NEJM 2003;349:868–74.

142 Alzheimer's Research and Prevention Foundation. Tuscon AZ, Shankle W. International conference on the integrative medical approach to the prevention of Alzheimer's disease. October 11, 2003.

143 Pizzo P. Letter from the Dean. Stanford Medical Magazine. Stanford: Stanford University School of Medicine; Fall 2002.

144 Begley S. "Too Many Patients Never Reap the Benefits of Great Research". Wall Street Journal, September 26, 2003.

145 "Science Know Best," Daily Policy Digest. National Center for Policy Analysis, September 26, 2003.

146 Choudhry NK, Fletcher RH, Soumerai SB, et al. Systematic review: the relationship between clinical experience and quality of health care. Ann Intern Med 2005;142(4):260–73.

147 Balas EA. Information systems can prevent errors and improve quality. J Am Med Inform Assoc 2001;8(4):398–9.

148 National Institute of Medicine Report, 2003b.

149 Bill Number: AB 592 amended bill text; amended in assembly April 4, 2005, Introduced by Assembly Member Yee FEBRUARY 17, 2005. An act to amend Section 2234.1 of the Business and Professions Code, relating to healing arts.

[150] The Principals of Medical Ethics adopted by the American Medical Association in 1980.

[151] Asch SM, Kerr EA, Keesey J, et al. Who is at greater risk for receiving poor-quality health care. NEJM 2006;354:1147–55.

[152] Johnson L, Stricker RB. The Infectious Disease Society of America Lyme guidelines: a cautionary tale about the development of clinical practice guidelines. Phil, Ethics, and Humanities in Med 2010;5:9.

[153] Kissam P. Antitrust boycott doctrine. Iowa Law Rev 1984;69:1165.

[154] McAlister FA, van Diepen S, Padwal RS, et al. How evidence-based are the recommendations in evidence-based guidelines? PLoS Med 2007;4:e250.

[155] Sniderman AD, Furberg CD. Why guideline-making requires reform. JAMA 2009;301(4):429–31.

[156] Lin KW. Identifying and using good practice guidelines. Am Fam Physician 2009;80(1):67–9.

[157] Toriello HV, Goldenberg P. Evidence-based medicine and practice guidelines: application to genetics. Am J Med Genetic 2009;151C:235–240.

[158] May T. Bioethics in a liberal society: the political framework of bioethics decision making Baltimore and London. Baltimore, Maryland. The Johns Hopkins University Press; 2002.

[159] American Medical Association Council on Ethical and Judicial Affairs. Decisions near the end of life. JAMA 1992;267:2229–33.

5

Wilson's Temperature Syndrome

Many people who are not taking thyroid medicine suffer from debilitating symptoms consistent with low thyroid function. Sometimes, their doctors don't think to check their thyroid blood tests. However, even when the doctors do check, the thyroid blood tests often come back normal. Nevertheless, many of these patients have low body temperatures and symptoms that respond very well when their body temperatures are normalized with triiodothyronine (T3) therapy. Furthermore, their symptoms and temperature often remain improved even after the treatment has been discontinued (usually after a few months of treatment). This "resetting phenomenon" is not seen with thyroxine (T4)-containing medicines. I began making these observations in my patients in 1988. Over time I used T3 to treat over 5,000 patients who had low body temperatures and normal thyroid-stimulating hormone (TSH) tests. Based on my observations I defined Wilson's Temperature Syndrome (WTS, Wilson's Syndrome) as low body temperatures and low thyroid symptoms in patients with normal TSH that is often completely reversible upon normalization of body temperatures with T3 and/or herbal and nutritional support. The symptoms often come on or worsen together under periods of severe physical or mental stress, persisting even after the stress has passed. Treatment of WTS usually involves a few months and WTS often remains improved even after treatment has been discontinued.

In addition, many people who are taking T4-containing medicine and who have normal thyroid blood tests also have low body temperatures and suffer from debilitating symptoms consistent with low thyroid function. Many of these peoples' symptoms will respond very well when they are weaned off their T4-containing medicine and treated with T3 for a time in order to normalize their body temperatures. If they do need to stay on thyroid medicine and prefer going back to a T4-containing medicine, they are often able to maintain their normal temperatures on lower dosages of T4-containing medicine than they were taking before the T3 therapy.

> In my experience, about 80% of WTS patients are women.
> – Denis Wilson, MD

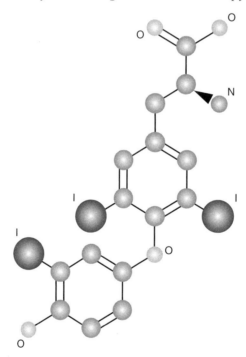

T3 molecule

Pathophysiology

The pathophysiology of the reversible hypometabolism of WTS is not fully understood and may be multi-factorial (see Chapter 1). However, a reversible endocrine dysfunction is not without precedent. For decades gynecologists have been using birth control pills to regulate irregular menstrual cycles. The diagnosis for irregular bleeding is a diagnosis of exclusion made entirely on history and ruling out other causes. Patients are often given a therapeutic trial of birth control pills even though their female hormone blood tests are normal. The cyclic oral contraceptives can re-establish a normal monthly cycle and the pills can often be discontinued after a few months with the patients able to maintain normal cycles on their own again. WTS exemplifies this same paradigm applied to the thyroid system.

The abundance of research presented in Chapter 1 and in this chapter shows that the TSH test is not a reliable indicator of thyroid status in the cells of the body. This means that not everyone experiencing low thyroid states will have an abnormal TSH. Then, it's even possible that MOST people experiencing low thyroid states will have normal TSH. In my experience, more than 90% of people that respond well to normalizing their body temperatures with T3 therapy have normal TSH. By focusing so much on the TSH in our medical system over the last few decades, we have been missing the forest for trees.

As we reviewed in Chapter 1, there are many processes involved in healthy thyroid hormone expression. The hypothalamus stimulates the pituitary gland, which stimulates the thyroid gland to make T4. T4 must be transported into the cells and then converted to T3. T3 must attach to the nuclear thyroid receptors to make complexes,

> *Most of the active thyroid hormone T3 (at least 80%) is produced outside the thyroid gland.[1]*

which directly interact with the DNA and affect transcription of DNA, resulting in RNA and then proteins. We know there are factors and signals that can affect thyroid hormone transport into the cell, T4 to T3 conversion, and the function of the thyroid receptors. Problems in any of these areas might be addressed better with T3 than with T4. It is apparent that normalizing body temperatures with T3 therapy somehow resets the body so that it can maintain normal temperatures on its own, although the exact mechanism is unknown. T4 to T3 conversion is inhibited by stress, fasting, illness, cortisol, and many other factors. Interestingly, excess T4 and reverse T3 (rT3) may down-regulate the thyroid system by increasing the destruction of the deiodinating enzyme by proteasomes.[2,3] It may be that T3 clears thyroid hormone pathways of TSH, T4, and rT3 such that the thyroid system is refreshed or rebooted so that it can maintain proper function on its own again once the T3 therapy is discontinued. Some patients benefit from, and tolerate well, being on T3 therapy on an ongoing basis.

Signs and Symptoms

The symptoms of WTS are those that have been seen to improve with normalization of body temperature (raised to 98.6°F orally, especially through the use of T3) and remain improved even after the treatment has been discontinued. The symptoms correlate very closely with the temperature so it is helpful to measure the temperatures when patients are experiencing the symptoms that are bothering them. For these purposes, oral temperature readings with glass/liquid metal thermometers are quick, accurate, and often more convenient than axillary or rectal temperatures. The symptoms of WTS are identical to the symptoms of

> *Patients and I have seen a strong correlation between body temperature and low thyroid symptoms. I wouldn't expect people with low temperatures to feel better until their temperatures improve.*

hypothyroidism,[4–6] but can also include some symptoms not typically associated with hypothyroidism (such as asthma, hives, and migraines). Sufferers may experience many, few, or even a single symptom (see Table 4.1). In addition to a low body temperature (<98.6°F), very typical symptoms of WTS include persistent or relapsing fatigue, anxiety, depression, headaches, insomnia, and muscle aches. Other common symptoms of WTS include cognitive dysfunction, dry skin, carpal tunnel syndrome, hair loss, an overall lack of well-being, and many others. A presumptive diagnosis of WTS requires the sign of low body temperature accompanied by at least one symptom associated with WTS. WTS is a diagnosis of exclusion that is entertained after other possible explanations have been ruled out (such as iron deficiency anemia, kidney disease, liver disease). Low body temperature is the most accurate biological indicator of WTS, consistently predicting its presence and progression.

One reason why body temperature is a good guide to thyroid hormone treatment is because the range of normal for body temperatures (in relation to randomness) varies far less statistically than do those of thyroid hormone blood tests. Therefore, it is easy to see how mildly depressed temperatures (1–1.5 degrees below 98.6°F) can have a significant downstream effect. If I had to guess which physical attribute was the most similar among all people, I would guess body temperature. No matter what age, height, weight, race, or gender, body temperatures are all quite similar (because body function depends on it).

Table 5.1 Signs and Symptoms of WTS

Average oral temperature <98.6°F	Depression	Dry hair
Fatigue	Decreased memory	Insomnia
Headaches	Decreased concentration	Falling asleep during the day
Migraines	Decreased sex drive	Arthritis and joint aches
Premenstrual syndrome (PMS)	Unhealthy nails	Allergies
Irritability	Low motivation	Asthma
Fluid retention	Constipation	Muscular aches
Anxiety	Irritable bowel syndrome	Itchiness
Panic attacks	Inappropriate weight gain	Elevated cholesterol
Hair loss	Dry skin	Stomach ulcers
Increased nicotine, caffeine use	Frequent urinary infections	Raynaud's phenomenon
Abnormal throat sensations	Lightheadedness	Poor coordination
Sweating abnormalities	Ringing in the ears	Inhibited sexual development
Heat and/or cold intolerance	Slow wound healing	Infertility
Low self esteem	Easy bruising	Hypoglycemia
Irregular periods	Acid indigestion	Increased skin infections/acne
Severe menstrual cramps	Flushing of the skin	Abnormal swallowing sensation
Low blood pressure	Frequent yeast infections	Prematurely gray hair
Frequent colds and sore throats	Cold hands/feet	Carpal tunnel syndrome
Excessive fatigue after eating	Dry eyes/blurred vision	Hives
Halitosis		

from pg. 102

It is clear there is a continuum of body function along the temperature gradient between the two extremes. For people with severely low temperatures, the warmer they get the better they feel, up to a point. For those with severely high body temperature, the cooler the better, up to a point. High fevers (107°F) can cause denaturing of the enzymes, brain damage, and even death. Severe hypothermia (<90°F) can also be a life-threatening medical emergency. A mild fever of 100°F can produce familiar symptoms of fever. It is easy to see how mildly depressed temperatures (1–1.5 degrees below 98.6°F) can also produce a very characteristic set of symptoms. This data shows that the proper functioning of the body vitally depends on it being at the right body temperature.

In the 1800s, the average temperature of 25,000 people was reported to be 98.6°F. In 1992, the average temperature of 148 people was reported to be 98.2°F. Perhaps the measurement technology has changed, or perhaps temperatures really are lower now. Interestingly, rather than thoroughly investigating this possible trend, some in mainstream medicine have suggested that we simply change our definition of normal.[7]

Typically, the symptoms of WTS come on together after some major physical or emotional stress [e.g., childbirth (#1 cause), abuse, divorce, death of a loved one, job or family stress, medical treatment (medication or surgery), accidents, excessive dieting, etc.]. It is not uncommon for WTS symptoms to persist even after the stressful event has passed.

Diagnosis

WTS is a diagnosis of exclusion and is best confirmed by a therapeutic trial of normalization of body temperatures with Wilson's T3 (WT3) therapy or herbal and nutritional support. WT3 therapy is the T3 therapy described in this chapter. As opposed to other methods of using T3, it is usually aimed at resetting the thyroid system so that patients can remain improved after the treatment has been discontinued. Patients with normal TSH, high T3, and low rT3 levels may still respond well to normalization of low body temperatures with T3. Therefore, thyroid blood tests such as those indicating T3 deficiency or rT3 excess need not exclude patients from a therapeutic trial of T3 when indicated. Even hypothyroid patients who are supposedly well-managed on T4-containing medicines can develop WTS and may benefit from a trial of T3 therapy.

A history, physical exam, and laboratory tests can help identify other possible causes of fatigue including: anemia, chronic infections, blood sugar abnormalities, lifestyle factors, side effects of prescription drugs, toxicity, other endocrine disorders. If no more likely explanation can be identified for the patient's symptoms, a trial of WT3 therapy can be considered. WT3 therapy can also be a useful adjunct in the treatment of certain chronic illnesses such as Lyme disease and diabetes.

Workup

Part of the workup for WTS includes having the patient record body temperature patterns in a temperature log to document that they do in fact run below normal (on average). Evaluation of the numerous possible symptoms can often be facilitated through the use of a symptoms checklist the patient may fill out (see symptom checklist on **p168**). Once the patient has completed the symptom checklist, a thorough past medical history should be conducted in order to put the symptoms and chief complaint in the proper context. The past medical history should include questions about past acute and chronic illnesses, present illnesses, surgeries, accidents, and especially the maternity history. Because childbirth is the number one cause of WTS in women, it is important to take a careful history regarding miscarriages, abortions, ectopic pregnancies, infertility, and full-term pregnancies.

> *It is helpful to determine which complaint is bothering the patient most of all. I will frequently ask, "I know all these symptoms can be related, but if we could fix just one thing, what would it be? Which of them is bothering you the most?" It is sometimes difficult for patients to narrow it down to just one, but they can almost always narrow it down to two or perhaps three symptoms.*

It is important to evaluate the patient's current medications to see if any are no longer necessary, and to consider possible interactions (drug–drug or drug–disease or drug–nutrient). A complete family history should also be documented, and should cover stroke and cardiac problems, especially myocardial infarction, cardiac bypass operations, and at what ages these events transpired in the lives of family members. The thorough family history should investigate any possible familial link to thyroid disease.

All potential WTS patients should be asked the following 5 questions:

1. Did the symptoms seem to come on all at once, or gradually?
2. Since the onset of symptoms, has symptom intensity stayed the same, or has it worsened in stages (possibly precipitated by successive stresses)?
3. How long have the symptoms been present?
4. What is the patient's nationality?
5. What impact has past treatment (if any) had on symptoms?

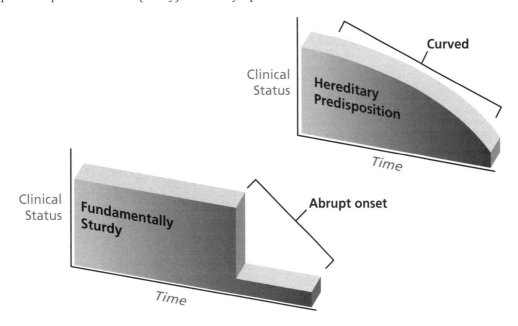

Patients who report an abrupt onset of symptoms tend to have a "sturdy" metabolism that is normally able to resist the development of WTS, until a precipitating event sends them over the edge.

WTS symptoms that suddenly appear early in life may have been brought on by a traumatic experience such as abuse, or the patient may have a profound predisposition.

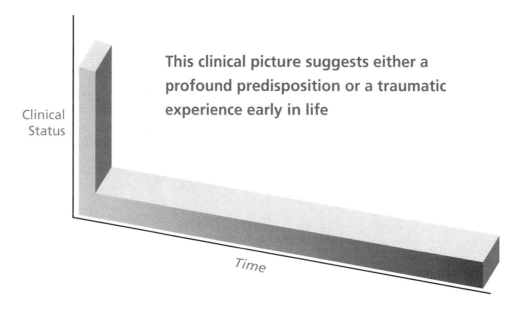

This clinical picture suggests either a profound predisposition or a traumatic experience early in life

Clinical Status

Time

In general, patients who report sudden symptoms require a much less complex management strategy with lower doses and less treatment cycles. They are also less likely to relapse after treatment has been discontinued.

A more gradual onset of WTS symptoms is an indication that the person may have a hereditary predisposition to developing WTS. Nationalities whose ancestors survived famine seem more prone to developing WTS, especially Irish and American Indian (but also Scottish, Welsh, Russian, and Polish). These patients frequently have reddish highlights in their hair, and a fair complexion with some freckles. When patients come in with such a gradual presentation that starts manifesting later in life, I sometimes say, "Wow, you must take good care of yourself." And they say, "Yes! That's what I've been trying to tell doctors, I eat right and sleep and exercise and I still feel bad!".

This picture suggests hereditary predisposition with symptom onset forestalled by good health habits

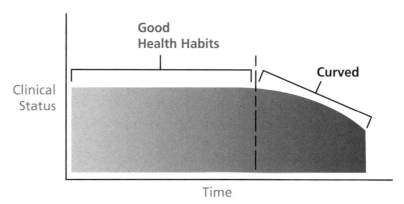

Good Health Habits

Curved

Clinical Status

Time

Patients with a more gradual onset of symptoms, or those who have had symptoms for a longer period of time (>6 months) often require more management (i.e., more T3 cycles, and higher doses) in order to correct the problem. On the other hand, patients who have only had WTS symptoms for 6 months or less can frequently be corrected with one cycle (3–6 weeks) on relatively low doses of medicine. For this reason, even mild presentations of WTS should be "nipped in the bud" rather than allowing them to become worse and more difficult to manage. When the symptoms have gotten worse in stages especially after successive stresses, generally, the more stages the longer it will take to correct the problem. For example, a person whose symptoms got worse in one stage may need only one cycle of WT3 therapy, while a person whose symptoms got worse in three stages may need three cycles of WT3 therapy. If a person's symptoms have improved with thyroid treatment in the past that's a good sign, but if the symptoms have worsened with thyroid treatment then the problem may take longer to correct. WTS symptoms can often get worse with cortisone shots, dieting, and stress.

Physical Exam

The physical exam should look for signs of thyroid system dysfunction:

- Thyroid gland – The thyroid gland should be examined for any nodules, goiter, or tenderness.
- Skin – The patient's skin may appear to be more dry, coarse, and wrinkled than might otherwise be expected.
- Fluid retention – The patient may present with subtle facial puffiness (i.e., "fuller facial features"), especially around the eyes. If more severe, patients may look like they just woke up because of the mild puffiness around the eyes.
- Nails – The patient may have artificial nails or peeling, splitting nails that break easily or that are soft.
- Hair – The patient's hair may appear dry and thin, such that you can see down to the scalp. May have thinning of the lateral 1/3 of the eyebrows.

Tests

from pgs. 142, 156
Body temperatures should be taken by mouth every 3 hours, 3 times a day, starting 3 hours after waking, and averaged for several days (not the 3 days prior to the menstrual period in women because it is higher then). Because the body temperature is normally lower upon rising, it seems that the temperature averaging low during the day when the temperature is supposed to be at its highest would be a more specific indication of a potential problem. Persons with WTS usually have a normal diurnal variation in their body temperature patterns, but these patterns are shifted down usually about a degree.

Laboratory tests can include complete blood count (CBC), multi-chemistry panel, T4, TSH, total T3 [radio immuno-assay (RIA)], total rT3 (RIA), antinuclear antibodies (ANA), and baseline electrocardiogram (EKG). The TSH test is done to rule out glandular hypothyroidism. Multi-chemistry and CBC help rule out other possible explanations for the patient's symptoms as well as conditions that can be exacerbated by thyroid treatment (e.g., cardiac arrhythmias and Addison's disease). Total T3 and total rT3 tests are not always diagnostic because some patients with high T3 levels and/or low rT3 levels can still respond very well to treatment, neither are they very useful in directing management. However, T3/rT3 ratios can provide interesting documentation. Because low progesterone and testosterone levels can also be a cause of low temperatures, these parameters can also be assessed.

Most people tolerate T3 therapy very well with no cardiac manifestations. WT3 normally involves using T3 that is compounded with a sustained-release (SR) agent **(p108)** with the aim of the T3 being slowly released over a 12-hour period. In my experience, it is important that such T3 be taken very much on time (not even 3 minutes late) every 12 hours. Sometimes, especially if the medicine is not taken properly on time, or if the T3 level becomes unsteady for some other reason, patients can notice an increased awareness of the heart beat/palpitations, and/or increased pulse rate.

The patients that are most likely to notice these manifestations with unsteady T3 levels, are those who already noticed heart flutters, PVC's, or the like, before ever starting T3 therapy. If the unfavorable conditions progress, a person could develop an arrhythmia, most commonly atrial fibrillation. In atrial fibrillation, the p-wave on the EKG of the atrial contraction is lost due to the disorganized electrical activity of the atria. Without the regular contraction of the atria and the regular conduction of the electrical impulses to the ventricles, the ventricles contract in an irregular pattern. Furthermore, the time between QRS complexes on the EKG is unpredictably different from contraction to contraction. This is referred to as the rhythm being irregularly irregular.

from pg. 161
In such cases, the baseline EKG might appear to be normal sinus rhythm at first glance, but with careful scrutiny with a pair of calipers, vestiges of irregular irregularities might be detected. It is good to review the baseline EKG carefully for such abnormalities, because their discovery allows one to advise a prospective candidate for T3 therapy that they may be more likely to develop such manifestations.

Such findings on the presenting EKG are not an absolute contraindication to T3 therapy, but serve to let one know what to watch out for. These types of manifestations can be avoided by watching carefully for any such signs, and then adjusting the treatment at the first sign of such problems to see to it that they resolve (this can include weaning completely off the T3 therapy).

Special care should be taken in elderly patients. And there are many patients who would not be good candidates for T3 therapy at all, because of their cardiac or cerebrovascular risk.

If TSH and T4 production appear to be within the normal range (in the presence of clinical symptoms), then a therapeutic trial of T3 therapy should be considered instead of a T4-containing medicine. T3 uptake, T3 RIA, and rT3 RIA levels are not helpful in predicting who will and will not respond well to T3 therapy. However, they can be useful as baseline and serial testing (tracking an individual's progress over time).

Why is WTS Overlooked?

Faulty assumptions (and sometimes even faulty education) have played a major role in this condition being overlooked by mainstream medicine for so long. One reason why this condition was not recognized in the past is because doctors did not have an easy way to identify and treat it. For example, many doctors assumed that because traditional thyroid medication dosing was not very effective for patients with normal TSH tests, the symptoms couldn't be remedied with thyroid medication. However, this is like looking through the wrong end of a pair of binoculars and concluding: "These are not useful for seeing long distances." Using the right thyroid medicine in the right way can be a game changer for many patients.

Another reason why WTS is often overlooked (or deemed insignificant) is because its symptoms are numerous and non-specific. However, the symptoms of WTS are no more varied, numerous, vague, or non-specific than those of hypothyroidism (because they are the same). Yet, no one would suggest that the symptoms of hypothyroidism are insignificant. Unfortunately, many doctors are not aware of WTS, and so they have difficulty thinking of anything that might be causing these symptoms. This leads to two common pitfalls: (1) the doctor attempts to treat each and every symptom individually, thus over-medicating the patient, or (2) the doctor assumes that the symptoms are psychosomatic, and thus refers the patient for psychological assessment.

> Just because a patient reports a large number of non-specific and varied complaints, does not mean that they are unlikely to have a significant clinical problem. Unfortunately, many doctors tend to overlook these "vague" symptoms, and instead preoccupy themselves with the problems that only show up on thyroid blood tests.

Finally, some doctors might overlook WTS because its diagnosis is based on clinical presentation rather than on "definitive" blood tests. However, it has been said that as much as 80% of medical diagnoses are made based on clinical parameters. Take antidepressants, for example; they are the most widely prescribed medicines in the United States, and yet they are prescribed and managed solely on a clinical basis. So when it comes to the thyroid, how did doctors ever get so preoccupied with the blood tests in the first place?

One explanation is that doctors have been concentrating only on the problems affecting the glandular portion of the thyroid system that they were able to correct using blood tests as a guide, but when the tests were normal, they (not surprisingly) were not able to improve low thyroid system symptoms reproducibly with conventional treatment strategies. Without the principles of management recently developed for WTS, or body temperature as a guide, they had virtually no way of effectively treating patients with low body temperatures and normal thyroid blood tests. Most doctors gave up on the possibility that some people with normal tests might greatly benefit from thyroid treatment, and thus mainstream medicine collectively turned a blind eye to the problem.

Conventional (Symptomatic) Treatments Commonly Given to WTS Sufferers

It is common for patients being treated with five or six different medications for five or six different symptoms to respond better to the single treatment of normalizing their body temperatures with the WT3 protocol. The other treatments can often be discontinued. Moreover, the symptoms often remain at bay even after the WT3 protocol has been weaned. Correcting the underlying problem rather than just treating the symptoms can make all the difference in a person's life.

The following list represents *just some* of the many treatments that are commonly prescribed in an effort to address symptoms that often respond completely to treatment for WTS.

- Allergy shots, antihistamines, and decongestants
- Antacids, histamine blockers
- Anti-dizziness medicines
- Anti-inflammatory medicines
- Antibiotics
- Antidepressants
- Appetite suppressants, liquid diets, gastric bypass
- Artificial nails, wigs/repeat perms
- Asthma medicines
- Birth control pills
- Carpal tunnel syndrome surgery
- Cholesterol lowering drugs
- Cortisone
- Diuretics
- Evaluation for ringing in the ears
- Fertility drugs
- Hypoglycemic diets
- Laxatives, antispasmodics, hemorrhoid preparations
- Marriage and family counseling
- Migraine and headache medicines
- Orthopedic and chiropractic therapies
- Progesterone and female hormones
- Sleeping pills
- Surgical revision
- Thyroid hormone medicines (T4 preparations and T4/T3 preparations)
- Tranquilizers and antianxiety medications
- Vitamins

The best way to tell if a given medication is being used symptomatically is if the symptom(s) being treated return shortly after discontinuation. Happily, many people who are struggling on these side effect-prone drugs often fare much better on proper thyroid hormone therapy (i.e., the WT3 protocol). One reassuring sign that the WT3 protocol is physiologic and not pharmacologic is that symptoms often remain improved after the treatment is weaned.

Recommended Treatment and Support for WTS

Because body temperature dictates the shape and function of the body's enzymes, a decrease in body temperature will undoubtedly reflect the body's metabolism. I have seen such a strong correlation between body temperature and low thyroid symptoms in my patients that I am satisfied that the low temperature (key sign of WTS) is actually the cause of low thyroid symptoms. I don't believe it is possible for a person to have thyroid-hormone-responsive symptoms (even from primary hypothyroidism) without having a low body temperature. The overarching goal of treatment for WTS is to raise the body temperature back to normal again. The body is designed to maintain normal body temperatures on its own, and with proper herbal and nutritional support it often can. However, sometimes thyroid hormone replacement therapy is necessary. Some people do well with herbal and nutritional and lifestyle support alone, some do well with T3 alone, some do well with both.

Sustained-Release Triiodothyronine (SR-T3)

In 1988, I began considering the use of T3 in patients with low body temperatures and normal thyroid blood tests. At that time, there was little to no emphasis in the medical literature or lay media about the importance of T3 and the peripheral cellular factors affecting actual thyroid hormone activity in the tissues, such as the peripheral conversion of T4 to T3. By 1990, I had refined the WT3 protocol for the treatment of a condition I identified as Wilson's Syndrome (now Wilson's Temperature Syndrome). Unlike hypothyroidism, this condition can often be completely reversed (with the patient remaining improved off treatment) in a matter of weeks, or months. I was the first doctor to use sustained-release T3 and I remember the day when we all gathered around and watched my receptionist swallow the first capsule of it. A few hours later she reported that she thought she was feeling a little better. The term WT3 protocol is used to identify the principles and methods for using T3 presented in this book as opposed to the way others use T3. T3 is like a paintbrush in that the results people get definitely depend on how it's used.

In 1991, I wrote the first version of this textbook you're now reading and then began speaking about WTS at medical conventions. Many physicians felt the approach made complete sense and explained a lot of what they were seeing in their patients. The WT3 protocol has gained widespread use among complementary and alternative medicine practitioners. WTS is taught in every naturopathic medical school; however, since 1995 the American Thyroid Association has said there is no evidence in the literature to support it or the use of T3 in patients that have normal TSH tests.

The considerations supporting WTS and the WT3 protocol have stood the test of time. As you can see from the abundant medical research presented in this manual the critical importance of what happens to T4 after it is delivered to the cells is becoming accepted as self-evident. Many current discussions on the thyroid system, whether in the medical literature or in the lay media, now acknowledge the importance of factors such as the peripheral conversion of T4 into the active thyroid hormone T3, thyroid hormone transport, and/or the function of the thyroid hormone receptors. Many are recognizing that signs and symptoms are more reliable than thyroid blood tests as indicators of thyroid hormone activity in the tissues. Just as estrogen and progesterone are prescribed to regulate menstrual cycles in patients who have normal serum hormone levels, the WT3 therapy can be used to regulate metabolism despite normal serum thyroid hormone levels.

The WT3 protocol involves the use of SR-T3 taken orally by the patient every 12 hours according to a cyclic dose schedule determined by patient response. The patient can often be weaned once he/she has maintained a body temperature of 98.6°F for about 3 weeks. However, some patients enjoy staying on T3 for months to years.

SR-T3 can be prescribed based on low thyroid symptoms and low body temperature in the presence of normal thyroid blood tests. Some hallmark symptoms of WTS include fatigue, anxiety, depression, headaches, insomnia, and muscle aches. Some people with low temperatures don't suffer from the symptoms of WTS, but for the ones that do their body temperature *is* a reliable biomarker for WTS, and can be used to consistently predict changes during the progression from illness to health.

Iodine

Iodine is an integral component of thyroid hormones and is essential to thyroid function. Iodine is critically important to the development of the fetus and newborn, and iodine deficiency is the leading cause of preventable mental retardation in the world. In 2008, at least 8.8% of the US population was severely iodine deficient.[8] Sadly, the incidence was even higher in pregnant women. While iodine deficiency in pregnancy and nursing can result in cretinism, congenital heart disease, reproductive problems, and a myriad of birth defects, there have been a few reports of high TSH and low T4 (though T3 levels weren't mentioned) in babies born to and nursing from mothers consuming excess iodine during pregnancy and nursing.[9] Maternal consumption of over 2–3 g iodine/day is associated with severe thyroid suppression.[10] Therefore, the current recommendation for pregnant women is 300 µg/day.[11]

Some people that are iodine deficient experience hypothyroidism and goiter while others develop autonomously functioning follicular cells, toxic nodular goiter, and hyperthyroidism.[12] Besides seaweed, rich sources of iodine are animal products such as milk (though only when iodine is used as a disinfectant on the udders), fish, and eggs. The iodine content of cow's milk can be increased by adding seaweed to the bovine diet.[13] Of note, strict vegan practitioners are at particular risk for iodine deficiency because of limited dietary sources.[14]

Some practitioners have reported anecdotally that high-dose iodine (6–48 mg/day as potassium iodide) greatly improves the body temperatures and low thyroid symptoms in a majority of their patients with normal thyroid blood tests. In addition, iodine supplementation is reported to help some people feel better on the T4-containing medicine they are taking and may help them reduce the dose. Some practitioners report that their need to prescribe thyroid medicine in general has dropped significantly (by about a third or more) when they began using high-dose iodine supplementation. Some practitioners report that autoimmune antibodies frequently improve significantly with high-dose iodine and sometimes go away completely. Unfortunately, no double-blind studies have yet been done to confirm these findings. Probably less than 10% of the general population responds adversely to excess iodine.[15] For example, a randomized double-blind placebo-controlled multi-center trial with 111 euthyroid patients showed no adverse effects in a group that took 6 mg of iodine/day for 6 months.[16]

One benefit of iodine is that it displaces other halides such as bromine and chlorine so that they can be excreted from the body. Bromine and chlorine can impair proper thyroid function. Moreover, some proponents of high-dose iodine feel that iodination of certain lipids and proteins can be very beneficial to thyroid function and require iodine levels 100 times higher (15 mg/day) than the RDA (150 mcg/day). Iodine has been well documented to help in fibrocystic breast disease. In one study, 70% of a group of fibrocystic breast disease patients responded well to iodine.[17]

Iodine can cause TSH levels to increase and T4 levels to decrease while at the same time T3 can increase. If patients are feeling very well on iodine and their T3 levels are not dropping, then they should not be considered hypothyroid even though TSH levels are increased and T4 levels are decreased. These changes in TSH are transient and usually resolve within 6–9 months. Even though less than 10% of people respond adversely to excess iodine, a small percentage of people can become and feel either hypothyroid or hyperthyroid even on doses less than 1 mg/day (including palpitations, high pulse rates, and general discomfort). Some people that are iodine deficient develop autonomously functioning thyroid cells and when they are supplemented with iodine can develop hyperthyroidism (especially the elderly, or those who are rapidly replaced). Iodine supplementation can lead to thyroid storm in patients with hot nodules.[18]

In all of this, it should be remembered that selenium and iodine work synergistically because selenium is at the heart of glutathione peroxidase (GPX) and the non-pituitary deiodinases. GPX prevents oxidative damage of the follicular cells by holding down the level of hydrogen peroxide.

It has been repeatedly documented that the incidence of thyroid autoimmunity can increase following salt iodination programs to eradicate iodine deficiency in populations.[19] However, although increasing doses of iodine have been shown to increase thyroid autoimmunity in mice, high dose iodine plus selenium has been shown to reduce it.[20,21] In addition, selenium supplementation has been shown to significantly reduce anti-thyroid antibodies.[22] Supplementing with iodine alone is very different than supplementing with iodine and selenium. Moreover, bioactive compounds in seaweed may be very helpful in thyroid-related disorders such as Hashimoto's thyroiditis.[23]

Although the incidence of thyroid autoimmunity has increased following iodination programs in iodine-deficient populations, it is not entirely clear how much of the increase in autoimmunity is due to iodine and how much might be due to increased goitrogens in the environment (toxins like perchlorate). The incidence of all forms of autoimmune disease has increased over the last 40 years. The incidence of autoimmune thyroid disease (ATD) is higher now in the United States than it was 40 years ago even though iodine levels in the population are lower now. However, one study showed an increase in antithyroid antibodies in some patients with ATD given low-dose iodine supplementation for about 4 months as compared to a control group.[24] Although increased antibodies due to iodine may be a transient effect in most people, it may be more lasting in a small number of predisposed individuals.[25]

Spot urine iodine testing and 24-hour urine collection testing after a 50-mg loading dose can provide some data. However, the most accurate assessment of iodine requires spot checking for 10 consecutive days. Because iodine tests don't rule out possible benefit from or possible hypothyroid/hyperthyroid reaction to iodine treatment, a therapeutic trial of iodine and selenium can be given. Iodine 6 mg/day (potassium iodide), selenium 100 mcg/day for 3 days can be given to see how the patient responds. If the patient is tolerating it well, consider increasing iodine gradually up to a replenishing dose of 12–48 mg/day as potassium iodide for up to 3 months and selenium 200–800 mcg/day, then reduce back to iodine 1–12 mg/day, selenium 100–200 mcg/day. These are maintenance levels that are being used by a number of practitioners who feel that they are well tolerated. If there is a worsening of signs or symptoms (hypo or hyper), then the treatment should be discontinued and further tests should be considered. If planning on staying on a maintenance dose, then consider TSH, T4, free T3, and thyroid peroxidase (TPO) antibodies every 6 months.

A possible benefit of long-term maintenance with iodine in the range of 1–12 mg/day of potassium iodide is continued protection against exposure to brominated compounds in the environment. In many instances, the benefits of high-dose iodine supplementation far outweigh the risks and with proper monitoring the risks can be minimized.[26]

A few patients can experience a papular rash, a metallic taste, and other minor complaints. This is not allergy. Reactions to seafood, radiocontrast agents, and iodine-containing antibacterial preparations should not be considered IgE antibody-mediated iodine allergy or sensitivity. (Position statement of the American Academy of Allergy Asthma and Immunology) Ref: http://www.sciencedirect.com/science/article/pii/S0091674904024819#cor1

Selenium

A deficiency of selenium (a constituent of selenoproteins) can increase the duration and exacerbate thyroid disease severity. It is possible that this is due to reduced activity of the selenoprotein GPX leading to increases in hydrogen peroxide production. Iodothyronine selenodeiodonases, D1 and D2, are another class of selenoproteins that produce active T3 through deiodination in peripheral tissues. During selenium supplementation, serum selenium has been reported to increase by 45%, plasma GPX by 21%, and TPO antibody decreased by 76%. On withdrawal of supplementation, a sharp decrease was seen in selenium and GPX accompanied by a marked increase in TPO. Extracellular GPX is secreted by thyrocytes and primarily modulates hydrogen peroxidase and organification of iodine. Its secondary function is to prevent oxidation damage to the thyrocytes themselves.

Iron

Iron deficiency is shown to significantly reduce T4 to T3 conversion, increase rT3 levels, and block the thermogenic (metabolism boosting) properties of thyroid hormone.[27-31] Thus, iron deficiency, as indicated by an iron saturation below 25 or a ferritin below 70, will result in diminished intracellular T3 levels. Additionally, T4 should not be considered adequate thyroid replacement if iron deficiency is present.[27,28,30,31]

Zinc

Zinc is a metallic chemical element essential for many biochemical processes such as cell proliferation. There are indications that zinc is also important for normal thyroid homeostasis. Its effects on thyroid hormones are complex and include both synthesis and mode of action.[32] For example, thyroid transcription factors, which are essential for modulation of gene expression, contain zinc at cysteine residues. Rats that are deficient in zinc have been shown to have 67% decreased type I deiodinase (D1) activity and 30% lower T3 levels as compared to zinc-sufficient controls.

Zinc deficiency can influence thyroid function through its effects on TSH and thyroid hormone levels. Conversely, thyroid hormones influence zinc metabolism by affecting zinc absorption and excretion. In patients with nodular goiter, serum zinc levels were significantly negatively correlated with thyroid volume.[33]

Bladderwrack

Bladderwrack (*Fucus vesiculosus*, a member of the Fucaceae family) is a genus of brown algae found in intertidal, rocky seashores of the temperate zone (especially the Pacific Ocean). Bladderwrack has been used for both dietary and medicinal purposes for centuries, particularly in Asian cultures. Fucus was termed "Bladderwrack" because little air-filled bladders (or flotation devices) keep it in the upper regions of the sea (i.e., close to the ocean surface). Fucus is often known as kelp, the name given to the alkaline ashes that were used as an alkali agent to make soap. *Fucus vesiculosus* contains the flavonoid fucoxanthin and is reported to have the highest antioxidant activity of the edible seaweeds.[34,35]

Seaweed, being high in numerous minerals and halides including iodine, may enhance thyroid function when consumed in appropriate amounts. In Japan, where seaweed is a dietary staple, the average daily intake of iodine has been estimated to be between 1 and 3 mg per day, which is well above the US Recommended Daily Allowance (RDA) of 150 µg for an adult male.[34,36]

In seaweed tests, iodine content was found to be highest in young, freshly-cut blades and lowest in the sun-dried form. In the 12 species tested, iodine levels varied from 16 µg per gram in nori (*Porphyra tenera*) to 8,165 µg per gram in processed kelp granules made from *Laminaria digitata*. Because of the variable and sometimes large doses of iodine in these natural products, physicians should ask patients with hyper/hypothyroidism about seaweed consumption in their diet and/or taken as supplements.

Fucus also has the ability to decrease trans-sialidase activity in the blood (an enzyme associated with cholesterol accumulation), which may benefit patients with low thyroid function because decreased metabolism is associated with hyperlipidemia.

While many forms of seaweed are a good source of iodine, be sure to only use and prescribe forms which have been screened for heavy metals. Unfortunately, some seaweeds are harvested from bays with significant industrial pollution.

Guggul

Commiphora mukul or Guggul can also support thyroid function. C. *mukul* (a relative of the myrrh gum tree in the Burseraceae family) is noted for its content of aromatic gummy resins that have many medicinal, culinary, aromatic, and spiritual uses. Guggul from C. *mukul* is currently at risk of being endangered due to overharvesting in India and Pakistan.

Germacrene (a volatile hydrocarbon found in the Burseraceae family) is a building block in the formation of resins.[37] C. *mukul*, a traditional Ayurvedic medicinal herb, has shown thyroid-stimulating effects in animals and is used to treat high cholesterol, obesity, and a sluggish metabolism.[38,39] *C. mukul* contains sterols (known as guggulsterones) that act on bile acid receptors to process lipids and contribute to its hypolipidemic effect.[40] It may also lower lipid levels by supporting the thyroid's basic metabolic functions. Animal studies have shown *C. mukul* to reduce the effects of thyroid-suppressive medications such as propylthiouracil (PTU) and may be helpful in the treatment of hypothyroidism.[41]

Ketosteroids in *Commiphora*, found in the oleoresin, are reported to increase the uptake of iodine by the thyroid gland and enhance the activity of TPO and protease enzymes.[38,42,43] T3 production was increased along with a healthy alteration in the ratio of T3 to T4 indicating a thyroid-supporting effect. Recent research found that guggulsterones may inhibit nuclear receptors involved with basic metabolic functions and cholesterol metabolism, contributing to the plant's hypolipidemic effect. Although guggulsterones are associated with several plausible mechanisms to reduce cholesterol, it is believed that Guggul's effects on thyroid regulation are responsible for the therapeutic effects seen in cholesterol levels.[44] However, results of clinical trials have been inconclusive.[45,46]

Iris Versicolor (Blue Flag)

Iris was utilized and written about extensively by an organized group of physicians (members of the American eclectic physician movement) who, from the 1830s to the 1940s, heavily relied on the use of carefully prepared botanical medicines. *Iris versicolor* (also called "Blue Flag"), is a small wild iris found in the marshy areas of North America. The plant contains volatile oils, resins, alkaloids, and the oleoresin iridin, but little molecular, cellular, or clinical research has been conducted on this plant. Nonetheless, this plant has a long history of medicinal use targeted at "moving the sluggish bodily fluids" (i.e., saliva, lymph, bile, digestive secretions, bowels, congested tissues) and has been used to treat hepatomegaly, splenomegaly, and thyroid dysfunction.

Iris is traditionally administered orally and/or topically. It is specific for the treatment of thyroid enlargement and goiters, making a valuable contribution to botanical medicine as well as acting as a synergist in herbal formulations to support the thyroid.

Supporting Adrenal Function with Adaptogenic Herbs

Stress appears to be the main contributing cause of WTS. Prolonged stress can also lead to adrenal fatigue over time. In my experience, patients with WTS often benefit from adrenal support. There is a lot of overlap between thyroid and adrenal hypofunction. Considering that Addison's disease is a contraindication for T3 therapy, it's easy to see how adrenal support can help some people tolerate T3 therapy much better. Some practitioners like to support the adrenals before treating with T3, some practitioners usually treat with T3 and add adrenal support if it seems warranted, and some practitioners like to start patients on both adrenal and thyroid support. The adrenal and thyroid systems work very closely together like two players on the same team. When one of the players is struggling, the other tends to struggle as well.

Adaptogens are herbs capable of restoring normal tone and function to the HPA (hypothalamic–pituitary–adrenal) axis and the SAS (sympatho-adrenal system), and therefore to the entire body. Adaptogens are considered safe agents that increase overall resistance to stressors, and normalize endocrine function through numerous broad and non-specific actions.

The adrenal glands underlie much of the body's response to external and internal stressors. Likewise, stress is a primary contributor to adrenal/HPA axis dysfunction. Adaptogenic herbs may improve resistance to stress as well as prevent some of the more common symptoms of stress (e.g., poor concentration, sleep disturbance, fatigue, decreased immune response, and decreased resistance to infections). Adaptogenic herbs modulate stress responses, prevent down-regulation of the adrenal glands, enhance energy production and sleep quality, and improve immune function.[47]

The three herbs described below (i.e., *Eleutherococcus*, *Ocimum*, and *Rhodiola*), all fit the classic definition of an adaptogen due to their influence on overall health via a variety of non-specific, broad-scope, normalizing mechanisms. By exerting an effect on the HPA axis and hormonal regulation, as well as mitigating the harmful effects of stress, these three adaptogenic herbs can improve energy, reduce stress symptoms, and improve hormonal balance as well as general well-being. Allergies, inflammation, nervousness, mood disorders, and poor physical stamina are among the many conditions that may respond to adaptogen therapy. Enhanced immune response, resistance to infection, and improved concentration are also among the more common benefits associated with the use of these adaptogenic herbs.

Eleutherococcus senticosus

Eleutherococcus (Siberian ginseng) is a member of the Araliaceae family. Not only is this adaptogenic herb commonly used in Russia (where the first studies were conducted in the 1950s), but also in North America and throughout the world. Native to Siberia and the northern regions of Russia, the Korean peninsula, and the northeast region of China, *Eleutherococcus* has *Panax ginseng*-like effects.

Eleutherococcus has demonstrated stress-relieving effects on the HPA axis, reducing excessive corticotropin release and optimizing adrenal response.[48,49] *Eleutherococcus* may act directly on the hypothalamus to regulate hormones, including mineralocorticoids, glucocorticoids, and reproductive hormones. Syringen, lignans, and sesamin found in this plant have been shown to exert immune-enhancing effects.[50]

Eleutherococcus contains coumarins, steroidal glycosides, and a group of polysaccharides, eleutherosides A, B, C, D, and E, which have significant immune-stimulating properties. Among the specific conditions where *Eleutherococcus* has shown possible effects are in treating immune depression (i.e., compromise), head colds, influenza, bronchitis, respiratory allergies, atherosclerosis, rheumatic valve lesions, arrhythmias, arthritis, chemotherapy side effects, and altitude sickness, as well as for general weakness, fatigue, stress intolerance, and nervous debilities.[51–54] Some of the anti-allergy and anti-inflammatory responses may relate to inhibition of nitric oxide synthase and cyclooxygenase during macrophage activation.[55]

Numerous studies have demonstrated the ability of *Eleutherococcus* to enhance physical stamina in athletes and also inhabitants of high altitudes. The herb may increase oxygen consumption and utilization and increases overall work performance,[56] although this effect is not seen in all studies.[57,58] The mechanisms identified include improved physical stamina via adrenal responses as well as improved glucose uptake/metabolism in muscle cells and prevention of nitrogen depletion.[59] Positive effects on fibrinogen and blood coagulation have been demonstrated and proposed as another mechanism of enhanced exercise performance.[60]

Eleutherococcus has been shown to improve general mental function, well-being, and quality of life in the elderly.[61] *Eleutherococcus* is reported to affect noradrenalin responses in the brain in a manner that helps to blunt the stress response, specifically, in the paraventricular and supra-optic nuclei (the regions of the brain found to be integral to stress responses).[62]

Ocimum sanctum

Ocimum sanctum (Holy Basil or tulsi) is a plant species from India. *Ocimum* is in the Lamiaceae (mint) family and has been used traditionally in the treatment of diabetes, stress, ulcers, and inflammation. Agrawal and colleagues showed its ability to reduce fasting and postprandial blood glucose levels in humans.[63] O. *sanctum* also has anti-inflammatory properties, and has been found to promote glutathione transferase, reductase, and peroxidase enzymes as well as promote superoxide dismutase.[64,65]

Ocimum contains common anti-inflammatory flavonoids such as apigenin, luteolin, and one unique to *Ocimum* (called ocimarin). Other constituents include ocimumosides and cerebrosides. Oil extracted from the seeds can reduce inflammation by lipoxygenase inhibition and histamine antagonism and can help to heal ulcers.[66,67] In addition to its antioxidant properties, modern research has shown *Ocimum* to be radioprotective, anticarcinogenic, and cardioprotective.[68,69] The ocimumosides in *Ocimum* have anti-stress effects in that they help to normalize hyperglycemia, corticosterones, and adrenal hypertrophy from chronic stress.[70] *Ocimum* has been shown to reduce serum cortisol and glucose.[71]

Numerous effects on the brain, neurotransmission, and stress response have been demonstrated by *Ocimum*. Ethanol extracts of *Ocimum* tend to blunt the stress response in animals, regardless of the experimental protocol. The plant extract reduced behavioral and neurochemical responses to stress in the swimming endurance test and gravitation, restraint stress, and noise stress.[72–75] In fact, noise pollution has been shown to be a real and significant stress causing changes in the central nervous system's neurotransmitter balance and activity. Exposure to constant, irritating noise can lead to increased dopamine and serotonin in the brain, with a simultaneous reduction in acetylcholine and an increase in acetylcholinesterase, presumably as a stress response to the noise irritation. Response to a noise stimulus may be used as a research tool to evaluate the effects of stress-alleviating herbs and medications. *Ocimum* has been shown to prevent the above changes in brain neurotransmitters suggesting an anti-stress effect directly within the central nervous system.[76,77] Animal studies have demonstrated a dopaminergic activity that promoted a calming and mood-stabilizing effect.[78] One study found that enhancement of γ-aminobutyric acid (GABA) neurotransmission enabled *Ocimum* to exert a normalizing effect on immune modulation.[79]

Like other adaptogens, *Ocimum* has been shown to prevent both humoral and cell-mediated responses associated with stress, and researchers point to calming mechanisms as underlying contributors. These calming effects may also extend to the vasculature because *Ocimum* has been shown to be both vasodilating and hypotensive.[80] It has demonstrated positive effects on cognitive ability and has possible application for dementia while animal studies have shown anti-convulsant effects.[81,82]

Rhodiola rosea

Rhodiola rosea (Rose Root or Golden Root) is a member of the Crassulaceae family. It is a widely used adaptogen and anti-stress herb for mood disorders, fatigue, and adrenal weakness. This plant is native to Russia, where most of the initial scientific and clinical research was conducted. *Rhodiola* contains rosavin, rosarin, rosin, tyrosol, and salidroside, and these are often used as markers to standardize *Rhodiola* extracts. The herb's main use is as an adaptogen for mood disorders, sleep difficulties, irritability, fatigue, poor concentration, headaches, vascular stress, and generalized deficiency states.[83] *Rhodiola* elevates serotonin levels in the central nervous system in animal models of depression and hippocampal suppression.[84] *Rhodiola* is also believed to exert antidepressant and anti-anxiety effects.[85]

Cardiac complaints that arise from stress (such as hypertension and arrhythmias) may respond to *Rhodiola* therapy.[86] As with other adaptogenic herbs, its cardio-protection may minimize ischemic injury.[53,87] Antiarrhythmic effects are due to its ability to block excessive epinephrine-driven stimulation and activation of opiate pathways in the central nervous system.[88]

In a rat model of acute stress, *Rhodiola* prevented changes in behavior, immunity, and hormonal regulation to the same degree as fluoxetine.[89] Certain stress-inducing paradigms can cause reproducible effects on serotonin, cell proliferation, and differentiation in the central nervous system. *Rhodiola* increased serotonin and had a normalizing effect on hippocampal stem cells, restoring them to levels seen in non-stressed control animals.[90] In one clinical study, *Rhodiola* supplementation improved energy, promoted mental focus, and increased concentration among chronic fatigue syndrome (CFS) patients while normalizing their cortisol levels.[91]

Diet

Here are a few dietary modifications that can benefit patients with symptoms of low thyroid dysfunction/WTS. For one, aspartame can exacerbate Graves' and Hashimoto's. Therefore, patients should consider the relatively simple strategy of cutting aspartame out of their diet before they undergo a more serious treatment intervention such as thyroid ablation. The mechanism by which aspartame interferes with thyroid function is yet unclear.[92–94] Likewise, Celiac disease is linked to subclinical hypothyroidism, therefore researchers have concluded that eliminating gluten might entirely reverse hypothyroidism in certain cases. Indeed, most patients with low thyroid function experience symptom improvement when gluten is avoided.[95]

Tyrosine is an amino acid to which iodine atoms are attached to form active thyroid hormones. Low plasma tyrosine levels have been associated with hypothyroidism, low blood pressure, low body temperature, and restless leg syndrome. As a precursor to catecholamine neurotransmitters, tyrosine is also helpful in treating depression. The following high-protein food products serve as rich sources of tyrosine:[96]

- Chicken
- Turkey
- Fish
- Peanuts
- Almonds
- Avocados
- Milk
- Cheese
- Yogurt
- Cottage cheese
- Lima beans
- Pumpkin seeds
- Sesame seeds
- Bananas
- Soy products

Lifestyle

Lifestyle modifications such as aerobic exercise and stress management all appear to support proper thyroid function and peripheral conversion. On the contrary, stress, sleep deprivation, and excess alcohol consumption seem to impair thyroid hormone function.[97]

WT3 Protocol

Rationale for T3 Therapy

One advantage to a therapeutic trial of T3 therapy is that there is one variable and one endpoint (give enough T3 to normalize the body temperature). With this clear endpoint, it's easy to see whether or not the treatment is helping. T3 is not foreign and has been present since birth in every person's body. The results can be very dramatic and some people can start feeling better within hours, days, or weeks. It is generally well tolerated. The symptoms of WTS can be very debilitating and many people respond well to treatment for WTS when many other approaches have failed. Herbal and nutritional support are often enough to help people begin to normalize their body temperatures within 3–4 weeks with very little risk. In more severe cases, T3 therapy may be necessary to normalize patients' temperatures but it also carries more risk of cardiovascular side effects such as palpitations and increased heart rate.

from pg. 153

When giving a therapeutic trial of thyroid hormone for WTS, one might ask, "why not use T4 instead of T3?" The main answer to this question is that with T3 therapy the symptoms often remain improved even after the treatment has been discontinued (i.e., the "resetting phenomenon"), which is not the case with T4 treatment strategies that utilize dessicated thyroid and/or levothyroxine products. Thus, patients who are biochemically euthyroid and clinically hypothyroid might improve with the use of T4-containing preparations, but their symptoms almost always return once the treatment is discontinued. Also, the symptoms

> Remember, T4 is 4 times less potent, and 3 times longer-acting than T3. So even though it stimulates the thyroid hormone receptor, it has a much weaker action here than T3. So if T4 occupies the receptor instead of T3, it results in decreased stimulation of the cell.

can often return even while patients are still taking the T4-containing medicine. The classic story is that the dose of T4 can be increased, and the patient may feel well for 2–3 months and then the symptoms will return. Then, the dose can be increased and the patient may feel well again for a similar period of time before feeling bad again. Finally, the dose can be increased and the symptoms can immediately get worse, without the usual transient improvement. This is likely caused by competitive inhibition of T3 at the level of the cell, and suggests that the patient is being pushed too far in the wrong direction with the wrong medicine. This is an all too common story, and such patients are typically more difficult to treat, requiring more cycles of T3 therapy in order to return to feeling well on less/no medicine.

Although the blood tests are not very useful in predicting who will respond to T3 therapy, those with the highest rT3/T3 (RIA) ratios are typically the same patients who were being pushed too far in the wrong direction with the wrong medicine (with T4 therapy as described above). The rT3/T3 ratio can be calculated by simply dividing the total rT3 by the total T3. The median of the normal range of rT3 divided by the median of the normal range of T3 can be used as a reference point; this usually works out to be approximately 2. Sometimes untreated patients have rT3/T3 ratios up to about 3 or 4. Patients who are inappropriately managed with T4 therapy can occasionally present with ratios of >6, however, this is rare.

These abnormally high rT3/T3 ratios can be explained by the observation that the enzyme 5'-deiodinase converts T4 to T3, as well as rT3 to 3,5-diiodothyronine (T2, which is considered an inactive metabolite). rT3 has been shown to competitively inhibit the conversion of T4 to T3. With less T4 being converted to T3 and more being converted to rT3, which generates more competitive inhibition of the T3, a vicious cycle can start and perpetuate WTS (rT3 and T4 can actually accelerate destruction of the activating deiodinase through the ubiquitin-proteosome pathway). It may get to the point that there is so much rT3

> Impaired T4 to T3 conversion can lead from a state of T3 preponderance to a state of T4 and/or rT3 excess, which we will label T4/rT3 preponderance. This can have two dire consequences: (1) it perpetuates decreased T3 production; (2) it competitively inhibits what little T3 is being produced.

present that increases in T4 dose no longer correlate with an increase in T3 stimulation, because of inhibition of the 5'-deiodinase enzyme. Instead, the added T4 just competes at the level of the cell with what little T3 is being produced, to actually decrease T3 stimulation of the cell.

from pg. 116 T4 therapy may temporarily improve symptoms via the transient increase in T4 to T3 conversion and subsequent T3 stimulation of the cell. However, the same factors that made it difficult for the patients to convert their own T4 will eventually begin to hinder the conversion of the orally supplemented T4 to the much needed T3 form. Thus, more of the supplemented T4 begins to go toward rT3, and the system gets bogged down again and the symptoms return. This theoretical backlog situation leads to what I call T4/rT3 preponderance, as opposed to T3 preponderance.

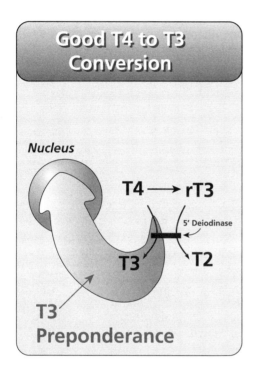

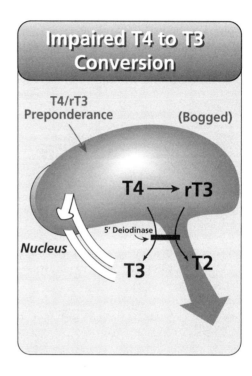

from pg. 144 T4/rT3 preponderance can be problematic in two ways. First, it perpetuates decreased T3 production. Second, it can compete with what little T3 is produced, at the level of the nuclear receptor. A T4/rT3 preponderance leads to insufficient T3 stimulation of the cells, and thus thyroid function is compromised. This all happens outside the blood stream on a cellular level and is not necessarily reflected in the thyroid blood tests.

The thyroid system typically bogs down again on T4 therapy within about 2–3 months of T4 therapy. If it happens sooner, say in about 3 weeks, this suggests the patient's system is bogging down rather precipitously. If it happens only after 6 months or a year, it is a more indolent process with outside stress usually playing a significant role in the impaired T4 to T3 conversion. As mentioned previously, WTS symptoms may improve while on T4 therapy, but because the underlying problem still exists, these symptoms will mostly likely reappear after T4 therapy is discontinued.

The drastic difference between T4 and T3 therapy is that T3 therapy can clear out the thyroid pathways to give the thyroid system a fresh start and an opportunity to "reboot". T3 decreases TSH resulting in decreased T4 and rT3 levels. This removes the T4/rT3 preponderance that bogs down the thyroid system. Then, when T3 therapy is weaned, TSH and T4 production recommence, exposing the 5'-deiodinase enzyme to primarily T4. With high rT3 levels no longer dominating the 5'-deiodinase enzyme, T4 to T3 conversion can once again proceed normally (i.e., T3 preponderance).

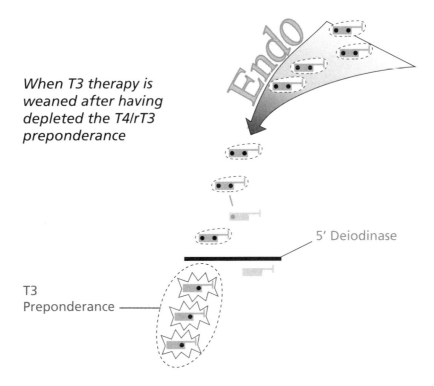

When T3 therapy is weaned after having depleted the T4/rT3 preponderance

5' Deiodinase

T3 Preponderance

Some skeptical patients have questioned how so many different problems could be treated with the same therapy (as if it's too good to be true). However, the idea that one specific treatment can be used to manage a variety of problems is relatively uncontroversial. Take insulin-dependent diabetes for example, where one therapy (i.e., insulin) is associated with a significant reduction in a wide range of symptoms. One important difference is that patients who do well with T3 can frequently wean off the medicine and continue to do well while remaining drug free.

T3 therapy can accomplish two separate goals. One is to deplete TSH, T4, and rT3 levels well enough to reset the patients' thyroid systems so that they are able to feel well when the T3 medicine has been discontinued. The other is for the patients to take the T3 so that their temperatures are high enough and steady enough for them to feel well while they are taking the T3. While these two goals can often be accomplished simultaneously, they can also be accomplished separately because they are dependent on different parameters. Different approaches with the T3 therapy can be used depending on a patient's priorities of cost, time, simplicity, convenience, symptomatic improvement while on the T3, and persistent resolution after discontinuing the T3. Specifically, there is an "Original WT3 Protocol" described below that focuses on titrating the T3 according to the patients' daily temperature readings. This approach is more focused on helping patients feel well while they are on the T3 therapy (which depends on having a normal and steady body temperature). There is also a "Simplified WT3 Protocol" which focuses more on convenience for doctor and patient in that patients don't need to track their temperatures every day. The T3 dose is increased according to a set schedule in order to deplete the TSH, T4, and rT3 levels with the patients monitoring their pulse rates every day to make sure they do not go too high. The Simplified WT3 Protocol is much easier for doctors to explain and easier for patients to do and works in about 80% of cases. The Original WT3 Protocol is more time-intensive for patients and doctors but it is helpful in about 90% of cases, and is often tailored to help patients feel well while taking the T3 therapy. We will discuss the Simplified WT3 Protocol first, and then explain the Original WT3 Protocol.

Simplified WT3 Protocol[98–100]

With this approach, patients check their temperatures before treatment to see if they are low. Then, if indicated, they are given a small starting dose, which is then increased every day as long as their pulse rates do not go above 100 bpm and as long as they are not having any complaints. They go up to a suppressive dosage of up to 75–90 mcg BID. Then, they gradually wean down off the T3 by reducing the dose a step at a time (using the same dosage levels they used on the way up) every 2 or 3 days. Patients check their temperatures after the cycle and report back to the doctor and the cycle is repeated as needed.

Directions for patients:

- Before starting T3 therapy:
  - Take your temperature three times a day for a couple of days. Average your daily temperatures by adding up the temperatures for each day and dividing by 3. Are your temps averaging <98.6°F?
  - Discuss with your doctors the benefits and risks of T3 treatment.
  - Can you run around the block? Do you feel ok when your pulse goes up?
  - Some people with low adrenal function benefit from adrenal support.

Day	AM	PM
1	7.5 mcg	7.5 mcg
2	15 mcg	15 mcg
3	22.5 mcg	22.5 mcg
4	30 mcg	30 mcg
5	37.5 mcg	37.5 mcg
6	45 mcg	45 mcg
7	52.5 mcg	52.5 mcg
8	60 mcg	60 mcg
9	67.5 mcg	67.5 mcg
10	75 mcg	75 mcg

- While taking T3 therapy:
  - Set alarms on your watch or phone to take your T3 doses every 12 hours at the same times each day (e.g., 7 am, 7 pm).
  - Always take your T3 on time! (Not even 3 minutes late).
  - Record your pulse reading every day.
  - Increase your dose each day according to the schedule below but stop increasing your dose and call your doctor if your pulse goes above 100 bpm or if you feel palpitations.
  - If you're a few hours late with a dose, go ahead and take the dose and keep following the schedule at your regular times.

- Weaning off T3 therapy:
  - Stay at 75 mcg twice daily for 2–3 days and then start stepping down through the T3 doses, one dosage level every 2–3 days (per your doctor).
  - Once you have stopped the T3, record your daily average temperature for 2–3 days and report to your doctor.

Original WT3 Protocol

Basic Principles of Treatment

from pgs. 145, 150

Feeling well on T3 therapy has everything to do with having enough T3 stimulation to get the temperatures back up to normal (i.e., 98.6°F), but that is also very steady. This involves providing T3 in a highly controlled manner, in order to generate smooth, steady, sufficient, and well-tolerated T3 stimulation of the cell. The significance of steady T3 delivery becomes obvious when one provides the patient with T3 directly rather than relying on the body to convert T4 to T3. For example, even though the half-life of T3 is 2.5 days, enough is gone within 3 hours of a missed dose that patients can often notice this little difference.

The notion of attaining and sustaining a stable, normal body temperature with T3 therapy can be referred to as "capturing the temperature." Sometimes, this cannot be accomplished until T4 and rT3 levels have been largely depleted, or in other words, until the T4/rT3 preponderance has been removed. While it is the depletion of rT3 levels that probably makes the most impact, the depletion of rT3 levels only occurs upon depletion of T4 levels. This would explain why T4-containing medicines are not useful in bringing about the resetting phenomenon.

from pg. 150

from pg. 157

Taking enough T3 to get the temperature up and delivering that T3 smoothly enough for the patients to feel well are two different matters. Although people may get enough T3 to achieve normal temperatures, they still may not feel quite right. For example, a patient's average temperature of 97.8°F is raised to 98.6°F by gradually increasing the dose (e.g., to 45 mcg BID). Yet, the patient notices no improvement in symptoms. However, as the patient is weaned off the T3 therapy, and she begins to steadily make her own endogenous supply of T3, the WTS symptoms begin to subside and eventually resolve. Although cases like this are not typical, some patients don't feel better until they are actually off the T3 therapy (because only then are their temperatures both normal AND steady).

A precedent for a "resetting" approach is the one that is commonly used in women who are having irregular menstrual cycles. Their female hormone blood tests may be in the normal range, but clinically, they're having irregular menstrual bleeding. Frequently, there is nothing anatomically wrong with the patient's ovaries or uterus, but her female hormonal milieu has established itself in such a functional pattern as to be problematic. So, control of the patient's menstrual cycles is taken over with exogenous hormones (i.e., oral contraceptive pills). This leaves the patient's own endogenous hormonal production suppressed, but only for a time. The patient is cycled for several months to artificially re-establish a pattern that her body can hopefully maintain on its own once the oral hormones are discontinued.

The Concept of Cycling

It sometimes takes more than one cycle of T3 therapy to even get the temperature up to normal. Just as patients must frequently be cycled on hormonal contraceptives several times, so too do WTS sufferers sometimes need to be cycled on and off T3 therapy. This cycling continues until the optimal thyroid hormonal milieu is fully re-established such that the symptoms are improved, and the patient's own body can maintain normal body temperature on its own. Patients who have a strong T4/rT3 preponderance will often need multiple cycles. The first cycle of T3 therapy (up to a dose of about 90 mcg BID) might not be able to break through the competition at the nuclear receptor well enough to normalize the patient's temperature; but only enough to deplete T4 and therefore rT3 levels, through negative feedback inhibition.

When the first cycle of T3 therapy is weaned, the patient's own T4 production begins to increase again. With less rT3 around to compete against it, T4 to T3 conversion may be improved, which favors a smaller T4/rT3 preponderance than before.

from pg. 156

At this point, if a second cycle is started, there is less of a T4/rT3 preponderance for the T3 to break through to stimulate the receptors than there was prior to the first cycle. So the second cycle of T3 will have a better opportunity at normalizing the temperature, or at least of further depleting the T4/rT3 preponderance as compared to the first cycle. In fact, higher temperatures and/or greater depletion might be accomplished with lower doses of T3 on the second cycle than on the first. Likewise, a third cycle (if needed) will often have a better opportunity than the second of getting more accomplished on lower levels of T3 therapy, and so on with subsequent cycles.

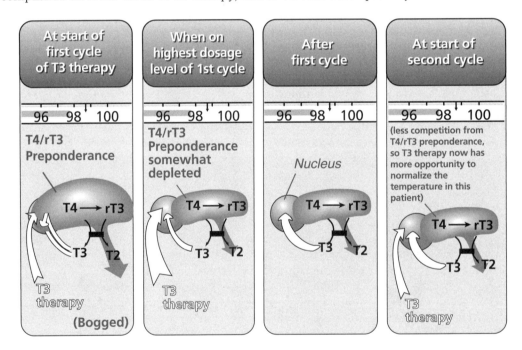

Some have wondered what kind of defect is at the heart of WTS. However, there may not be one specific WTS defect per se. If there was a structural enzymatic defect involved, it is unlikely that we would see such drastic improvement with T3 therapy as we do (as quickly as 10 days in some cases). Rather, based on its onset and response to T3 therapy, WTS appears to be a functional impairment.

Here's an analogy to illustrate the nature of WTS:

When you push a lawn mower into deep grass, it can become "overwhelmed" and begin to slow down. If you pull it out in time, it often speeds back up to normal on its own again. If you do not pull it out in time, it can slow down further and stop completely. Sometimes, the lawn mower has slowed down so much that it's just on the verge of stopping when you pull it out. When this occurs, the machine can keep chugging along neither speeding up nor slowing down, and you can't tell if it's going to return to normal speed or if it's going to stop completely. Sometimes, it can keep chugging along in this manner for a surprisingly long period of time. It seems to be just teetering on the edge, ready to lose its momentum and stall, or to gain the advantage and speed back up to normal. Here are three different and distinct modes of functioning: running normally, chugging along, and stopped. Yet in all three cases, in our example, there is nothing mechanically wrong with the lawn mower. The blade, gas line, carburetor, and spark plug are all fine. It's just that it's a system in motion that has operational limits and an optimal operating speed. The machine can handle efficiently only so much grass per unit time.

Likewise, our bodies have operational limits and an optimal operating speed. To further the analogy, if the lawnmower was chugging along, and there was some way you could give it a little push or advantage, you could help it to speed back up to normal (let's imagine you had some sort of drill attachment you could use to speed up the top of the engine as it was spinning around). But if the engine stops, the drill attachment is not going to have enough power to start the engine, so you're going to have to pull the starter cord. If the engine just stopped a few moments earlier, it may take only one pull of the cord. If it has been sitting there stopped since yesterday, it may take several attempts. And if it has been in the garage since last season, it may take quite a few more.

This is very much like the way the thyroid system behaves. When people are under enough physical and/or emotional stress, their metabolisms can slow down. When the stress goes away, they frequently come back up to normal on their own again. But sometimes they don't, and their system stays depressed, chugging along even after the stress has passed (remember, a functional impairment does not necessarily mean that there is an anatomical or mechanical impairment). It may be possible to give them a little push (via T3 supplementation) to help restore them to normal speed without suppressing their systems completely. In more long-standing and severe cases, however, supplementation will often not be enough. In such cases, restoration must "start from scratch," by suppressing the patient's own thyroid system completely for a short time (via T3 replacement). This is akin to pulling the starter cord. When the person is being replaced with T3, their T4, TSH, and rT3 may be close to the lower limits of detection. Indeed, in more severe cases, one pull of the cord may not be enough, and the patient's system may have to be completely suppressed more than once by cycling on and off T3 replacement therapy in order to reset the system well enough for it to begin functioning properly on its own again. Also, it is not uncommon for diminishing cycles of T3 supplementation to be needed after one or more cycles of T3 replacement in order to fine-tune or coax the system all the way back to normal.

In mild cases, the system can be reset without requiring extreme suppression; by reset I mean that the patient is left with a net gain in endogenous T3 stimulation. However, because of negative feedback inhibition of the pituitary gland, as more T3 is given by mouth, less is being naturally made by the body (i.e., endogenous T3 production is suppressed), and the temperature may drop back down again. At such a time, the T3 dosage can be increased to bring the temperature up again. In such mild cases, the system is chugging along on its own well enough (because it is not too bogged down by T4/rT3 preponderance) that the T3 therapy can get through and capture the temperature before the system is very suppressed (this is T3 supplementation and is likened to the little push with the drill attachment in the analogy).

When the T3 therapy is weaned, the endogenous system comes back up again, often being able to maintain the normalized temperature on its own by virtue of a net gain in endogenous stimulation of the cell (i.e., resetting phenomenon).

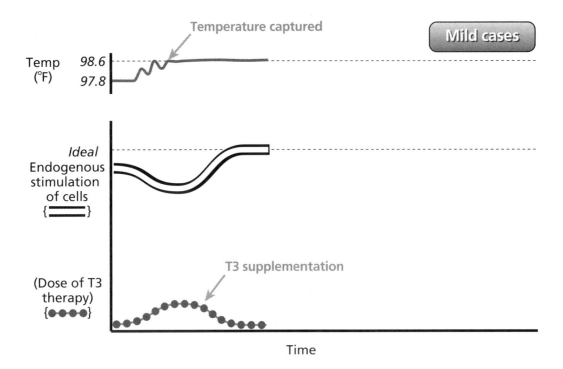

In less mild cases, higher doses of T3 (which cause greater suppression of the system) may be needed to capture the temperature. Furthermore, the body may not be able to maintain the temperature on its own after the first cycle of T3 therapy is weaned. The system might be reset to a degree, but perhaps not enough to remain normal after only one cycle. Thus, a second cycle (usually of lower doses) may be required for fine-tuning.

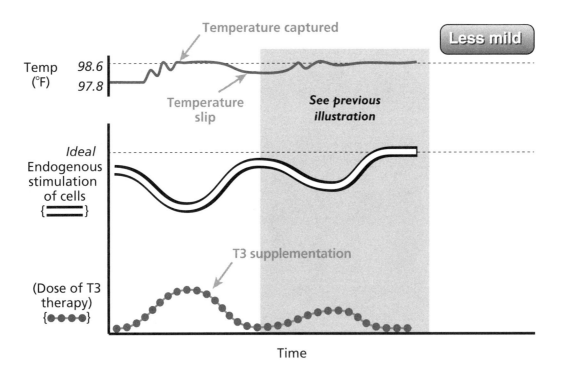

This situation can occur for a number of reasons such as the severity of the case, weaning the first cycle too fast, because of outside stress, or unsteady T3 levels due to higher dosage levels/decreased compliance with dosage times. In rather difficult cases, the system is so bogged down that T3 supplementation is not enough, and T3 replacement is needed. In these patients, the system must be completely suppressed in order to remove the T4/rT3 preponderance before the temperature can be captured (this is likened to pulling the starter cord in the analogy). Once the temperature is captured, the patient is likely to need less medicine to get their temperature up on subsequent cycles.

Because T3 stimulation needs to be sufficiently steady to be very effective, the system can sometimes be completely suppressed with the temperature still not being captured. This is primarily due to T3 unsteadiness. The T3 may first need to be weaned (to let the T3 levels steady down) and then started back up again on the next cycle before the temperature can be captured. Lower doses, which are easier to keep steady, may then be able to capture the temperature because higher doses on the previous cycle removed the obstructing T4/rT3 preponderance.

Before the temperature is captured, one cannot be very sure that the patient will need less medicine on subsequent cycles. But capturing the temperature marks the turning point in the resetting process such that one can then be very confident that the patient will be able to make progress by increasing their temperature with less and less medicine upon each subsequent cycle (if any are needed) until the process is complete.

In difficult cases, the first cycle (with a maximum dose of about 90 mcg BID) is not enough to capture the temperature or to completely suppress the system. However, this first cycle is not useless because it may pave the way so that the next cycle can accomplish the task. In cases like this, it is usually more effective to wean off the T3 and to start another cycle than it is to increase the dosage level much higher. This is because increasing the T3 level much more just tends to make the T3 level more and more unsteady. When weaning, the goal is to proceed slowly enough that the temperature does not drop any lower than it is, even if it hasn't been captured (c12).

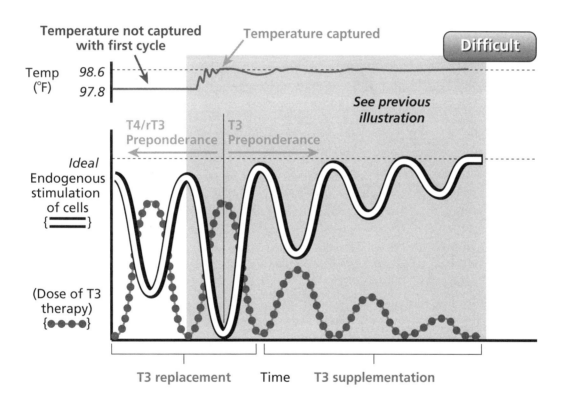

In more difficult cases, it may take several cycles to completely suppress the system and capture the temperature (p101). Once the system has been suppressed completely, reducing the T4/rT3 preponderance, it is not uncommon for diminishing cycles of T3 supplementation to be needed (although they may not be) to fine-tune or coax the system to maintain the temperature on its own. Therefore, sometimes the endogenous system must be suppressed down, down, down before it can come up, up, up and maintain things on its own after the treatment has been discontinued.

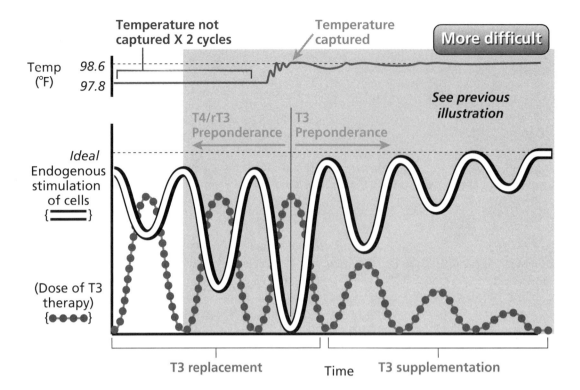

Temperature not captured X 2 cycles

Temperature captured

More difficult

Temp (°F)   98.6
            97.8

T4/rT3 Preponderance ←   T3 Preponderance →

See previous illustration

Ideal Endogenous stimulation of cells {═══}

(Dose of T3 therapy) {●●●●}

T3 replacement   Time   T3 supplementation

The benefits of T3 therapy are obtained by passing control of the thyroid system from endogenous control to exogenous control, and then back again (via one or multiple cycles). Passing control of the thyroid system from endogenous control to exogenous control involves beginning the patient on the starting dose, and increasing the dose by 7.5 mcg/dose/day if the patient is without complaints until the temperature remains 98.6°F on average (which is almost always when the patient's symptoms are most improved) or until the dose is up to about 90 mcg BID (in which case the T3 may be weaned off for a time, and another cycle can be started).

> For T3 therapy, I recommend a T3 preparation that is compounded with a sustained release agent (p108). The starting dose is usually 7.5 mcg p.o. every 12 hours, and it is increased in 7.5 mcg increments from 7.5 mcg up to about 90 mcg BID.

When patients are treated with a cycle of T3 therapy, they often retain what symptomatic improvement they do get from that cycle, even if it is not complete. For example, a patient with a percentage index of 40% (patient feels 40% of what the patient imagines a normal person to feel like) may improve to 60% with the first cycle (c5). This improvement to 60% often persists indefinitely, even if a second cycle is not started right away. With another cycle, that patient may improve to 80%, and with the next cycle to 100%. There is a possibility, however, of factors pushing progress backward: if such a patient has progressed to a percentage index of 80%, and undergoes some stress, then his/her percentage index might slip back a step to 60%.

Compensation and Compensation Time

from pgs. 105, 150, 156

Once the patient's temperature reaches 98.6°F under exogenous control on a given dose of the T3, that dose can be continued for a time. If, while on that dose, the temperature drops back down again, this is most likely because the body is taking back control endogenously through negative feedback inhibition (I refer to this as compensation). Exogenous control of the system is then regained and maintained by raising the dose to the next increment to bring the temperature back up to 98.6°F.

The patient may compensate to the T3 therapy again, in which case, the exogenous dose can be increased again (incrementally as needed up to about 90 mcg BID). As this process continues, less and less T3 is produced endogenously, and more and more is supplied exogenously. The period of time from when a person's temperature goes up to 98.6°F with a 7.5 mcg increment to the time it drops back down again is what I refer to as a person's compensation time.

If a person compensates to each of several increments of T3, the compensation time usually repeats itself. For example, let's say a lady's temperature went up on 30 mcg BID and averaged 98.6°F only for it to go back down on the 5th day. Then, her temperature went back up the next day when the dose was increased to 37.5 mcg BID, and then dropped back down again 5 days later. We could say that she has a 5-day compensation time or that she is a 5-day compensator. This pattern of increased dose and compensation will frequently repeat itself until the temperature doesn't drop back down again. Although compensation times vary among patients (from less than 1 day to about 3 weeks), the average compensation time is about 4 days.

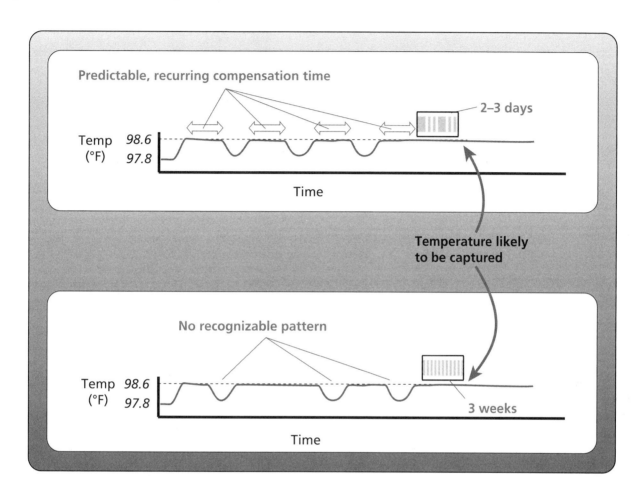

Capturing the Temperature

from pgs. 140, 142, 155, 156 When a person's compensation time (or 3 weeks, if compensation time is not obvious) has passed by a couple of days, and the temperature has not dropped back down again, I refer to the patient's temperature as being captured. The benefit of a cycle has been pretty well obtained once the temperature has been captured, but it is often preferable to allow the patient to remain on that plateau of T3 therapy for a time before weaning. This is the point at which control of the thyroid system has been completely passed from endogenous to exogenous control. However, this does not necessarily mean that a person's thyroid system has been completely suppressed.

The Importance of Steady T3 Levels

 It's important to remember the differences between endogenous and exogenous T3 stimulation, and it's ideal to strive
from pg. 141 for the best of both. The endogenous system is the indisputable world champion at generating steady T3 levels, but
sometimes has trouble generating sufficient T3 stimulation. On the other hand, the exogenous T3 therapy is excellent
at providing sufficient T3 stimulation, but it is sometimes difficult to keep very stable. The ideal situation of course is
when the patient's own system has been reset to provide sufficient T3 stimulation that is endogenously steady. And,
as discussed previously, this can often be accomplished by the passing control of the thyroid system from endogenous
control to exogenous and back again, once or more than once.

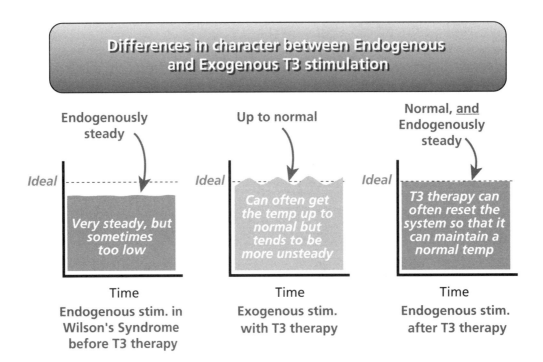

It is important to keep the T3 levels steady, because there are temperature thresholds above which or below which
patients can experience temperature-mediated problems, even if their temperatures average normal. The whole trick
is to keep the T3 levels as steady as possible during this process of passing control from endogenous to exogenous and
back again. One of the reasons for this is that patients can develop temperature-mediated problems when their temperatures are too high, or when they are too low (p80). Thus, there is a range (or window) of temperatures within
which people are less likely to experience temperature-mediated problems.

This temperature window is bounded on either side by temperature thresholds above or below which temperature-
mediated problems (or side effects) become more likely. So even if a temperature pattern averages about normal, if it
is ranging so widely that it breaks through these thresholds, the patient may experience decreased benefits and some
complaints.

 Another reason that steadiness is so important is that rapid changes in body temperature seem to lead to decreased
from pg. 145 benefits and some complaints, even if the thresholds are not broken (p115).

This is probably due to the fact that different enzymes change conformation, in response to temperature change, at
different speeds, and because the reactions they catalyze have different rates. If the temperature swings through the
optimal temperature too quickly, some of the quickly-responding enzymes and reactions may start becoming less efficient again just as some of the more slowly-responding enzymes and reactions are beginning to function well. But when
the temperature transitions are more gradual, then more enzymes are able to function well at the same time, so that
the patient is left with a more settled feeling.

When patients' temperatures are fluctuating more rapidly (even if not beyond the thresholds), less time is spent by the system as a well-functioning unit, at the optimal temperature. This also leaves patients unsettled, or feeling on edge. Take this illustration for example, suppose you were a passenger in a car traveling 55 mph down a four-lane highway (divided by a wide median, two lanes on either side). No other cars are in sight. As long as the car drives in one of the two lanes going your direction, and doesn't drive off the road, you should be all right. But which do you think you would find more comfortable: for the car to swerve from edge to edge every 50 feet, or for it to drift from lane to lane every mile? If it were to swerve every 50 feet, you wouldn't be able to travel as far in the same amount of time (less benefit), and you'd probably not feel as well.

from pg. 157
from pgs. 105, 144, 145
from pg. 154, 157

In pharmacology, when patients are given a maintenance dose of a drug without a loading dose it takes 3–5 half-lives of the drug for the blood level to reach steady state. This shows that each dose can have a bearing on the blood levels for longer than just a single half-life. The half-life of T3 is 2.5 days. Some patients who have not been taking the medicine on time for weeks can correct the resulting unsteadiness by taking the T3 very much on time for a couple of days. However, once the T3 level becomes unsteady due to not taking the T3 very much on time (within minutes of the dosing time), it usually takes 4–5 days to settle down again when proper dosing resumes. So it's best to keep things steady from the start, especially because improvement can be lost before any side effects are experienced. Evidence for this settling effect can be seen clinically. Suppose a person has a temperature averaging 98.6°F on a T3 dose of 45 mcg BID, and is feeling very well. If that person began missing his dosing time, and noticed some of his symptoms returning, and then started taking his medicine on time again, it would usually take about 4–5 days for his T3 levels to steady back down, and for his symptoms to improve again. Sometimes this steadying takes up to 2 weeks, but not usually any longer. This potential 2-week settling period is a major reason why one should not make unnecessary changes to the T3 dosing schedule. For example, women doing well on a certain T3 dose, whose temperatures go up on the 2 or 3 days prior to their period, should not change their T3 dose. Likewise, people don't need to change their doses due to a temporary fever from a cold or virus. It's better not to destabilize T3 levels for 2 weeks for an issue that will only last a few days.

Fast Compensators vs. Slow Compensators

from pgs. 147, 156, 160

Interestingly, how well T3 levels can be kept steady is not only a function of how the medicine is administered, but also of how a patient's body compensates to it. About one out of ten people compensate to a 7.5 mcg increase in the T3 in less than 1 day. These patients would be considered 1-day compensators. Some patients will compensate so quickly that they can even over-compensate, causing their temperatures to drop lower than they were before treatment!

While only about 10% of patients will be 1-day compensators, if not managed appropriately they can easily account for 50% of the WTS management problems. Generally speaking, the more rapidly patients compensate, the harder it is to keep their T3 levels stable. This notion can be visualized by thinking about a father pushing his daughter on a swing. If he steps forward under her, such that just as she swings back about 16 inches he can stop her and push her up again. This way, he can keep her swing path within a 16 inch range. On the other hand, if he steps back, allowing her to swing all the way through baseline and to the zenith of her swing before pushing her forward again, she swings through a much broader range (maybe 16 feet). Likewise, if dosage increases are not made quickly (often) enough, the system can over-compensate (swinging through the baseline of total T3 stimulation), and the body temperature can actually be lower the day after starting T3 than it was the day before. If people tell you that their temperatures are going down on T3, that is your first indication that they might be 1-day compensators. Rapid compensation often results in a larger amplitude of T3 unsteadiness (especially if the delayed increases are made at times that resonate with the swings in the T3 level). For example, increasing the T3 dose every 3 days in a 1-day compensator could cause the body temperature to swing through a wider range, resulting in a higher risk of related side effects.

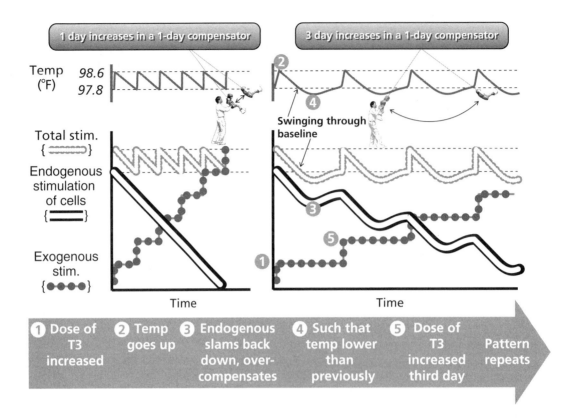

| ① Dose of T3 increased | ② Temp goes up | ③ Endogenous slams back down, over-compensates | ④ Such that temp lower than previously | ⑤ Dose of T3 increased third day | Pattern repeats |

In contrast to the case described above, slow compensators tend to tolerate T3 therapy being rapidly increased quite well. That is to say, they often exhibit temperatures that are quite steady with small ranges of displacement.

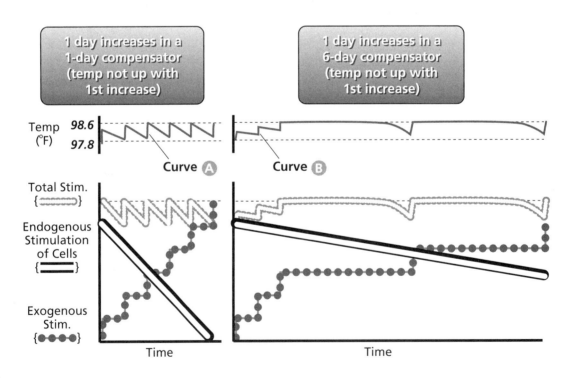

Because you cannot tell the difference between fast and slow compensators by looking at them, I recommend gearing the T3 therapy towards the fast compensators by increasing the T3 dose by 7.5 mcg/dose/day in all patients. By increasing the dose each day as needed to keep the fast compensators steady and in good shape, you'll avoid a lot of problems and disappointment, and the slow compensators will likely tolerate this just fine. Remember this is only when the T3 needs to be increased; when the average temperature is 98.6°F, there is no need for the dosage to be increased.

The question behind a therapeutic trial of T3 therapy is: "How would a given patient feel with a normal and steady temperature, generated by a steady level of T3?" Even if the combination of the two conditions of normal temperature and steady temperature can only be accomplished for a short time (hours or days) at first, it could answer a lot of questions. The longer that combination of conditions can be accomplished, the better the therapeutic trial. If the patient's symptoms significantly improve (even for the short time that the temperatures are steady), it would strongly suggest that the symptoms are temperature-mediated and that the T3 therapy is likely to be on the right track. At that point, resolving the patient's complaints may very likely be just a matter of getting things regulated such that the temperature stays normal and steady.

from pgs. 141, 152, 156, 157

When one starts a patient on T3 therapy to increase the temperature, the level of endogenous T3 often drops in compensation, and along with it, the temperature **(p100)**. As the endogenous portion of the T3 level becomes smaller and the exogenous supply becomes larger, this alone will tend to make the T3 level more unsteady, even if the T3 doses are taken properly and on time. So to maximize the amount of time spent with the combination of a normal and steady temperature, it is often best to get the temperature up to normal, with endogenous T3 making up as great a proportion of the T3 level as possible. Thus, the main goal is to quickly increase the T3 therapy on top of a steady endogenous platform before that platform recedes too much. This is why a steady platform of endogenous T3 is ideal, and why it is so important to start each cycle with a stable T3 level (by allowing at least 2–3 days between cycles) **(Q13)**. Keeping an exact dosing schedule is also important to ensure that the T3 level is as steady as possible **(p103)**.

If the patient's T3 levels do become unsteady on the T3 therapy, it may take several weeks to regain that steadiness, which may involve having to wean the patient off the treatment for a time to get a fresh start, and then starting it back up again **(p103)**. If you don't increase fast compensators quickly enough, then when they compensate their temperatures will go back down, and be as low as they ever were. But then, not only will their temperatures be too low but they will also be unsteady (because the higher the dose of exogenous T3, the harder it is to keep the T3 level steady), and they may feel worse than when they started. Therefore, if you are going *from pgs. 142, 145* to give people T3 therapy, you need to give them sufficient T3 quickly enough to get their temperature close to normal. Otherwise, you are only giving them enough to make their T3 levels unstable, which increases their chances of side effects.

from pgs. 156, 160

You and the patient may choose to increase the T3 more slowly each day, which in some cases may work out quite well. But if you do, you must accept the 10% risk that this patient might be a 1-day compensator, and may not do very well. In which case, the first sign of side effects should be addressed promptly **(p112)**, and the patient may need to be weaned off the T3 for a couple of days to let the T3 level settle back down. At this point, it may need to be decided to increase the T3 each day (or even every 12 hours) or not at all.

from pg. 116

Another good reason to increase the T3 dose every day (when appropriate) is that in more severe cases it may take a few cycles before the patient notices much improvement. Even if the dosage is increased every day, going on and off one cycle could easily take over 4 weeks. In some cases, it could be over 3 months before the patient reports an improvement! Increasing the T3 dose every 3 days (rather than every day) could lengthen this time to 6 months. This is why everyday dose increases are recommended.

Cycle Up, Cycle Down, or Plateau?

To avoid the pitfalls of T3 therapy, one should make deliberate (not tentative), and gradual (not necessarily slow, but they should be gradual) one-way transitions between endogenous control and exogenous control. For example, let's say a woman has captured her temperature for a month on 75 mcg BID and she is weaning down by 7.5 mcg/dose every 2 days and her temperature begins to slip. It's usually best to decelerate the wean and keep weaning than it is to try and increase the dose back up again in an attempt to recapture the temperature, because sometimes the temperature will not go back up even on doses higher than 75 mcg/dose. This is probably due to unsteady T3 levels and can be very disconcerting to the patient and somewhat difficult to explain. On the other hand, by gradually weaning off the present cycle and maintaining as much temperature as possible, allowing the system to steady down between cycles, and starting another cycle, the patient is more likely to capture her temperature on less medicine than 75 mcg BID.

from pg. 148

Remember, once a patient compensates to a dose of T3 it is unlikely that the temperature will go back up again on that dose. Thus, it is typically more effective to continue increasing the dose of T3 until the patient's temperature is normal, rather than to leave the patient on a smaller dose of the T3 for longer periods of time. This is especially true in more severe cases that require several cycles of therapy to be corrected. If one hesitates in such a case, a patient could be treated for 6 months with very little improvement, and very little being accomplished. On the other hand, I have heard of cases where people have taken small doses (even a 7.5-mcg, 12-hour sustained release capsule every morning) over long periods of time (6 months) and their temperatures did normalize.

Sometimes, when a patient's temperatures are normal on a certain plateau dose of the T3, their temperatures will begin to increase with no further increases in dosage, requiring their dosages to be decreased. This process can continue until the patients are "automatically" weaned as their own systems resume normal function.

When patients don't take the sustained release T3 on time, they can put gaps and overlaps into their T3 levels that can cause symptoms to return or side effects to appear. These symptoms and/or side effects may resolve within 4–14 days of resumed exactness with dosing times. Patients can be given a T4-test dose **(p112)** or weaned off the T3 and restarted to help their T3 levels steady down, but it's ideal to keep the T3 dosing on time in the first place.

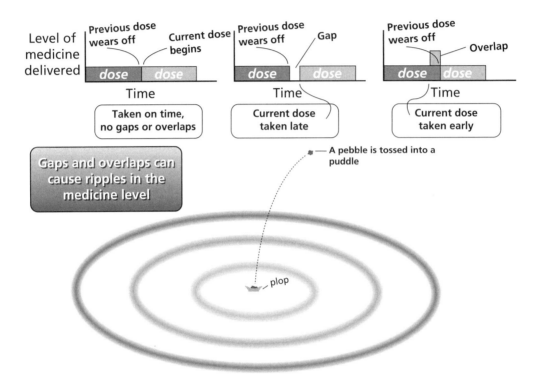

Overview of Resetting the Thyroid System

from pg. 144
To summarize, the process of resetting patients' thyroid systems, and therefore their metabolisms, is like moving the position of a croquet ball on a sandy beach. The thyroid system has a great deal of inertia, and once it has settled into a certain position it tends to stay functioning in that same way. Imagine a croquet ball that has been sitting in the moist sand for a time. It has become embedded there. It takes more effort to dislodge it from its position, but once it is free, it is relatively easy to roll along the sand. However, its position is more easily influenced by the wind and other forces as it rolls along the top of the sand, than it was when it was embedded. Once you have let it roll to a new position, and held it there for a time, it will again begin to settle in and get embedded. Once it has become embedded in a new position, it will have a tendency to stay there.

Likewise, it may take some decisive and deliberate effort to begin to reset a person's thyroid system, but once her temperature has been captured, it is frequently relatively easy to cycle it with diminishing cycles of T3 until her temperature is normal without medicine. However, during the cycling process, her temperature and symptoms may be more easily influenced by changes in sleeping habits or work habits, traveling through time zones, emotional stresses, and timing of doses. This is why it is best during the cycling process to take great care to keep everything else in life as steady as possible while her system is being reset. Once the patient's symptoms are completely corrected, it is sometimes preferable to leave the patient on the same dose of T3 for several weeks after the temperature has been captured to give her system more time to "settle in" to its new mode of functioning before weaning the T3. Once off treatment, the patient might consider not making any drastic changes in her life for 3–6 months, to allow further embedding, and to decrease the chance of relapse. Once settled in, the patient should again be less influenced by the vicissitudes of daily life.

Timing of Doses and Compliance

If 100 patients were on T3 therapy and were missing their doses by 15 minutes here and 20 minutes there, about 60% of them would be responding fairly well to the treatment. However, if those same 100 patients took their T3 doses on a strict schedule (within a few minutes of the dose time), then about 85% would be responding very well to the treatment. It may be surprising how much of a difference it makes to take the medicine on an exact schedule, until one considers the physiology involved.

The body makes T3 (from available T4), a little at a time, around the clock, 24 hours a day. So ideally, it would be best if the T3 taken by mouth could also be delivered a little at a time, around the clock, 24 hours a day. Although this is not currently possible, T3, compounded with a sustained release agent like that used in many sustained-release medications on the market, does a much better job at approaching this than does traditional or instant-release T3 therapy (e.g., Cytomel™). While the sustain-release technology available is not perfect, it nevertheless is associated with very satisfactory results. This is particularly true if the T3 compound (designed to be taken every 12 hours) is taken on time – not even 3 minutes late.

If the patient misses the dose by an hour, they will more than likely not notice any difference at first. Thus, they might assume that it does not really matter very much how they take the medicine. But if the patient misses the dose by 10 minutes here and 20 minutes there, that can add up over a period of a week or two, and the therapy may not work as well. It is true that about 6% of patients seem to do better when they don't take their doses so much on time, or when they use Cytomel™ instead of the sustained-release T3 compound (p108). However, a vast majority of patients do better when they are taking the T3 compound on an exact schedule.

from pg. 145

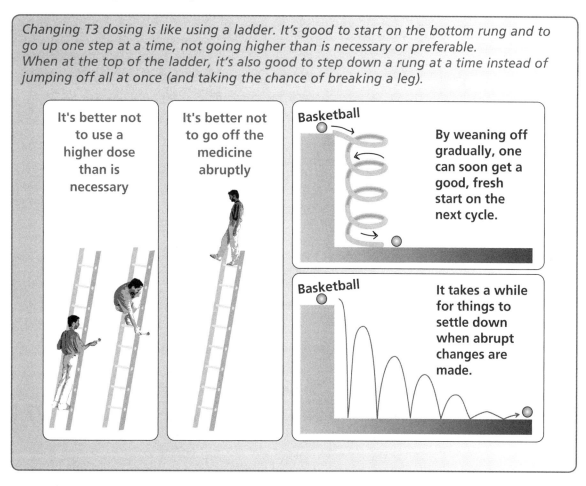

Changing T3 dosing is like using a ladder. It's good to start on the bottom rung and to go up one step at a time, not going higher than is necessary or preferable.
When at the top of the ladder, it's also good to step down a rung at a time instead of jumping off all at once (and taking the chance of breaking a leg).

It's better not to use a higher dose than is necessary

It's better not to go off the medicine abruptly

Basketball

By weaning off gradually, one can soon get a good, fresh start on the next cycle.

Basketball

It takes a while for things to settle down when abrupt changes are made.

Given that the WT3 protocol requires T3 to be dosed every 12 hours exactly, it is good to ask new patients what is the latest time they wake up on the weekends. If they wake up at 9 am on the weekends, and 7 am on weekdays, they might consider taking the medicine at 9 am and 9 pm every day, so that they do not have to wake up at 7 am on weekends. Alternatively, they may take the medicine at 7 am and 7 pm everyday if that is easier, but they will then have to set a 7 am alarm on the weekends (they can go back to sleep if they like). Of course, "weekends" here represents the days the patient usually gets up the latest, which may or may not be Saturday or Sunday.

It's best to start low and then to increase the T3 dose gradually, in order to use the smallest effective dose. The lower the exogenous dose, the easier it is to keep the T3 level steady. If one uses a large starting dose, or increases the dose in large increments, one may overshoot the lowest effective dose, thereby waiving progress and benefits by using an unnecessarily high dose.

Not only may patients poorly tolerate the abrupt discontinuation of T3, but doing so can also squander benefits obtained in the cycle by not giving the system enough time to effectively maintain endogenously what may have been re-established artificially. Moreover, stopping the medicine abruptly can also create a disturbance that could take 2 weeks to settle down before one could get a fresh start on the next cycle (if needed). Whereas, if things are let down easy with the cycle being weaned gradually and smoothly so that the endogenous system has enough time to come up steadily, then one should be able to get a relatively fresh start on the next cycle about 2 or 3 days after being completely off the present cycle. Finally, there is no need to "wean gradually" off the medicine when one is taking the smallest dose. When one is on the bottom rung of a ladder, one simply steps off.

There are two classes of pharmaceutical preparations in use today. One is manufactured pharmaceuticals, and the other is compounded pharmaceuticals. Manufactured pharmaceuticals are mass-produced by drug companies and are therefore regulated by the FDA. Compounded pharmaceuticals are prepared with pharmacies according to a doctor's prescription, and the pharmacists are regulated by their state boards of pharmacy. Relatively few pharmacies are interested in specializing in compounded pharmaceuticals for financial and regulatory reasons. However, specialized compounding pharmacies are not uncommon, and may be called upon in situations when the desired dosage or route of administration of a specific drug is not available on the market (e.g., forming a suppository out of an oral pill or capsule).

from pgs. 83, 100, 107, 155

At first, I used only traditional T3. However, I noticed that patients would often get more benefit and less side effects if they took the traditional T3 every 3 hours, 6 times a day, instead of only once or twice a day. It became very apparent that a little medicine taken at intervals, throughout the day, worked much better than a lot of medicine all at once. What I needed was a T3 preparation incorporating a sustained-release agent, but no such preparation was available on the market. So I asked a com-

from pg. 152

pounding pharmacist to prepare such a product for some of my patients. What we came up with was a T3 compound that utilizes a hydrophilic matrix system, designed to dissolve and release the

> *Proper T3 therapy is a comparatively deliberate approach. If one wants to be serious about T3 therapy, I would not recommend that it be done with instant release T3, but with a T3/HPMC compound made in the following doses: 3.75, 7.5, 15, 22.5, 30, 37.5, 45, 52.5, 60, 67.5, 75, 82.5, and 90 micrograms (higher doses are sometimes used).*

active ingredient slowly. At first, patients reported that the medicine was typically wearing off about 30 minutes before the next dose. We increased the polymer in the formula. Then, many patients reported that it seemed to wear off 15 minutes before the next dose. Each time we increased the polymer in the formula till we finally got it to last as close as possible to 12 hours (based on clinical observation). This process also revealed that patients can detect/feel small changes in their T3 levels; which is why (regardless of the particular T3 formulation), I recommend routine assessments of "how the patient is feeling."

The only mass-produced T3 medicine currently on the market (Cytomel™) is instant release. Cytomel is liothyronine sodium, which is the sodium salt of T3. Therefore, a skilled and experienced compounding pharmacy will be required in order to create a T3 product (liothyronine) that is time released [using HydroxyPropylMethylCellulose (HPMC)]. This necessitates specialized equipment (accurate scales and a v-blender) capable of precisely measuring and mixing very small quantities of pure T3 powder. This product is not best made by mixing by hand.

Although it might be difficult to obtain, I feel that the compounded T3/HPMC preparation is about 20 times more effective in the treatment of WTS, while the incidence and severity of side effects is about 20 times less as compared to instant release T3. When I first started treating WTS, Cytomel (instant release) was all I used. When I had about 300 patients at a time on Cytomel, I would get about 6–8 calls over the weekend from patients having complaints and 2–3 of those calls would be about some pretty worrisome side effects. After I switched to the compounded T3 product, it was not uncommon for me to go 6 months without an after-hours call.

I recommend a starting dose of 7.5 mcg (3.75 mcg may be used in the very rare patient for whom 7.5 is a little too high). The dose should be increased in 7.5 mcg increments by having the patient go up to the next highest strength each day, as needed. For financial reasons, it is usually best to use an assortment of doses. For example, taking five 7.5 mcg capsules each dose instead of one 37.5 mcg capsule can be almost 5 times more expensive. Also, the more capsules that are taken each dose, the more gel-forming polymer is introduced into the gut, and some patients have reported diarrhea when larger numbers of capsules are used.

Because the patient may be changing the dose every day, it is important that they have enough of the medicine to maintain or increase their dose as needed without running out before the next appointment (usually 2 weeks after starting). This minimizes the chances of the patient experiencing a hold-up in the progress of therapy, or even a setback. If her progress is disturbed, a couple of weeks of progress can be lost. Not to mention the aggravation and inconvenience to the patient and the office in having to call in another prescription, or perhaps even having to make arrangements for the office to give her a few capsules to hold her over.

Monitoring, Compliance, and Steadiness

It is usually best for the patients to have a return office visit 2 weeks after starting the T3 therapy. Body temperature patterns, as well as patient response, help guide T3 therapy. Thyroid blood tests do not direct therapy per se.

One morning temperature does not give a good feel for the steadiness of the temperature patterns, nor really do two. For this reason, I recommend that patients take their temperatures 3 times during the day while on the treatment. This gives three points on the curve, which gives one an idea of the steadiness of the body temperature patterns. I would prefer a 24-hour temperature map, but three oral temperatures is what I would consider a minimum. This is mostly because of how difficult it is to have patients comply with more than three temperature measurements per day.

It's true that we cannot make too much of these three temperatures because of possible variations in relation to meals, exercise, dosing of the T3, etc. But I view these temperature logs the way one may view the ocean. Looking out over the ocean, one can tell whether it is high tide or low tide. One can also tell whether it is choppy or calm. And just because disturbances are made by a fish jumping, or by a bird plunging in, or by the wind blowing a whitecap onto the top of a swell, that doesn't change it from being

> For the Original WT3 Protocol, I recommend new patients get a 96-capsule "starter pack" of T3/HPMC that contains 30 capsules of the 7.5's and 30 of the 15's, with 12 each of the following strengths: 22.5, 30, and 37.5 mcg.

high tide or low tide, or in general, choppy or calm. I don't make too much out of each individual temperature, but look more at the overall pattern to see how high the temperature is on average, and to get a feel for how steady it is. This analogy helps the patient see rather clearly the importance of taking the medicine and temperature measurements properly.

I strongly advise the patients to take the medicine (liothyronine sodium compounded with a sustained-release agent), every 12 hours to the minute, not even 3 minutes late, and to purchase a timer or set alarms on their cell phones to make it easier. It is best to set two recurring alarms that go off automatically at dosing times. It may be worthwhile to have an alarm that vibrates as well as sounds (so patients can perceive the alarm discreetly or in noisy environments). Alarms can be set to remind patients of temperature times as well as doses.

A temperature range (highest minus lowest) of about 0.6°F is what I consider pretty steady. A range of 1°F is getting to the point of being rather unsteady, and where symptoms more frequently begin. Ranges of 1.5–2.0°F can frequently be symptomatic, and rarely, I have seen patient's temperatures range as much as 3°F during the day.

Body temperature patterns are more useful for comparing intrapersonal data than they are for comparing one person to another. For instance, one patient might enjoy a great improvement when temperature improves from 96.5°F to 97.8°F. However, because another patient's temperature is not below 97.8°F does not mean that they will not benefit from the treatment. This is because their symptoms might resolve completely with a temperature improvement from 98.0°F to 98.6°F. I've had a few patients (very few, because usually patients temperatures are less than 98.0°F) who were symptomatic at 98.4°F and whose symptoms resolved when their temperatures were raised to 98.6°F. Mild cases can sometimes take only on the order of days to correct, from start to finish. Moreover, one person with a temperature of 98.3°F and a range of 1.0°F might not be feeling as improved as another person with a temperature averaging 98.0°F with a range of 1.5°F (who had improved from 97.0°F and a range of 1.5°F). But if the first person's temperature improves to 98.6°F with a range of 0.6°F, they are likely to feel better than they did at 98.3°F with a range of 1.0°F.

 It appears that lower levels of T3 that are more steady can often provide greater T3 stimulation of the cell than higher levels. One example of this is when a patient is doing well for 6 weeks on a dose of 45 mcg BID. Then the patient *from pg. 145* misses the timing of their dosing significantly for a couple of days resulting in unsteady T3 levels and temperatures. Let's say that in this case, the temperature drops from 98.6°F down to about 97.8°F. The patient then increases her dose, but instead of the temperature returning to normal, it simply becomes more and more unsteady as she takes more and more T3. It is only after the patient weans off the T3 therapy, allowing the T3 levels to stabilize (as the endogenous *from pg. 157* T3 production resumes), and then starts the T3 again, is she able to get her temperature back up to 98.6°F on 45 mcg *from pg. 150* BID. This kind of crumbling of the temperature is rare, but it does happen. Steadiness can often be regained without weaning off the T3 medicine (e.g., by increased compliance, or by a T4 test dose), but sometimes it is preferable to wean completely off to get a fresh start **(p112)**.

As an analogy, suppose you were participating in a contest, where the object is to carefully stack metal blocks so as to reach a certain height. The catch is that you must stack the blocks atop a small (2" × 2") platform mounted on the *from pg. 157* top end of a 3-foot long spring standing on end, and mounted to a table top. Below the 2" × 2" platform, the spring passes through the center of a broad plexiglass bowl, which is attached to the spring so that it forms a sort of "crow's nest". If done very carefully, you might be able to stack up seven blocks. The difficulty is that the more blocks that are stacked up, the more the spring tends to sway, and the more likely the blocks are to topple over. If the spring starts swaying a little, perhaps you may only be able to build up four or so blocks before they begin to topple over. So you might think, "I need to build it up higher than 4, so I'll add more blocks." But as the blocks topple over and fall into the bowl, more and more weight is added to the system, destabilizing it further if anything. So adding more blocks to a less stable system often does not increase one's chances of getting the stack any higher, and can actually decrease them. At that point, you may need to remove all the blocks, let the spring straighten up and settle down, and start again before having another good shot at stacking the blocks sufficiently high.

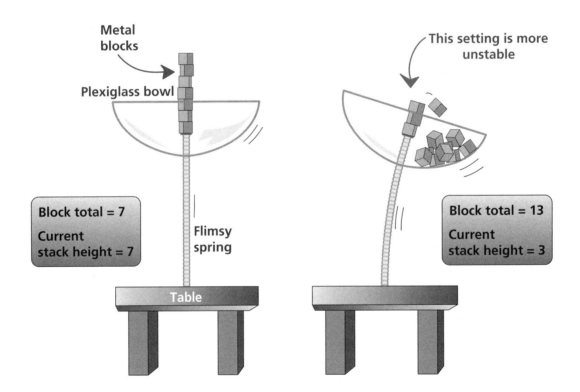

To further the analogy, let us suppose that the contest is won by reaching the desired height while having the least amount of swaying (or displacement from vertical) of the spring and stack. But one thing makes it easier to keep steady: once you are able to build the stack up to the desired level, you are allowed to remove all the blocks and start over, except this time, the table top is raised a few inches so that fewer blocks have to be stacked to reach the height line. With fewer blocks, there will tend to be less swaying/displacement. If, with with fewer blocks, you are able to reach the height line again, then you can start over again with the table being raised another few inches. And so on, until perhaps the spring reaches the height line all by itself, and with no blocks there would be minimal swaying/displacement.

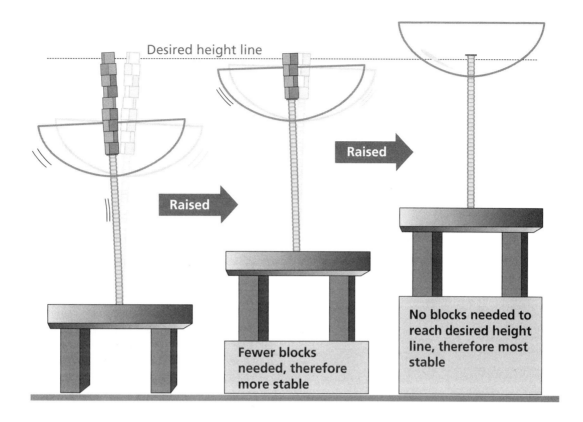

Desired height line

Raised

Raised

Fewer blocks needed, therefore more stable

No blocks needed to reach desired height line, therefore most stable

 Likewise, the smaller the dose of T3, the easier it is to keep the T3 levels steady. So the patients who always do the best on T3 therapy are those who are lucky enough to get their temperatures up on the smallest doses of T3, whether on the first cycle or a subsequent one. This is because the greater the proportion (at any given time) of a patient's T3 level that is exogenous, the more difficult it is to keep the T3 level steady. Thus, patients who are lucky enough to get their temperature up on a smaller amount of exogenous T3 have a greater proportion of endogenous T3, which is more stable. This often leads to the ideal combination of normal temperatures with a T3 level that is 100% endogenous (endogenously steady), which is the goal of treatment.

from pg. 145

As mentioned previously, this goal is accomplished by passing the thyroid system from endogenous control to exogenous control, and then back again (once or more than once). Some patients may need more than the smallest dose of the T3 therapy to get their temperatures up, so the T3 can be gradually increased until their temperatures are normal.

However, for reasons discussed previously, if a patient does need more T3 on previous cycles to achieve a normal temperature, they can often be weaned gradually while retaining benefit. This is likened to the tabletop being raised a few inches when the blocks are removed to start over.

Thus, by cycling from endogenous to exogenous and back again, a patient can often get closer and closer to normal (T3 preponderance and normal temperatures) on less and less medicine until their temperatures remain normal and their symptoms remain improved even after the treatment has been discontinued completely.

 Because the higher the doses of T3 the harder it is to keep the T3 levels steady, we want to balance between two principles: (1) the need to give more T3 to reset things, and (2) the need to give less T3 so that it is easier to keep T3 levels steady. Fortunately, one can usually get to the point of using less T3 by resetting things through this process of cycling. Based on the above analogy, it's a little harder to reach the height line on the first cycle, because the table is so low; but once the height line is held the first time (temperature captured) benefit is achieved and during the wean benefit is retained (the table is raised), so it tends to get easier and easier on subsequent tries.

from pg. 158

from pg. 150 Because more medicine is commonly used in the first cycle, this is when patients are more likely to experience side effects (due to T3 unsteadiness). Sometimes, patients may not notice much if any improvement on the first cycle. This is why I consider a therapeutic trial to encompass at least two cycles. It is common for patients to notice that half as much medicine the second time around can often bring their temperature up and improve their symptoms more as compared to twice as much medicine used during the first cycle. Because a lot of corrective work is often accomplished in the first cycle (even if it's not very obvious), I refer to the 1st cycle as the "reset" cycle, and the subsequent cycles as "fine-tuning."

Although it is difficult to be as optimistic after two cycles of T3 with no change, if the patient is not having any complaints, attempting more than two cycles can sometimes pay off. In the case of one patient, we both felt that there was a good chance we were on the right track and had exhausted other treatment options, so she went up and down on the medicine 10 times without noticing much improvement. But on the 11th cycle, her temperature finally came up, and her symptoms improved.

Also, some patients who can't seem to get their temperatures up on T3 alone can often normalize their temperatures when they take T3 plus thyroid herbal and nutritional support (such as iodine, selenium, Guggul, Bladderwrack, Blue flag iris). Apparently, the differing mechanisms of actions of these substances can be synergistic.

Unsteadiness and the T4 Test Dose

The most common side effect is fluid retention, not severe pedal edema, but a little bit of fluid retention and puffiness in the hands that can cause some achiness (e.g., rings may fit tighter). Patients may also complain of dull headache, edginess, irritability, and increased heart rate. Sometimes patients report feeling flu-like symptoms. It is easy to confuse these symptoms with those of T3 toxicity, as opposed to the real cause, which is usually the unsteadiness of T3 levels. This distinction can be made pretty well by determining if the person's temperature is above or below normal, and by use of a T4 test dose.

from pgs. 105, 110, 144, 145, 152, 156, 160 The litmus test for T3 unsteadiness is a T4 test dose, which involves giving the patient 0.0125 mg of T4 (i.e., levothyroxine/Synthroid™). Because the smallest strength typically made is 0.025 mg, I recommend giving the patient just half of this tablet (nail clippers work well for halving the tablet). Patients who complain of symptoms of T3 unsteadiness such as achiness, shakiness, or irritability, can often have their symptoms dramatically resolve about 45 minutes after the T4 test dose. Most doctors would not expect such symptom resolution upon the addition of more thyroid hormone. None-the-less, this is often the case.

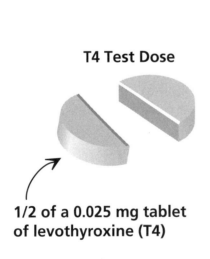

T4 Test Dose

1/2 of a 0.025 mg tablet of levothyroxine (T4)

45 minutes

The half-life of T4 is 7.5 days, so very little happens to the T4 itself within 45 minutes. This time frame is just enough for the T4 to get absorbed from the gut, enter the bloodstream, and travel to the appropriate cells of the body. T4 is a thyroid hormone receptor agonist, but it is four times less potent, and three times longer acting than T3. Therefore, I believe that by floating a little T4 into the system, one can coat the receptors, to provide some impedance against the unmitigated stimulation of the receptors by unsteady T3 levels. In this way, the T3 and T4 stimulation statistically average to provide for a steadier stimulation of the cells.

Characteristically, a T4 test dose does not negatively affect temperatures, energy levels, or overall well-being. In fact, the T4 test dose is so often effective that it can almost be considered an antidote for T3 unsteadiness (which is why it is used as a litmus test for unsteadiness). If a person's side effects are coming from T3 therapy, then the patient is absorbing the T3 therapy. If so, then the patient will absorb the T4, which will enter the bloodstream, attach to the receptor site, and ultimately level out erratic T3 concentrations. If, after 45 minutes or so, the patients' symptoms resolve or significantly improve, this strongly suggests that the patient was experiencing T3 unsteadiness. If the T4 test dose is not successful at relieving symptoms, then it is more likely that the symptoms are due to some other influence (e.g., the flu, or common cold), rather than due to the T3. The silver lining to these side effects is that they often go away quickly (with T4) and they give the patient an experience of what "not feeling well" is like. Thus, the next time the patient feels this way, they will know to take T4 again.

Taking too many rescue doses of T4 can ultimately work against the grain of this protocol. This is because the resetting of the thyroid system seems to be triggered by the depletion of rT3 levels, which requires depletion of T4 levels. In addition to slowing the depletion of T4, the regular use of T4 also appears to increase patient susceptibility to their low thyroid symptoms worsening under stress (as compared to patients who are taking T3 alone). This may be due to the fact that the T3 supply of patients taking more T4 is more dependent on the enzymatic conversion of T4.

Therefore, the T4 dose should be taken as needed for circumstances suspicious of T3 unsteadiness, and NOT on a continual basis. As it turns out, the odds that a particular person will ever require a T4 test dose is small. However, in the event that it is a reoccurring problem, it usually manifests on a reoccurring time interval. If this is the case, then T4 can be given ahead of that same time interval in order to stave off the T3 unsteadiness-related symptoms. For example, a patient taking 60 mcg of T3 BID may find she needs 0.0125 mg of T4 every 4 days. Incidentally, if her dose of T3 goes up to 75 mcg BID she may find she needs the 0.0125 mg of T4 every 3 days.

This effect also varies from person to person. Some patients may find that on their current dose, they need to repeat the T4 test dose every day while others may need it every week. But again, most patients probably won't run into this problem.

Patients whose side effects are not very significant should avoid taking the T4 test dose, unless they absolutely need relief. Patients experiencing side effects should be reeducated about the importance of strict dosing time adherence. Sometimes, improved compliance alone will enable their systems to stabilize on their own. If so, it usually only takes 4–5 days for things to settle down, but may take as long as 10–14 days for some patients.

from pg. 153 In some cases, the 0.0125 mg dose only provides partial relief. This most often occurs when patients are taking more than about 45 mcg of T3 twice a day. In this situation, a second (but not 3rd or 4th) 0.0125 mg dose of T4 can be given about 1.5 hours later, in the hopes of full resolution of symptoms. If this strategy is successful, the next time the patient requires T4 while taking the same dose of T3, he can start with a T4 dose of 0.025 mg.

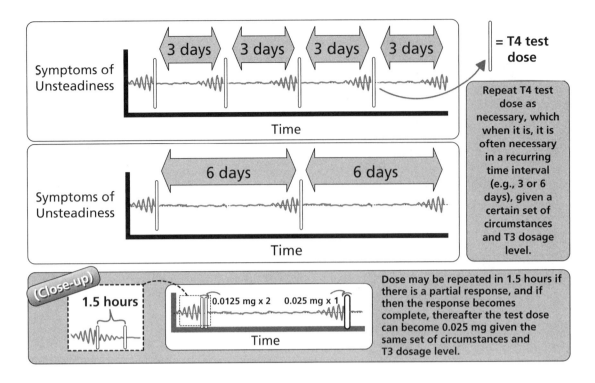

When the side effects are severe, or continue in spite of T4 test dosing (because T4 test dosing is sometimes not enough to "recapture" the steadiness of very unsteady T3 levels), it is usually best to wean from T3 therapy to let things steady down again. In such cases, side effects usually resolve before the cycle has been completely weaned, so 2–3 days between cycles should be sufficient.

from pg. 158

On the other hand, the side effects may not resolve until after the patient has been weaned completely off the cycle for a couple of days. When this occurs, it is usually best to have the patient stay off therapy another couple of days after the side effects have resolved, and before starting another cycle (if another is started). This allows things to settle down sufficiently to get a nice steady start on the next cycle.

from pg. 157

How long before next cycle, if this cycle is being weaned because of side effects?

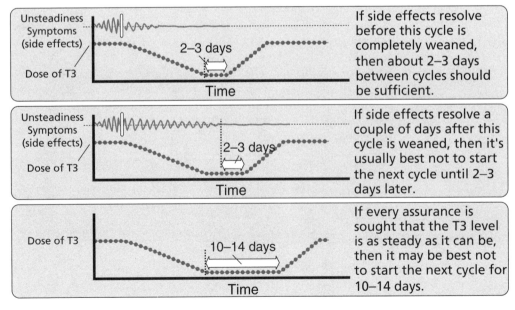

If every assurance is being sought that the patient's T3 level is as steady as it can possibly be, then it may be advisable to stay off the T3 cycle for 10–14 days before starting the next cycle. However, in most circumstances it is not necessary to wait that long. It is important for the level to be as steady as possible, but it is also good for the treatment to not go on unnecessarily, so usually 2 or 3 days between cycles is sufficient.

This case study illustrates the point above:

A patient starts a cycle of T3, but does not respond as well as one might expect based on presentation. Upon questioning the patient, it seems there may be T3 unsteadiness due to poor compliance on dosing times. The patient responds somewhat to a T4 test dose, but it is decided to wean and restart. She weans off the T3 and restarts and still does not do very well, but she only stayed off the T3 for 2 days between cycles, which may not have been enough time for the treatment to settle down. The patient is disillusioned, and it is not clear whether the T3 will not help her or whether she didn't adequately settle down between cycles. So to be sure, the patient weans off the T3 and waits 12 days before starting the next cycle. This time she achieves success. These results suggest that T3 unsteadiness was in fact the underlying problem.

T3 therapy should not be considered a "no pain, no gain" scenario. With T3 therapy, patients should only feel better, and not have to "just deal" with uncomfortable symptoms. Therefore, any complaints should be considered indicators that the T3 therapy needs to be adjusted. Remember, it is easier to manage any potential side effects, by "nipping them in the bud" as soon as they appear, rather than letting them develop into harder to manage problems.

A patient may experience decreased symptomatic improvement (clinical status) due to T3 unsteadiness before she ever develops any side effects. When this may be the case, a T4 test dose can be very illuminating.

from pg. 102

The T4 test dose is useful not only with regard to side effects but it is also valuable to see if unsteady T3 levels may be hindering a patient's resolution of low thyroid symptoms. For instance, if a patient's body temperature is averaging 98.6°F, but her symptoms are not as improved as one might expect they should be, it may be because of unsteady T3 levels (from inconsistent dosing times, strange sleep, or work hours, etc.).

This problem is easily checked, because if the patient's low thyroid symptoms improve significantly within 45 minutes of a T4 test dose, then it is likely there was some T3 unsteadiness that can be addressed accordingly. The T4 test dose is extremely useful in many situations, and can give one a great deal of information, as well as guidance in situations where T3 unsteadiness is suspected.

Summary of Original WT3 Protocol Concepts

T3 is being produced, having its effect, and being dissipated continuously. The body responds to T3 therapy through negative feedback inhibition. There are two important forces at work: (1) T3 therapy, and (2) the body's response to that therapy. Both must be taken into account to keep things steady.

Patients tend to feel best on the T3 therapy when the temperature is not only high enough but also steady enough for the system to work well. Usually, the steadier the better.

Exogenous T3 therapy is a somewhat unsteady source of T3 (as compared to endogenous production). The higher the dose of T3 therapy the harder it is to keep it steady. Sometimes less stimulation that is more steady can result in more progress than more stimulation that is less steady (i.e., steadiness is everything). It's not just a matter of quantity, it's also a matter of how steady that quantity is being supplied. So when the T3 dose is increased a "notch", it is not so static as that sounds.

The active form of thyroid hormone is being used, not a prohormone that must be converted, and that's a huge distinction, and should make a difference in the way one approaches thyroid treatment. T3 can be thought of as providing the power of the thyroid system while T4 can provide a lot of stability. The T4 test dose can be used to stabilize unsteady T3 levels/stimulation. Cycling off and on the T3 therapy is often necessary for patients to make progress toward complete recovery. Once the thyroid system becomes destabilized with unsteady T3 levels, it can take a while to settle back down again, especially if left on its own.

When weaning off a cycle of T3 it is best to do so gradually to help keep T3 levels as steady as possible.

It's best to allow the thyroid system to settle down between cycles (by staying off the T3 for at least 2–3 days or as long as 10–14 days between cycles). If the next cycle is started while the thyroid system is still unsteady, then that cycle may start unsteady and stay unsteady. Thus, it's important to strive on each cycle of T3 therapy to start steady (steady T3 levels) and stay as steady as possible right from the start.

Patients frequently need less T3 on subsequent cycles than they did on previous ones.

If the T3 therapy is weaned slowly enough that the temperature doesn't drop then the body is more likely to retain and maintain naturally what the cycle re-established artificially; that is, if the body is given enough time to come up endogenously to take back good control of the system and run with it. Weaning a cycle too fast can squander some or all of the benefit of that cycle. On the other hand, one doesn't want to wean cycles unnecessarily slowly, otherwise, they last unnecessarily long **(p105)**.

With T3 therapy, the system can often be reset well enough to remain functioning even after the treatment has been discontinued. This brings up a frequent choice: when an attempt is going well, do you stay with what you're doing, to enjoy the benefits and not rock the boat? Or, do you wean off the cycle to see if you will need lower doses on the next cycle (if another cycle is needed at all) to normalize the temperature? Remember, the lower the dose of T3, the easier it is for T3 levels to be steady. See Q9 for a discussion that will help you decide when to choose one option, and when to choose the other.

T3 Therapy in Hypothyroid Patients

In this section, the term "hypothyroid" is meant to describe those patients who actually have low thyroid gland function. Not everyone who has been diagnosed as hypothyroid is in fact hypothyroid, and even if they were hypothyroid at one point does not necessarily mean that they are hypothyroid now. Patients who have been diagnosed as hypothyroid in the past based on clinical parameters may have been suffering from WTS and not hypothyroidism. By far, most people who are clinically hypothyroid and who have thyroid-responsive symptoms are suffering from WTS and not hypothyroidism. So patients who present on T4-containing medicines with a past diagnosis of hypothyroidism may not actually be hypothyroid. However, some people *are* hypothyroid, and so it is helpful to obtain as much of the past medical information and tests upon which the patients' diagnoses have been made, so that nothing gets lost or changed in the translation. If these are no longer available, always take thyroid diagnoses with a grain of salt.

Patients who are hypothyroid and who are well replaced with T4-containing medicines to the satisfaction of blood tests may still be suffering from WTS. If their temperatures are low, and they are still suffering from their familiar symptoms of hypothyroidism, they may have peripheral thyroid transport, T4 to T3 conversion, or receptor resistance issues **(p93)**. For instance, I had one patient who presented to the office taking 0.3 mg of T4. She had a T4 level of 18 mcg/dl and a TSH of 0.2 mIU/ml, yet her temperature ran more than a degree below normal, and she had severe symptoms of low thyroid function. This patient was weaned off the T4 and started on T3 therapy. Her symptoms resolved when her temperature was brought back to normal. This type of presenting history and response to treatment is very common.

from
pg. 157
When a patient presents with a low body temperature and symptoms of low thyroid system function, in spite of being treated with a T4-containing medicine, and a therapeutic trial of T3 being contemplated, it is usually best to wean the T4-containing medicine before beginning the T3 therapy. Ideally, patients should not begin T3 therapy until they have been off T4-containing therapy for at least 10 days. However, if they begin to worsen clinically, the T3 therapy will be started before the 10 days have passed. After the 10-day period has passed, one may "chase" the patients' temperatures by increasing the T3 therapy as often as every day according to the protocol in an attempt to normalize their body temperature patterns.

Weaning off T4-containing medicine for 10 days before pursuing T3 therapy

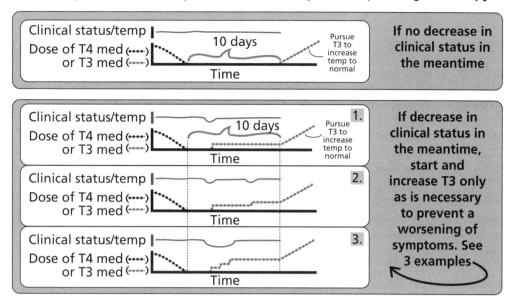

The rationale for these recommendations is that when patients present with WTS, they are in T4/rT3 preponderance. This is even more the case if the patients have been pushed too far in the wrong direction with the wrong medicine (i.e., T4).

If there is a T4/rT3 preponderance, the T4 and the rT3 will compete with any exogenous T3. So from the start, more T3 will be needed to generate the same amount of thyroid stimulation of the cell than would be needed if there was no T4/rT3 preponderance. This would call for higher doses of T3, which are harder to keep steady. However, the people that always do the best on T3 therapy are the ones that are lucky enough to get their temperatures back up on the smallest amounts of the medicine.

Generally speaking, the patients who have had their temperatures captured on smaller doses of the T3 are closer to being finished with the treatment. This is because T3 therapy involves cycling the patients on and off the medicine to get them closer and closer to normal, on less and less medicine, until they do not need medicine at all. Thus, some patients who are put on higher levels of medicine will just have to cycle on and off one or more times to be as far along as they would have been had they not needed such high doses. And cycling on and off the medicine takes time (each cycle can take over 1 month).

By weaning off T4, while staying on the smallest dose possible of T3 (preferably none) for 10 days before "chasing" the temperature, T4 and rT3 are given a chance to go out of the system, thereby depleting the T4/rT3 preponderance, and the competition against T3. Looking at the half-life of T4, this process is not complete within 10 days, but I feel it is sufficiently complete for therapy to be started (if you go strictly by half-life, one may want to wait 14–17 days or more).

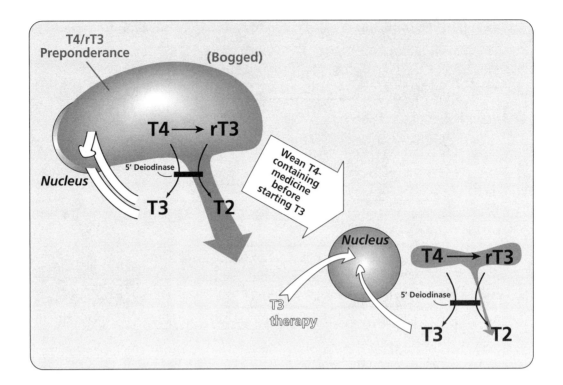

By allowing the competition against T3 to diminish, the patients are often able to capture their temperatures on much lower doses than if they had started increasing the T3 therapy sooner (against more competition). This strategy can save a patient from undergoing additional cycles and months' worth of treatment. Thus, even though it is often hard for the patients to hold off chasing the temperature with T3 for the 10 days while T4 and rT3 levels are being depleted, it is important for them to know that by doing so, they can often be as far along in 3 weeks as they otherwise might be in 6 months. Note that the 10-day period does not begin until the patient is actually off the T4-containing medicine, which may itself need to be weaned in stages over a few days, depending on how much the patient is taking.

If the patient is on 0.075 mg of T4 (a low dose), it can probably be stopped in one step (if the patient does not appear to be brittle). Otherwise, you can cut the dose in half for 2 days and then discontinue it. If the patient is on around 0.3 mg, it is recommended that they go down a third (0.1 mg) every 2 days until it is discontinued. Generally, the less constitutionally resilient a patient appears to be (use clinical judgment), the more gradually I wean the T4-containing medicine. However, there is a delicate line that must be walked here, because the longer it takes to wean the patient off the T4, the longer it will be before the 10-day period begins.

Patients should be reminded and reassured that should they clinically worsen during the weaning process (before T3 therapy is used to chase the temperature), that the T3 can be started to support them if needed. But again, it should be stressed that it would be in their best interest to remain off the T3 for 10 days, if possible. However, if during this 10-day period, the patient's symptoms are giving them a hard time with normal daily functioning, they should start on the smallest dose of T3 sooner, and increase it as needed to prevent them from getting worse.

Far more people are able to stay comfortably off all thyroid medicine for the 10 days than you might expect. Many patients are surprised that they are able to stop all thyroid medicine and stay off for 10 days and tolerate it as well as they do. Most patients don't need to start any T3 during the 10-day period, but are able to hold their own.

It is worth emphasizing the degree of progress that is often made during the 10-day period. By starting the treatment in this manner, the patient can almost completely reverse in a matter of 3 weeks what has perhaps taken years to develop, thereby giving the patient a virtually fresh start.

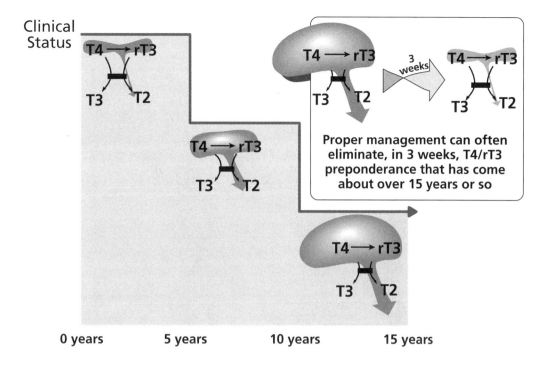

Clinical Status

Proper management can often eliminate, in 3 weeks, T4/rT3 preponderance that has come about over 15 years or so

0 years   5 years   10 years   15 years

This is especially encouraging in cases where patients have been pushed too far in the wrong direction with the wrong medicine. If the treatment is started in this manner, all the negative progress can be all but eliminated in a few weeks, so the patient is better prepared to make positive progress.

If it is not perfectly evident whether or not the patient is hypothyroid, when one weans the T3 therapy, one may do so without adding back any T4 supplementation to see if perhaps the patient can maintain normal body temperature patterns without T4 or T3 supplementation (c11) (Q16).

If the conditions are not favorable to challenge the patient, or it is clear that the patient definitely does not have any thyroid gland function (e.g., thyroid gland has been surgically removed), then while the patient is being gradually weaned off a cycle of T3 therapy, he or she must be supported with T4 supplementation.

One exception to the above principle is in cases where another cycle of T3 therapy is to be started once the present cycle is weaned, one may be able to avoid adding back any T4 between cycles (if the patients remain comfortable) even in patients who are somewhat hypothyroid. The reason one might want to consider this is because if one *does* add back T4 while one cycle of T3 is being weaned, it is usually best (once that T3 cycle has been weaned) to have the patients wean back off that T4, and not start the next cycle of T3 for 10 days (as described above), if comfortable. Thus, one may be able to save some treatment time if one is able to comfortably avoid having to add back the T4 between cycles in the first place.

Having said all that about it usually being better to wean T4 before starting T3, some doctors prefer to start the T3 while weaning the T4. This is easier to explain to patients. The doctor may have the patient start the T3 dosing tomorrow, while weaning off the T4 in the next day or so. This is not necessarily a bad way to go. The T4 and rT3 are going out of the system and T3 is coming into the system, and that's the main objective. Patients tolerate this approach well. The only downside is that the patient may not make as much progress as quickly, however, even that is theoretical, because no double-blind studies have been done.

As stated previously, many patients who have been diagnosed as being hypothyroid in the past, may never have been, or if they were, may no longer be. After cycling through T3 therapy, this type of patient may feel better off all thyroid medicine than they ever did while on it. However, even the patients who are hypothyroid, and who need some sort of T4 support (after cycling through T3 therapy), can often get more T3 stimulation out of less T4 than they were previously taking. For this reason, when T4 supplementation is added back, it is best to try lower levels first, before returning to the patient's original level of T4 supplementation.

For example, if a patient presented on 0.2 mg/day of T4, it would be good to add back only about 0.025 mg/day of T4 when you start weaning the T3, and increase the T4 only as needed to support the temperature (especially if she has a history consistent with being pushed in the wrong direction). Many patients who present on doses as high as 0.2 mg of T4 can often enjoy much better temperatures and clinical status on 0.05 mg of T4 than they ever did on 0.2 mg, after they have been cycled through T3 therapy. Presumably this is because the T3 therapy eliminates the T4/rT3 preponderance such that the T4 conversion and T3 stimulation of the cells is much "cleaner," or more efficient.

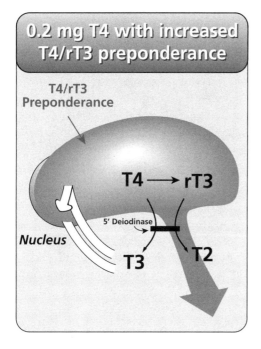

0.2 mg T4 with increased T4/rT3 preponderance

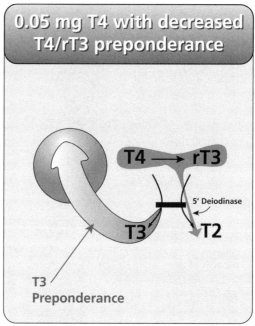

0.05 mg T4 with decreased T4/rT3 preponderance

The reasoning behind replacing T4 with the smallest dose possible is because the higher the T4 level, the more opportunity there is for stressful circumstances to shunt much of it to rT3, and the more opportunity there is for the shunting to get stuck that way due to T4/rT3 preponderance.

Interestingly, the most precipitous onsets of WTS have often been in patients who had been on large doses of T4-containing medicines, and then experienced a triggering stress. Also, if patients relapse when they are on 0.2 mg of T4 when 0.05 mg would have been sufficient, those relapses are likely to be more severe, and more difficult to correct, than they would have been if they were on 0.05 mg.

A patient who is being supplemented with a combination of T4 and T3 therapy is more likely to experience a decline in clinical status when presented with a physical, mental, or emotional stress than is a patient who is well replaced on T3 therapy alone. This is because a patient's T3 supply is more dependent on T4 to T3 conversion by the deiodinating enzyme when the patient is taking some T4 as well. Given these observations, some might wonder if it would be better to leave hypothyroid patients on T3 therapy, rather than to put them back on T4. Not usually. When T4 is 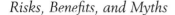 from pg. 158 working (temperature's normal, patient feels well), it's an excellent choice. It's once-a-day, ubiquitous, inexpensive, well-tolerated, familiar to all, and has a long half-life. For these reasons, I generally prefer T4 for long-term maintenance of hypothyroid patients, but I think long-term T3 therapy is fine for those that prefer it. Also, if hypothyroid patients ever notice that the T4 is not working for them, they can always consider going on T3 therapy for a time to "clean out" or reset their systems.

Risks, Benefits, and Myths

 As with all medical treatments, it is important to carefully weigh the potential risks and benefits of T3 therapy before initiating. The major consideration in terms of risk of T3 therapy is the impact it can have on the heart. Cardiovascular from pg. 146 disease is a major problem in our country. Every day many people who are not on thyroid medicine have heart attacks, strokes, and develop arrhythmias. Unsteady T3 levels can increase a patient's chances of increased heart rate and palpitations. If a patient is already on the verge of having a heart attack or a stroke, these cardiovascular side effects could aggravate the situation.

Cardiac support herbs like Crataegus (protective cardiac effects) and Convallaria (helps maintain healthy normal sinus rhythm) can provide useful support for patients taking T3 therapy.

Crataegus and *Convallaria* have been used for centuries by herbalists in the treatment of certain cardiac dysfunctions. *Convallaria* has been used for congestive heart failure and cardiomyopathy, while *Crataegus* has been used as an all-purpose cardiac and vascular tonic.

Crataegus (Hawthorne Tree) species are actually several varieties of the Hawthorne tree, and is known in Europe as the "Mayflower." *Crataegus* does not contain cardiac glycosides, but rather a group of flavonoids. These flavonoids have anti-inflammatory, anti-oxidant, and protective cardiac effects. Extracts of *Crataegus* leaf, flower, and berry have been shown to promote calcium influx via effects on sodium and potassium ATPase mechanisms, and to promote calcium concentrations affecting myocontractility.[101,102] *Crataegus* constituents also act as natural angiotensin converting enzyme (ACE) inhibitors, and are not only helpful in treating high blood pressure, but also elevated cholesterol levels, angina pectoris, and atherosclerosis.[103–105]

Convallaria majallus (Lily of the Valley) contains cardiac glycosides. For centuries, many herbalists and medical practitioners considered *Convallaria majallus* to be safer than *Digitalis*. The *Convallaria* plant transforms convalloside (the basic metabolic glycoside) into convallatoxin and other cardiac glycosides.[106] Convallatoxin affects vasoconstriction and vasodilation,[107] and cardiac stroke volume, pulse pressure, and cAMP activity are all enhanced by *Convallaria*.[108] *Convallamaroside* may reduce angiogenesis and have anti-tumor effects.[109] *Convallaria* has also been shown to be a lipoxygenase inhibitor.[110]

The risks of T3 therapy are more short-term (during treatment) than they are long-term (see myths below, as well as a discussion of osteoporosis in Q17). It is sometimes difficult to avoid unsteady T3 levels, and so it might not be advisable to implement T3 therapy in those patients who may not have the cardiovascular endurance to tolerate an increase in T3-level-unsteadiness (e.g., certain elderly patients). For the most part, one should not expect any drastic problems if T3 therapy is administered properly (i.e., no drastic changes, strict dosing time adherence, and swift side effect management).

Another risk is that some practitioners or medical personnel may not understand the importance of taking the T3 therapy on time, and not stopping it abruptly. They may not understand the significance, clinical presentation, or management of unsteady T3 levels. They may also attribute the symptoms of unsteady T3 levels to excess T3 levels in terms of quantity (as opposed to quality of steadiness), or to some other cause. All of these misconceptions can have a negative effect on outcome.

This issue would probably be most significant in the emergency medical setting. If the patient was in a serious accident and was unconscious, then the doctors might not know that the patient was taking T3. As the hours and days passed, the T3 level and metabolism might drop without the doctors even knowing it. This could adversely affect recovery.

T3 therapy will not work for everyone. So, it is important to think of T3 therapy as a therapeutic trial, and not a cure-all panacea. However, it is amazing to observe the drastic difference that normalizing a low body temperature can make on a patient's quality of life.

If patients symptoms resolve with T3 therapy, does that prove they had a thyroid system disorder? Not necessarily. However, it is clear that proper T3 therapy (based on the WTS protocol described in this book) does provide reproducible and predictable results.

The results I have observed since providing the WT3 protocol are very encouraging. Patients often enjoy complete resolution of very debilitating complaints, with that resolution persisting even after treatment has been discontinued. This is a much better result than is delivered by virtually all the symptomatic therapies to which these patients are routinely subjected.

What percentage of reasonable candidates will respond well to the T3 therapy described in this textbook is difficult to quantify precisely because of semantics of terms, and because it depends on the condition of the patients in question. I have been willing to treat relatively mild cases, as well as more severe ones. Many of the patients that respond most easily to the treatment are the ones who have been caught in the earlier stages of the condition. However, in my experience, at least 65% of patients could be characterized as being very happy with this treatment approach.

If the treatment is not administered carefully, only about 75–80% of patients will notice some clear improvement. If the treatment is administered carefully, the yield can be increased to at least 90% of patients noticing some unequivocal improvement in their symptoms. That is, there will be, at minimum, some improvement in at least one symptom. Only about 10% of patients experience discouraging results.

What is not conveyed in these numbers is what a profound difference is made in the lives of those people who do respond well to the treatment. Imagine a patient who has suffered with debilitating symptoms of fatigue, migraines, PMS, depression, and anxiety, lumbering along for years with little relief. Then, T3 therapy is initiated and all the symptoms completely resolve (the salient word here being *completely*) almost as if they were never really there, when other treatments have helped very little, if at all. When such patients see how simple it was to resolve their symptoms, they often are upset that they had to suffer with the symptoms for so long. Patients are often incredulous that something so simple has been overlooked for so long.

How many patients remain improved even after the treatment has been discontinued? It's not clear whether patients who have finished treatment do not return because they stay normal, or for some other reason. Official follow-up studies have not been done, but would be very interesting.

What I have observed is that many of the patients that do experience a relapse of symptoms similar to those that resolved with T3 therapy have come back for repeat treatment. These relapses very typically occur after a major stress event (usually emotional or mental pressure), many months after the treatment has been discontinued. Such patients are often quite anxious to begin treatment again. Remember, the earlier a relapse is caught once it occurs (e.g., 2 weeks vs. 1 year), the easier it is to correct it. The T3 therapy can be repeated as needed throughout a person's life.

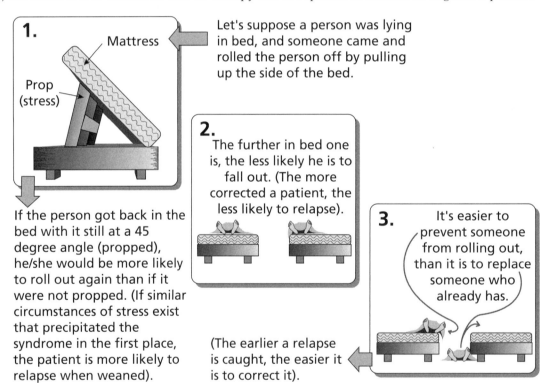

1. Mattress / Prop (stress)

Let's suppose a person was lying in bed, and someone came and rolled the person off by pulling up the side of the bed.

If the person got back in the bed with it still at a 45 degree angle (propped), he/she would be more likely to roll out again than if it were not propped. (If similar circumstances of stress exist that precipitated the syndrome in the first place, the patient is more likely to relapse when weaned).

2. The further in bed one is, the less likely he is to fall out. (The more corrected a patient, the less likely to relapse).

(The earlier a relapse is caught, the easier it is to correct it).

3. It's easier to prevent someone from rolling out, than it is to replace someone who already has.

I have enjoyed a very good rapport with my patients, and I can see little difference in the type of patients that return (after relapse) and the ones that do not. This leads me to believe that the large majority of patients do not readily relapse, because if they did, I would expect many of them to return for repeat treatment. And only a relatively small percentage of patients return for repeat treatment. In fact, some patients have come back after more than one relapse on the order of a year apart. For example, one patient did well with treatment and stayed well for about a year off treatment. She experienced a relapse when her son totaled her car. She was more easily corrected after this relapse than originally, and she stayed well for another year. She relapsed again when someone was trying to persuade this same son to go to the Bahamas to traffic in drugs. She again responded well to treatment, and is doing well off treatment as far as I am aware.

If the purpose of T3 therapy is to leave a person more endogenously T3-rich after therapy than before, then the question arises: Is it possible that a person can be left with an endogenous thyroid milieu that is too T3 rich? Of the many thousands of patients I have treated, I have wondered if this were not the case in about three of the patients (some symptoms of T3-level unsteadiness, with temperatures a few tenths above 98.6°F after treatment had been discontinued). These patients were not very uncomfortable but did not seem as well adjusted as they should have been. There are some natural circumstances that tend to slow a person's T4 to T3 conversion down below normal (stress, fasting). So at least the circumstances in the world tend to correct a slightly rich milieu rather than promulgate it. And one can always recommend fasting for a few days (as I did in those three cases) in order to increase the shunting of T4 toward rT3. The patients did not have persistent complaints, and the fasting seemed to help, although the patients were lost to long-term follow-up.

Myths

A considerable number of myths have been generated about the thyroid system in general, and the T3 molecule in particular. These myths seem a lot like those stories that change a little each time they're passed from one person to another, until they are no longer accurate and are without basis, but are still enthusiastically and authoritatively presented as fact.

Myth #1: *T4 is good, but T3 is a bad molecule; it damages the body, and its only clinical effects are negative.*

T3 is a molecule that is present from birth in every human's body, and is absolutely necessary for good health. The difference between exogenous T3 and endogenous T3 is not a chemical one, but how they are delivered to the body. It is important for exogenous T3 to be delivered as well as possible to limit adverse side effects, but it cannot and has not directly damaged heart, brain, or other tissues. Also, T3 does not expose the body chemically to anything more than exogenous T4 does, because T4 is T3 waiting to happen. In fact, T4 has to be converted into T3 in order to have its maximum effect. Before the principles of management of WTS were developed, T3 was being used in ways that did not make pharmacologic or physiologic sense, and so far more side effects were experienced. But that is no fault of T3, and is to be expected from any medicine that is being administered improperly. With appropriate T3 therapy, there should be very little side effects, and patients should only feel better. However, there is a chance side effects can develop (as with any treatment). The occurrence of side effects is an indication that the T3 therapy is not ideally adjusted, and that fine-tuning is required to make those side effects go away.

Myth #2: *T3 will atrophy the gland and cause a permanent dependence on thyroid hormone.*

Of course exogenous thyroid hormone therapy will suppress endogenous function for a time, but no evidence has ever shown that it can damage a previously healthy gland to prevent it from functioning normally again after the medicine is discontinued. There are many euthyroid (normal gland function) patients that have been on thyroid hormone therapy for years because somewhere along the line, someone felt it was reasonable in their cases. Many of these patients' own thyroid functions have been almost completely suppressed for over 20 years, having very low TSH (a normal T4 level in a patient on a T4-containing medicine cannot hide the fact that the patient's own system is virtually completely suppressed). And yet these patients, when weaned off T4-containing medicine and cycled properly on and off T3 therapy, often do better *off all* thyroid medicine, with regard to their previously partially-responsive low thyroid symptoms, than they ever did while *on* T4-containing medicine. Their systems come back up easily after 20 years of suppressive therapy, much less after a few months' worth.

Myth #3: *Once a person starts on thyroid treatment, they will need it for the rest of their life.*

Persons who have had all the thyroid tissue in their bodies removed or destroyed, will need some form of supplementation all of their lives. But that does not mean everyone else will. Even glandular insufficiencies of the thyroid system can be temporary. But especially, people without glandular insufficiencies can frequently be weaned off treatment successfully, after their symptoms have resolved with treatment.

Myth #4: *T3 is like cocaine or amphetamines (i.e., 'speed') and is thus very addictive.*

Perhaps the biggest thing that amphetamines and T3 have in common is that they were both abused decades ago in weight-loss treatments. Perhaps this is why some doctors remember them in their minds as being similar, and maybe the doctors who subscribe to this myth have simply confused what the similarity was (weight loss also comes to mind for some with cocaine). It's a little like saying that water and arsenic are just alike because they both have been used to commit murder. The difference though is that you can live without arsenic, but you cannot live without water. Likewise, you can live without cocaine and amphetamines, but T3 is physiologically necessary. Of course T3 therapy is not candy, and it is not for everyone (everyone needs exogenous water, but only for some do the potential benefits of T3 therapy outweigh the risks). Like any medical treatment, T3 therapy does have its risks, but addiction is not one of them.

T3 is naturally found in the body, while amphetamines and cocaine are not. T3, cocaine, and amphetamines are totally different pharmacologically, and in their mechanisms and sites of action. Cocaine is an alkaloid, while amphetamines are sympathomimetic amines, and both have their actions on the central nervous system. T3, on the other hand, is an amino acid derivative that has its action only on thyroid hormone receptors, which are found in all the tissues of the body.

Cocaine and amphetamines might give a normal person a "high" of some sort, but excess T3 makes normal people feel worse if anything, not better. If a person is very thirsty, then there's nothing quite like a long drink of water. But if a person's not thirsty, a long drink of water is not that enjoyable. Likewise, the purpose of proper T3 therapy is to eliminate classic symptoms of low body temperature and low thyroid function to bring a person's clinical status up to normal, not above normal.

When people are weaned off cocaine and amphetamines, they often have withdrawal symptoms (a characteristic of physical dependence). But when people are properly weaned off T3 therapy, they often retain a benefit. It is not wise to stop any routine drug treatment abruptly, because this does not give the patient's body enough time to bounce back. The weaning process is comfortably accomplished in days without withdrawal, rather than with great discomfort over months.

Other Considerations

Because there is no molecular difference between exogenous and endogenous T3, true allergic reactions are very rare. However, T3 therapy can interact indirectly with other medicines in that all medicines can have side effects, and those side effects can be additive. For example, T3, caffeine, decongestants, antihistamines, antidepressants, and asthma medicines can lead to nervousness, jitteriness, and palpitations. So when taken together, the chances of those side effects occurring may increase. Likewise, beta-blockers can suppress some of the mechanisms the body uses to adjust to T3 therapy (increased sympathetic tone in response to a drop in blood pressure in a patient who has over-compensated to an increment in dose of T3). Thus, patients whose blood pressure is being controlled with an ACE inhibitor or diuretic are more likely to acclimate very easily to T3 therapy.

Because the body is a complex, interrelated system, a drug that has its direct effect on one part of the system can indirectly affect another part. So, the effects of two drugs working on slightly different parts of the system can have indirect effects that enhance or diminish the effects of the other (i.e., synergism vs. antagonism). For example, the direct and indirect effects of the administration of estrogens, progesterones, and adrenal hormones may enhance or diminish a patient's responses to T3 therapy. If progress in T3 therapy seems to be impeded, a change in the dosage of other medications sometimes frees up the system enough for progress to continue (e.g., decreasing a conjugated estrogen dose from 0.625 mg/day to 0.3 mg/day).

It is much more important to take the T3 therapy exactly on time than for it to be taken on an empty stomach (which might provide a little more consistency in the dosing conditions from dose to dose). For this reason, I do not instruct that the medicine should be taken on an empty stomach because when such counsel is given, patients will frequently miss their dosage times by hours at a time trying to accomplish it.

Interestingly, if a patient changes time zones, then he may experience symptoms of unsteadiness even if his T3 therapy dose stays on the time schedule of his original time zone. One explanation for this phenomenon is the changes in the influence of the adrenal hormone system on body temperature patterns that results from a mild change in diurnal variation as influenced by the stimulation of the retinae by light, and perhaps also because of consequent changes in dietary patterns.

If the patient is not having any complaints with T3 therapy, then he or she may exercise normally. Generally, if the patient was going to have much difficulty while exercising, the patient would likely be able to notice some warnings or symptoms of unsteadiness prior to exercise. It is generally recommended that the patient follow a moderate exercise program to help encourage his/her body to return to normal health.

Alcohol, caffeine, and smoking can influence proper T3 therapy because they can influence body temperature patterns, and it is generally best to avoid these substances during treatment. There is, however, no direct chemical interaction with thyroid hormones and alcohol, caffeine, and smoking. But because the side effects of caffeine, smoking, and alcohol can be similar to the side effects of thyroid hormone therapy, their effects can be additive.

For patients who have inconsistent sleep and work hours (e.g., changing work shifts every other week), it is sometimes more difficult for them to respond as easily to T3 therapy because of their tendency toward unsteady T3 levels.

The thyroid system is dynamic and not static. If the patient responded in a certain way to a thyroid medicine given a certain way in the past, that does not necessarily mean he or she will respond in the same way if that medicine were to be given again using a different dosing schedule. Also, how a person has responded to medical therapies, stresses, lifestyle changes, diets, and other influences before proper T3 therapy doesn't necessarily predict how that person will respond to such influences during or after T3 therapy.

from
pg. 145
It is not wise to stop the medicine abruptly. If 100 patients stopped their T3 therapy abruptly, about 90% would not have complaints, about 5% would notice significant fatigue and achiness, and about 1% might feel exhausted, light-headed upon standing, and/or clammy, even to the extent of being rather incapacitated for several days or even a few weeks.

Thyroid medicine is pregnancy category A, which is the safest category for medicines that can be taken during pregnancy. In fact, it can be instrumental in helping a woman to conceive and carry a pregnancy to full-term. Although patients have stayed on T3 during their pregnancies, I usually recommend that patients wean slowly off (one increment every 7–10 days) the T3 therapy if they become pregnant while taking it. This is because, if for some reason (e.g., natural disaster) a patient ran out of medicine abruptly and did not have access to more, there would be a small chance she could miscarry. Remember, at the present time many physicians are still not familiar with the principles of management of T3 therapy, so if the patient was involved in a car accident out-of-town, the doctors treating her might not know she was taking T3 therapy, and might not know the significance of proper management (with respect to T3 levels/body temperature pattern considerations) even if they did. These same concerns would apply to a patient with severe complications during her pregnancy or at the time of delivery. Fortunately, many women with WTS feel their best while they are pregnant. Unfortunately, they will frequently go downhill again after the pregnancy, sometimes being worse than they were prior to the pregnancy. I suspect that WTS sufferers frequently improve during pregnancy because the developing fetus produces human chorionic gonadotrophin (HCG), which can increase the patient's body temperature patterns and function. Also, great care must be used to ensure the pregnant woman has adequate levels of iodine because low iodine is especially damaging to the fetus. Recent research shows that 50% of pregnant women in the US are deficient in iodine.[111]

Likewise, I generally recommend that patients wean off T3 therapy before undergoing general anesthesia. This reduces the number of variables with which the physicians involved need to contend. Also, it is good for T3 levels to be steady, and they are more steady when endogenously produced. If the time is short before surgery, and there is insufficient time to wean the T3 therapy normally, then the patient can be supported with exogenous T4 while the T3 is weaned quickly, or stopped abruptly for some reason.

How T3 therapy is managed depends, in part, on what one is trying to accomplish. T3 can be employed as symptomatic, therapeutic, or prophylactic therapy. That is, T3 therapy can be used in an attempt to treat symptoms, to correct symptoms, or to prevent symptomatic relapse. Ideally, we would like to see patients enjoy persistent resolution of their symptoms even after they have been weaned off the T3 therapy. However, if some other factor is preventing a person from remaining normal when the treatment is discontinued (e.g., stress, lifestyle, or some other hormonal imbalance, or nutritional deficiency), some patients are grateful that they can at least enjoy resolution of their symptoms while they are on the T3 therapy. One patient who was doing well off the T3 therapy noticed that she could prevent small relapses by taking the smallest dosage level of T3 therapy the day before, the day of, and the day after events she knew were going to be stressful.

Modules, Caveats, and Questions

In this section, there are six interrelated flowcharts called modules:

> Module 1: Wean T4-Containing Medicine Before Cycling On T3
> Module 2: Cycling Up
> Module 3: Plateau
> Module 4: Unsteadiness
> Module 5: T4 Test-Dose
> Module 6: Wean

The modules take a task-oriented approach to actually treating WTS. They take the principles and techniques explained in the chapters and organize them so that one can easily see how and when they are brought to bear under various circumstances.

The treatment begins in Module 2: Cycling Up. By following the branching of this module, you will be led to a box surrounded with chain links that will tell you to jump to one of the other modules. For example:

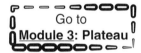

Start at the beginning of each module you jump to and follow its branching, jumping to subsequent modules as indicated, until finally the treatment is discontinued.

Each module may accommodate more than one path, which means that not all the choices presented at a given branch point may apply to where your patient is in the treatment, simply follow the ones that do.

Following the **Modules** is a convenient **directory** for the **Caveats** and **Questions**. The directory is then followed by the **Caveats** themselves, which are followed by the **Questions** and their answers. If you happen to have a question that is not on the list, review the answer to the question that is phrased most closely to yours because yours might be answered as well.

Many of the **Caveats** and **Questions** will be needed to understand the modules. As you progress through the modules, you will encounter links that will direct you to some of the pertinent **Caveats**, **Questions**, and pages.

For example:

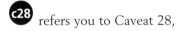 refers you to Caveat 28,

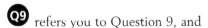 refers you to Question 9, and

 refers you to page 109.

Notes on the Modules

The symptoms of a low-thyroid state, and the side effects of T3 therapy can be very similar. The patients' symptoms are related to improper (in this case insufficient) T3 stimulation of the cells. There can also be improper T3 stimulation of the cells if the T3 therapy is not adjusted properly, and so in this way the *side effects of treatment* are often the same as the *symptoms of WTS*. But nevertheless, in the modules, the word "symptom" is used to refer to complaints related to the condition, and the word *side effect* is used to refer to complaints related to the treatment, even though it is sometimes difficult to make the distinction.

In T3 therapy, the overall treatment is made up of one or more cycles. It is not necessary for everything to be accomplished in one cycle. And so one might make progress that could be considered satisfactory for a given cycle, but that would not be considered satisfactory for the overall treatment. You will come across words like "sufficient", "sufficiently", and "satisfactory" as you proceed through the modules. These words usually refer to the present cycle, but may also refer to the overall treatment. For example, a patient's symptoms may be sufficiently improved for now, or for a given cycle, but still not sufficiently improved overall. So when you see words like "sufficient", don't become concerned if the patient isn't yet completely better from an *overall* standpoint, just consider if the patient is doing sufficiently well in the given *cycle* or setting. As the treatment progresses through one or more cycles of T3 therapy, it is hoped that the patients can also eventually become sufficiently improved *overall*.

M O D U L E   1

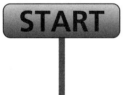

Consider whether the person has or has had poor gland function or whether the T4 was started for clinical reasons only

Wean the T4-containing medicine to zero over about 1–4 days depending on the presenting T4 dose

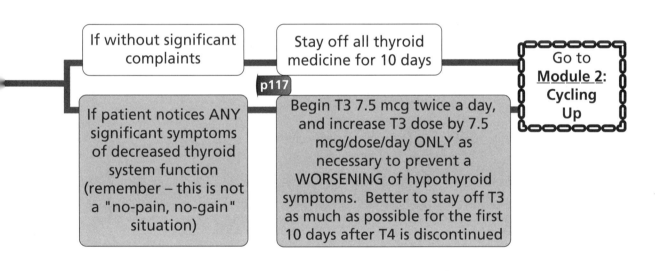

If without significant complaints

Stay off all thyroid medicine for 10 days

Go to **Module 2:** Cycling Up

p117

If patient notices ANY significant symptoms of decreased thyroid system function (remember – this is not a "no-pain, no-gain" situation)

Begin T3 7.5 mcg twice a day, and increase T3 dose by 7.5 mcg/dose/day ONLY as necessary to prevent a WORSENING of hypothyroid symptoms. Better to stay off T3 as much as possible for the first 10 days after T4 is discontinued

Module 2: Cycling Up

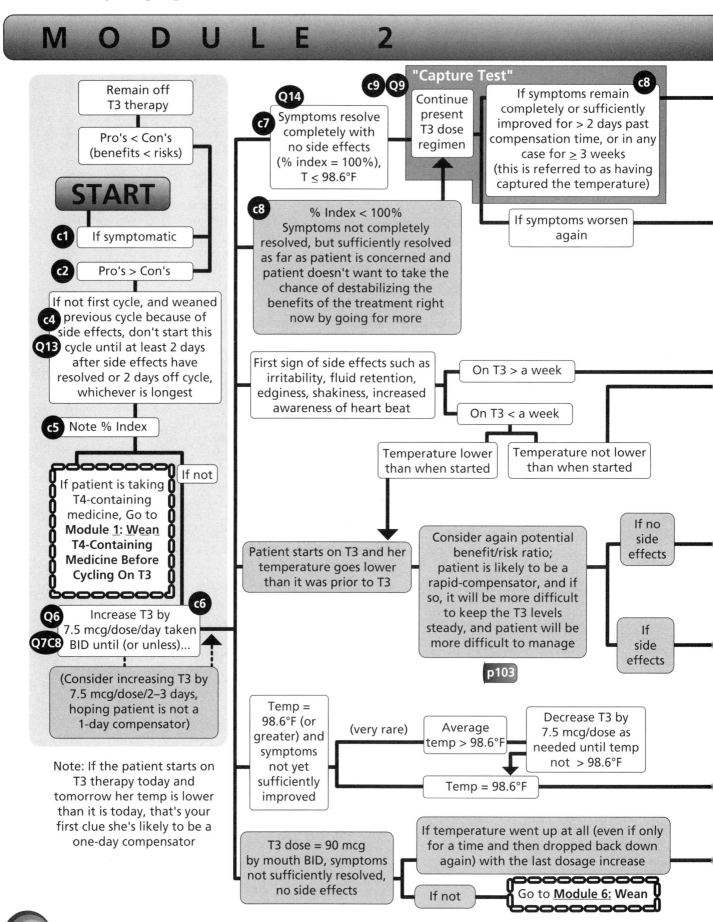

MODULE 2

Remain off T3 therapy

Pro's < Con's (benefits < risks)

START

c1 — If symptomatic

c2 — Pro's > Con's

c4, Q13 — If not first cycle, and weaned previous cycle because of side effects, don't start this cycle until at least 2 days after side effects have resolved or 2 days off cycle, whichever is longest

c5 — Note % Index

If patient is taking T4-containing medicine, Go to **Module 1: Wean T4-Containing Medicine Before Cycling On T3** | If not

Q6, Q7C8, c6 — Increase T3 by 7.5 mcg/dose/day taken BID until (or unless)...

(Consider increasing T3 by 7.5 mcg/dose/2–3 days, hoping patient is not a 1-day compensator)

Note: If the patient starts on T3 therapy today and tomorrow her temp is lower than it is today, that's your first clue she's likely to be a one-day compensator

Q14, c7 — Symptoms resolve completely with no side effects (% index = 100%), T ≤ 98.6°F

c9 Q9 — "Capture Test" Continue present T3 dose regimen

c8 — If symptoms remain completely or sufficiently improved for > 2 days past compensation time, or in any case for ≥ 3 weeks (this is referred to as having captured the temperature)

If symptoms worsen again

c8 — % Index < 100% Symptoms not completely resolved, but sufficiently resolved as far as patient is concerned and patient doesn't want to take the chance of destabilizing the benefits of the treatment right now by going for more

First sign of side effects such as irritability, fluid retention, edginess, shakiness, increased awareness of heart beat

On T3 > a week

On T3 < a week

Temperature lower than when started | Temperature not lower than when started

Patient starts on T3 and her temperature goes lower than it was prior to T3

Consider again potential benefit/risk ratio; patient is likely to be a rapid-compensator, and if so, it will be more difficult to keep the T3 levels steady, and patient will be more difficult to manage

p103

If no side effects

If side effects

Temp = 98.6°F (or greater) and symptoms not yet sufficiently improved | (very rare) Average temp > 98.6°F | Decrease T3 by 7.5 mcg/dose as needed until temp not > 98.6°F

Temp = 98.6°F

T3 dose = 90 mcg by mouth BID, symptoms not sufficiently resolved, no side effects

If temperature went up at all (even if only for a time and then dropped back down again) with the last dosage increase

If not | Go to **Module 6: Wean**

Go to
Module 3: Plateau

If the temperature was higher and the symptoms improved with the present dose, but now the temperature is dropping again and the symptoms have worsened `p100`

Note compensation time

Go to beginning of
Module 2: Cycling Up

If the temperature and symptoms have improved with treatment, but now the symptoms have worsened again, even though the temperature has not dropped back down any lower `p106` `p115`

Go to
Module 4: Unsteadiness

Go to
Module 4: Unsteadiness

Go to
Module 6: Wean

If benefits < risks

If benefits > risks

Consider weaning patient back down off the T3 for a couple of days to get a fresh, steadier start

It is recommended that the medicine be increased smoothly, deliberately, rapidly (7.5 mcg/dose/day) or not at all `p105`

Go to beginning of
Module 2: Cycling Up

Give T4 test dose of 0.0125 mg

Wean patient back down off T3 (one increment each day, or every two days based on clinical judgment) for a couple of days

If benefits > risks

If benefits < risks

Remain off at least 2 days longer than when side effects resolve

Remain off T3

Go to **Module 4: Unsteadiness** in anticipation of going to **Module 6: Wean** to cycle up again in **Module 2: Cycling Up**

Q8 Consider going to **Module 2: Cycling up**, continuing to cycle up, increasing T3 7.5 mcg/dose/day if T<98.6°F, except using 112.5 mcg p.o. BID as a limit instead of 90 mcg; otherwise, go to **Module 6: Wean**

M O D U L E   3

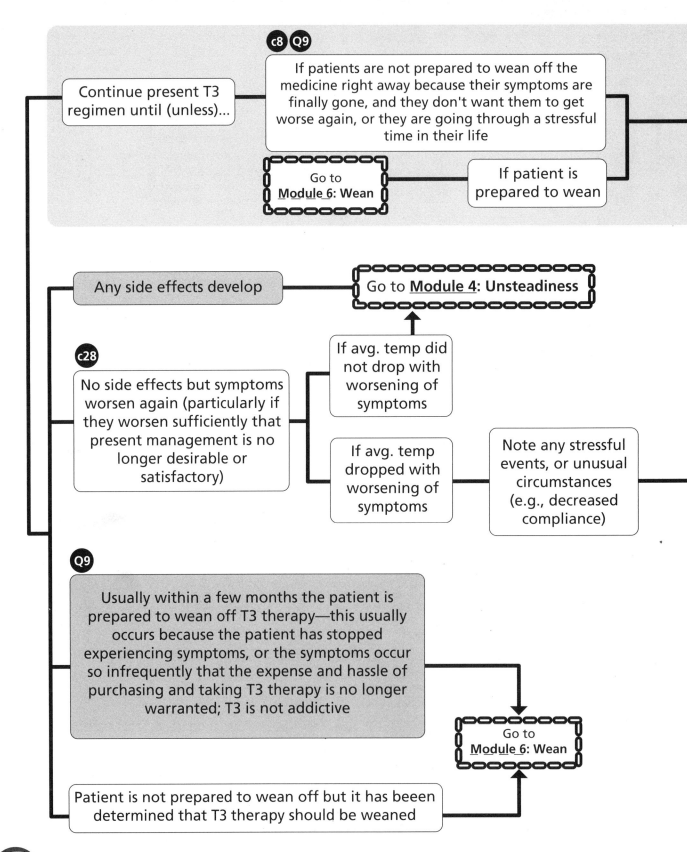

c8 **Q9**
If patients are not prepared to wean off the medicine right away because their symptoms are finally gone, and they don't want them to get worse again, or they are going through a stressful time in their life

Continue present T3 regimen until (unless)...

Go to **Module 6: Wean**

If patient is prepared to wean

Any side effects develop

Go to **Module 4: Unsteadiness**

If avg. temp did not drop with worsening of symptoms

c28
No side effects but symptoms worsen again (particularly if they worsen sufficiently that present management is no longer desirable or satisfactory)

If avg. temp dropped with worsening of symptoms

Note any stressful events, or unusual circumstances (e.g., decreased compliance)

Q9
Usually within a few months the patient is prepared to wean off T3 therapy—this usually occurs because the patient has stopped experiencing symptoms, or the symptoms occur so infrequently that the expense and hassle of purchasing and taking T3 therapy is no longer warranted; T3 is not addictive

Go to **Module 6: Wean**

Patient is not prepared to wean off but it has beeen determined that T3 therapy should be weaned

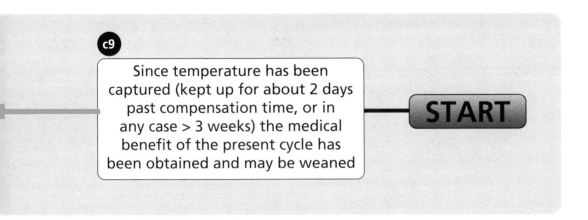

c9 Since temperature has been captured (kept up for about 2 days past compensation time, or in any case > 3 weeks) the medical benefit of the present cycle has been obtained and may be weaned

START

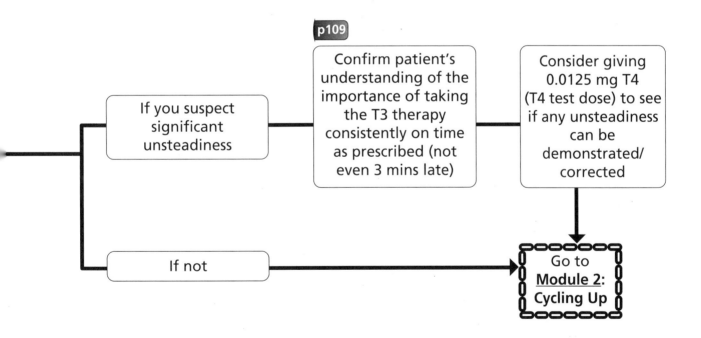

p109 Confirm patient's understanding of the importance of taking the T3 therapy consistently on time as prescribed (not even 3 mins late)

If you suspect significant unsteadiness

Consider giving 0.0125 mg T4 (T4 test dose) to see if any unsteadiness can be demonstrated/ corrected

If not

Go to **Module 2: Cycling Up**

M O D U L E 4

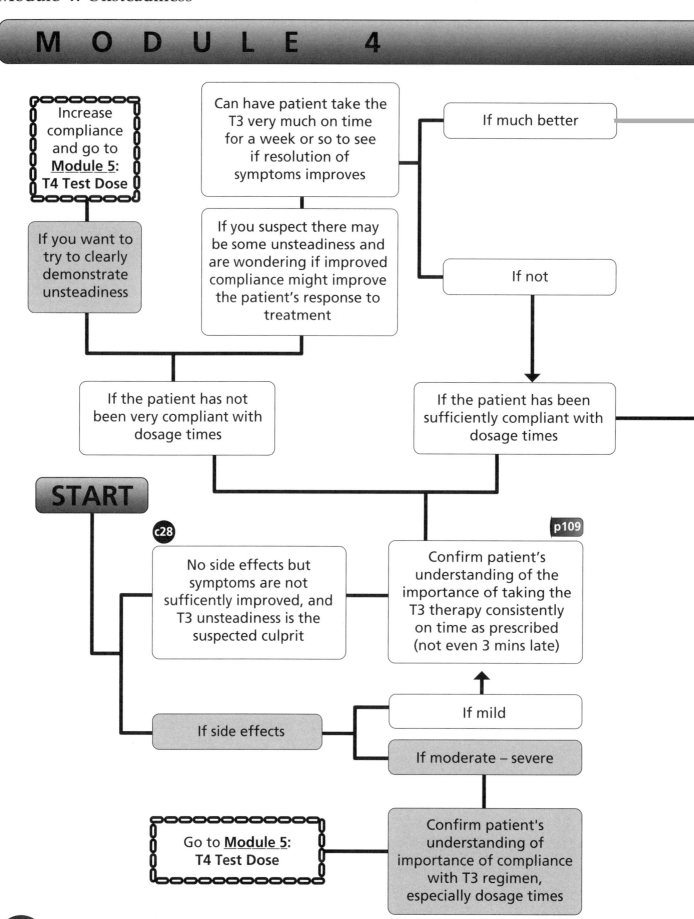

Increase compliance and go to **Module 5**: T4 Test Dose

If you want to try to clearly demonstrate unsteadiness

Can have patient take the T3 very much on time for a week or so to see if resolution of symptoms improves

If you suspect there may be some unsteadiness and are wondering if improved compliance might improve the patient's response to treatment

If much better

If not

If the patient has not been very compliant with dosage times

If the patient has been sufficiently compliant with dosage times

START

c28

No side effects but symptoms are not sufficiently improved, and T3 unsteadiness is the suspected culprit

p109

Confirm patient's understanding of the importance of taking the T3 therapy consistently on time as prescribed (not even 3 mins late)

If mild

If side effects

If moderate – severe

Go to **Module 5**: T4 Test Dose

Confirm patient's understanding of importance of compliance with T3 regimen, especially dosage times

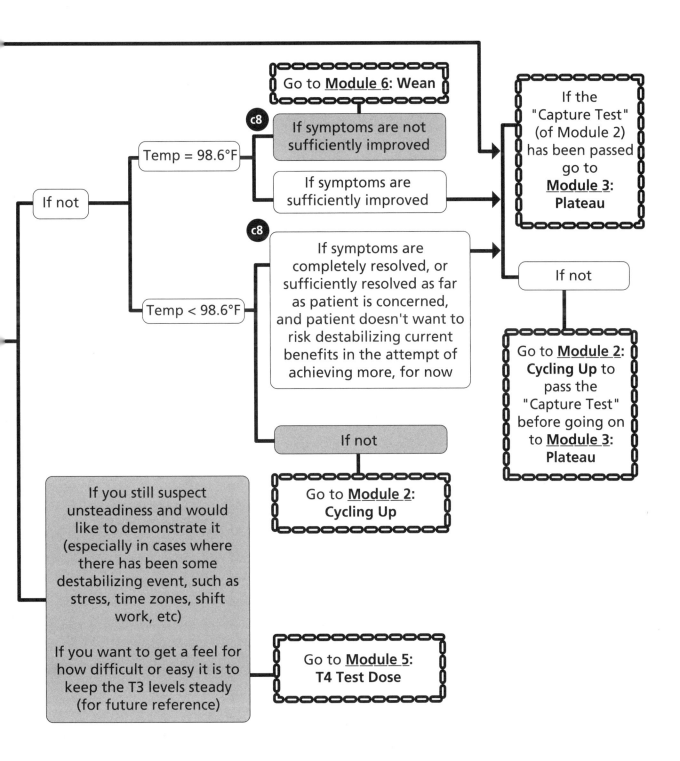

If not

Temp = 98.6°F

c8 If symptoms are not sufficiently improved

Go to **Module 6**: Wean

If symptoms are sufficiently improved

If the "Capture Test" (of Module 2) has been passed go to **Module 3**: Plateau

If not

Go to **Module 2**: **Cycling Up** to pass the "Capture Test" before going on to **Module 3**: Plateau

Temp < 98.6°F

c8 If symptoms are completely resolved, or sufficiently resolved as far as patient is concerned, and patient doesn't want to risk destabilizing current benefits in the attempt of achieving more, for now

If not

Go to **Module 2**: **Cycling Up**

If you still suspect unsteadiness and would like to demonstrate it (especially in cases where there has been some destabilizing event, such as stress, time zones, shift work, etc)

If you want to get a feel for how difficult or easy it is to keep the T3 levels steady (for future reference)

Go to **Module 5**: **T4 Test Dose**

M O D U L E 5

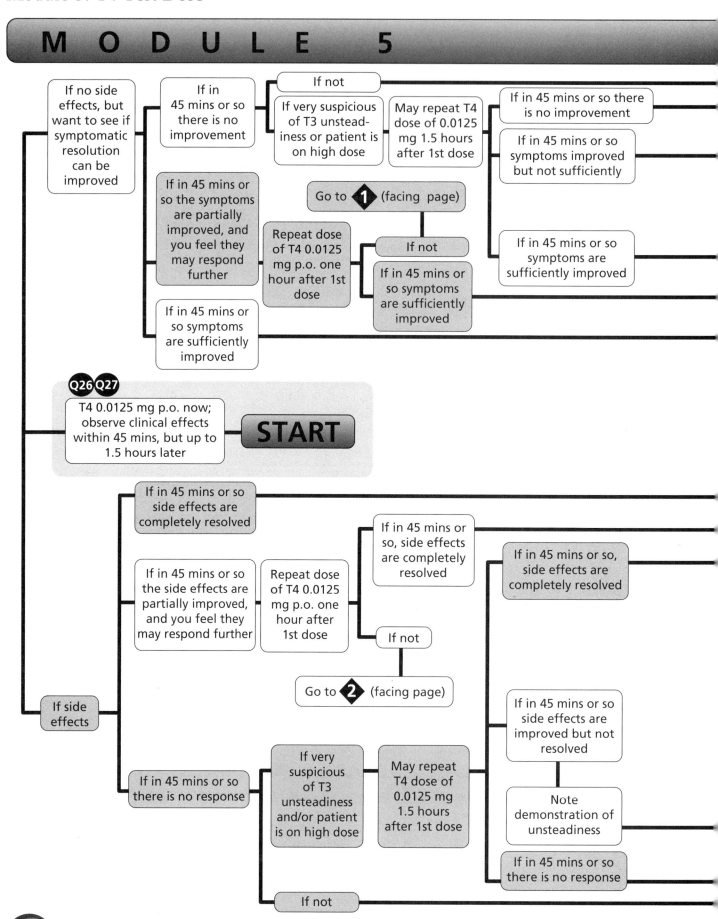

If no side effects, but want to see if symptomatic resolution can be improved

If in 45 mins or so there is no improvement

If not

If very suspicious of T3 unsteadiness or patient is on high dose

May repeat T4 dose of 0.0125 mg 1.5 hours after 1st dose

If in 45 mins or so there is no improvement

If in 45 mins or so symptoms improved but not sufficiently

Go to ◆1 (facing page)

If in 45 mins or so the symptoms are partially improved, and you feel they may respond further

Repeat dose of T4 0.0125 mg p.o. one hour after 1st dose

If not

If in 45 mins or so symptoms are sufficiently improved

If in 45 mins or so symptoms are sufficiently improved

If in 45 mins or so symptoms are sufficiently improved

Q26 Q27

T4 0.0125 mg p.o. now; observe clinical effects within 45 mins, but up to 1.5 hours later

START

If in 45 mins or so side effects are completely resolved

If in 45 mins or so, side effects are completely resolved

If in 45 mins or so, side effects are completely resolved

If in 45 mins or so the side effects are partially improved, and you feel they may respond further

Repeat dose of T4 0.0125 mg p.o. one hour after 1st dose

If not

Go to ◆2 (facing page)

If in 45 mins or so side effects are improved but not resolved

If side effects

If in 45 mins or so there is no response

If very suspicious of T3 unsteadiness and/or patient is on high dose

May repeat T4 dose of 0.0125 mg 1.5 hours after 1st dose

Note demonstration of unsteadiness

If in 45 mins or so there is no response

If not

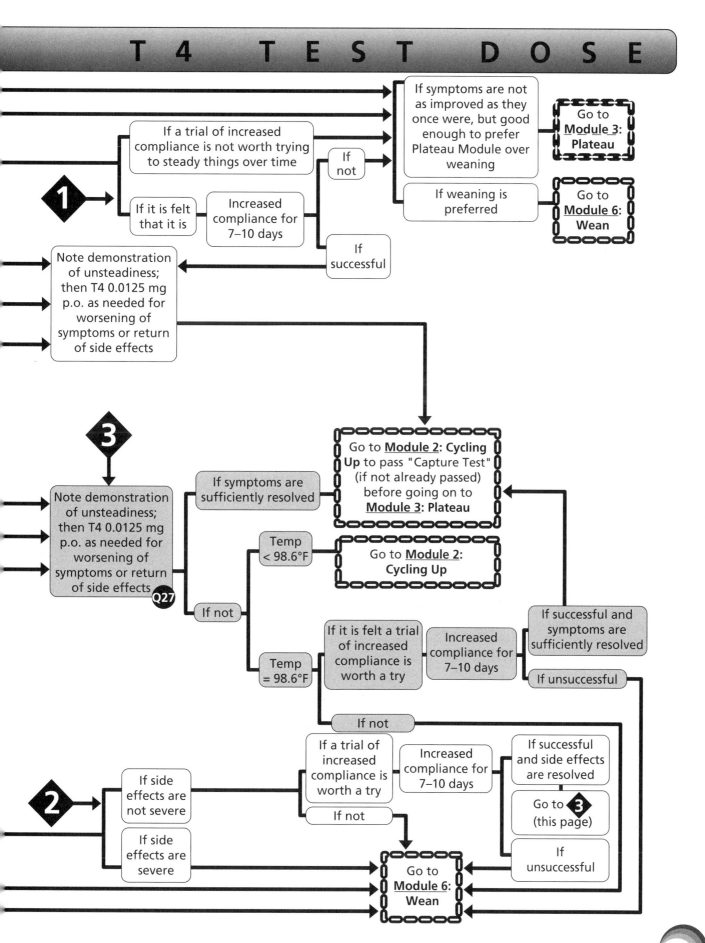

If a trial of increased compliance is not worth trying to steady things over time

1

If it is felt that it is

Increased compliance for 7–10 days

If not

If successful

If symptoms are not as improved as they once were, but good enough to prefer Plateau Module over weaning

Go to **Module 3: Plateau**

If weaning is preferred

Go to **Module 6: Wean**

Note demonstration of unsteadiness; then T4 0.0125 mg p.o. as needed for worsening of symptoms or return of side effects

3

Note demonstration of unsteadiness; then T4 0.0125 mg p.o. as needed for worsening of symptoms or return of side effects **Q27**

If symptoms are sufficiently resolved

Go to **Module 2: Cycling Up** to pass "Capture Test" (if not already passed) before going on to **Module 3: Plateau**

Temp < 98.6°F

Go to **Module 2: Cycling Up**

If not

Temp = 98.6°F

If it is felt a trial of increased compliance is worth a try

Increased compliance for 7–10 days

If successful and symptoms are sufficiently resolved

If unsuccessful

If not

2

If side effects are not severe

If side effects are severe

If a trial of increased compliance is worth a try

Increased compliance for 7–10 days

If not

If successful and side effects are resolved

Go to **3** (this page)

If unsuccessful

Go to **Module 6: Wean**

MODULE 6

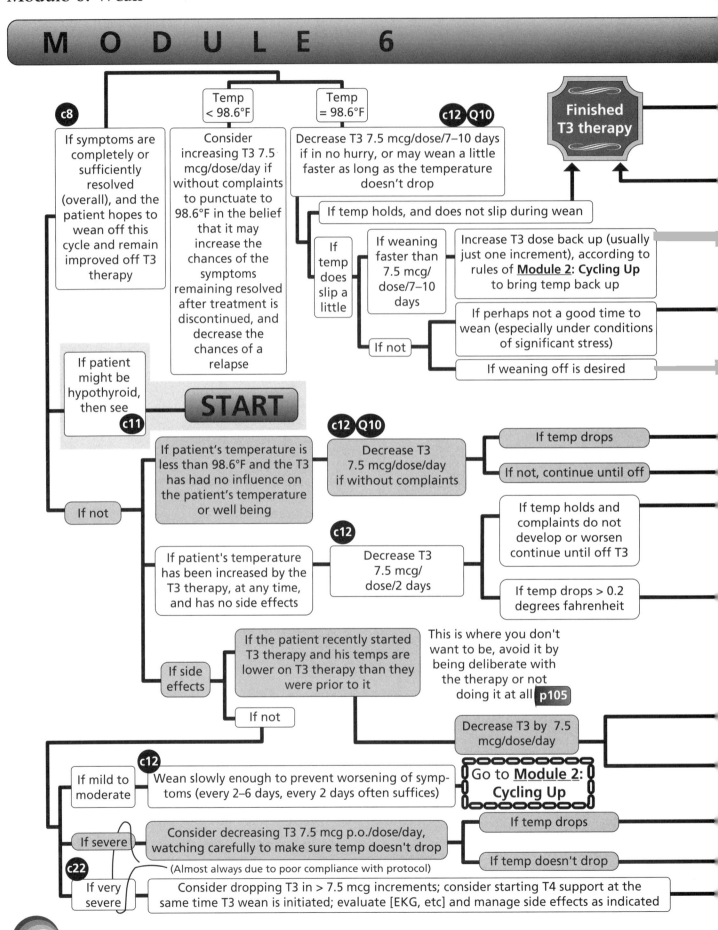

c8 If symptoms are completely or sufficiently resolved (overall), and the patient hopes to wean off this cycle and remain improved off T3 therapy

Temp < 98.6°F Consider increasing T3 7.5 mcg/dose/day if without complaints to punctuate to 98.6°F in the belief that it may increase the chances of the symptoms remaining resolved after treatment is discontinued, and decrease the chances of a relapse

Temp = 98.6°F **c12 Q10** Decrease T3 7.5 mcg/dose/7–10 days if in no hurry, or may wean a little faster as long as the temperature doesn't drop

Finished T3 therapy

If temp holds, and does not slip during wean

If temp does slip a little | If weaning faster than 7.5 mcg/dose/7–10 days | Increase T3 dose back up (usually just one increment), according to rules of **Module 2: Cycling Up** to bring temp back up

If not | If perhaps not a good time to wean (especially under conditions of significant stress)

If weaning off is desired

If patient might be hypothyroid, then see **c11**

START

If patient's temperature is less than 98.6°F and the T3 has had no influence on the patient's temperature or well being | **c12 Q10** Decrease T3 7.5 mcg/dose/day if without complaints | If temp drops

If not, continue until off

If not

If patient's temperature has been increased by the T3 therapy, at any time, and has no side effects | **c12** Decrease T3 7.5 mcg/dose/2 days | If temp holds and complaints do not develop or worsen continue until off T3

If temp drops > 0.2 degrees fahrenheit

If side effects | If the patient recently started T3 therapy and his temps are lower on T3 therapy than they were prior to it | This is where you don't want to be, avoid it by being deliberate with the therapy or not doing it at all **p105**

If not

Decrease T3 by 7.5 mcg/dose/day

c12 If mild to moderate | Wean slowly enough to prevent worsening of symptoms (every 2–6 days, every 2 days often suffices)

Go to **Module 2: Cycling Up**

If severe | Consider decreasing T3 7.5 mcg p.o./dose/day, watching carefully to make sure temp doesn't drop | If temp drops

If temp doesn't drop

(Almost always due to poor compliance with protocol)

c22 If very severe | Consider dropping T3 in > 7.5 mcg increments; consider starting T4 support at the same time T3 wean is initiated; evaluate [EKG, etc] and manage side effects as indicated

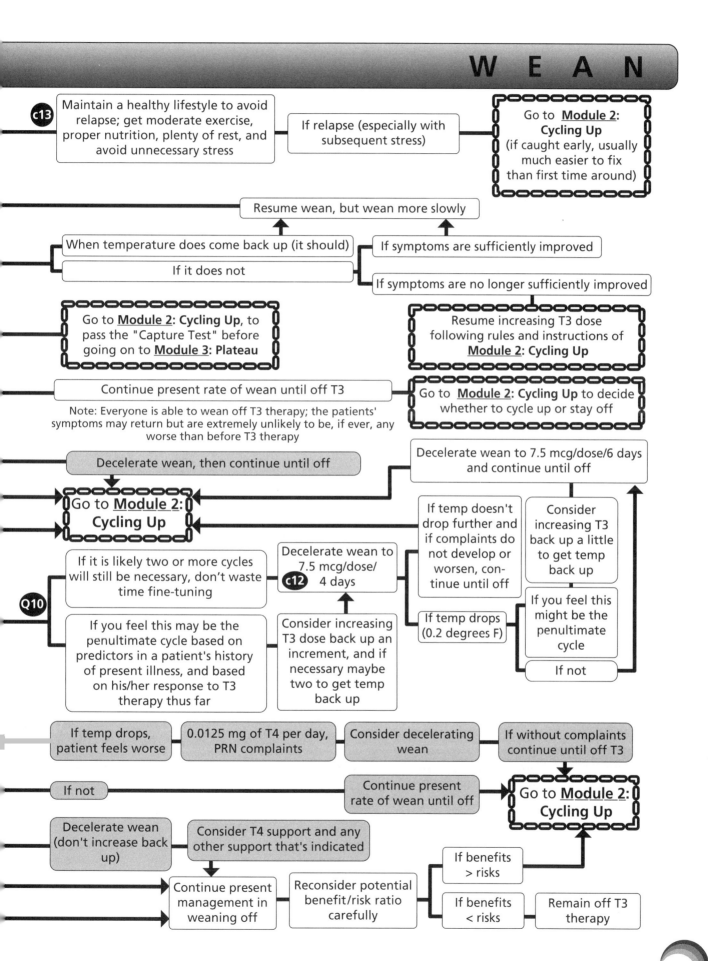

C13 Maintain a healthy lifestyle to avoid relapse; get moderate exercise, proper nutrition, plenty of rest, and avoid unnecessary stress

If relapse (especially with subsequent stress)

Go to **Module 2: Cycling Up** (if caught early, usually much easier to fix than first time around)

Resume wean, but wean more slowly

When temperature does come back up (it should)

If it does not

If symptoms are sufficiently improved

If symptoms are no longer sufficiently improved

Go to **Module 2**: Cycling Up, to pass the "Capture Test" before going on to **Module 3: Plateau**

Resume increasing T3 dose following rules and instructions of **Module 2: Cycling Up**

Continue present rate of wean until off T3

Go to **Module 2**: Cycling Up to decide whether to cycle up or stay off

Note: Everyone is able to wean off T3 therapy; the patients' symptoms may return but are extremely unlikely to be, if ever, any worse than before T3 therapy

Decelerate wean, then continue until off

Decelerate wean to 7.5 mcg/dose/6 days and continue until off

Go to **Module 2: Cycling Up**

Q10 If it is likely two or more cycles will still be necessary, don't waste time fine-tuning

If you feel this may be the penultimate cycle based on predictors in a patient's history of present illness, and based on his/her response to T3 therapy thus far

Decelerate wean to 7.5 mcg/dose/ **C12** 4 days

Consider increasing T3 dose back up an increment, and if necessary maybe two to get temp back up

If temp doesn't drop further and if complaints do not develop or worsen, continue until off

If temp drops (0.2 degrees F)

Consider increasing T3 back up a little to get temp back up

If you feel this might be the penultimate cycle

If not

If temp drops, patient feels worse

0.0125 mg of T4 per day, PRN complaints

Consider decelerating wean

If without complaints continue until off T3

If not

Continue present rate of wean until off

Go to **Module 2: Cycling Up**

Decelerate wean (don't increase back up)

Consider T4 support and any other support that's indicated

Continue present management in weaning off

Reconsider potential benefit/risk ratio carefully

If benefits > risks

If benefits < risks

Remain off T3 therapy

Caveats Directory

c1   If the patient has no symptoms before treatment (just a low temperature).
c2   Weigh pros and cons of treatment (see Q2).
c3   Some symptoms are more predictably responsive than others.
c4   The whole trick is to start with a steady level of T3 and keep it steady (see Q13).
c5   Use the percentage index to get a quick start on clinical assessment.
c6   Slow compensators tolerate rapid increases better than rapid compensators tolerate slow ones (see Q6, Q7).
c7   If the patient's symptoms resolve completely with a temperature less than 98.6°F (which is very seldom the case), it is not necessary to push the temperature higher (see Q14).
c8   The word "sufficiently" pertains to the present cycle, and may or may not also pertain to the treatment in general.
c9   The full benefit of a cycle, in terms of resetting the system, is obtained once the temperature has been captured (p101).
c10 The closer patients' temperatures are brought to 98.6°F, the less medicine they'll need on subsequent cycles (if such cycles are needed at all) (see Q14).
c11 If the patient may be hypothyroid (low thyroid gland function), it may be necessary to support the patient with T4 as she is being weaned off a cycle of T3 therapy.
c12 When weaning, the goal is to wean slowly enough that the patient's temperature doesn't drop.
c13 T3 therapy can be used as symptomatic, therapeutic, or prophylactic treatment.
c14 The more corrected a patient's WTS is, the less likely it is to relapse.
c15 Once people have been successfully treated, and are doing well off treatment, it is usually much easier to correct their symptoms, should they relapse, than it was the first time around.
c16 Patients' symptoms can often improve in stages that stick, just as they often have worsened in stages that have stuck.
c17 Subsequent cycles are promising if there is a net clinical improvement from a previous cycle.
c18 Periods of great stress and/or stringent dieting are not generally the best times to wean cycles of T3 therapy.
c19 Any side effects indicate less than optimal management and should be addressed.
c20 It is best to address side effects early so that they can be easily nipped in the bud.
c21 Patients should check their pulse rates daily and call if they go above 100 bpm.
c22 The best treatment of severe side effects of T3 therapy is prevention, but...
c23 Side effects can be caused by T3 levels that are too high, too low, or unsteady.
c24 The higher the dose of T3 therapy the harder it is to keep T3 levels steady.
c25 Steadiness is everything.
c26 Unsteady T3 levels are the most common cause of side effects and poor clinical results.
c27 It is not wise to stop the T3 medicine abruptly.
c28 T3 level unsteadiness can result in decreased clinical improvement, before it results in side effects.
c29 Side effects from T3 therapy are dependent mainly on how well the molecule is delivered.

Questions Directory

Q1   How do you know it's thyroid?
Q2   What are the substantive risks of T3 therapy?
Q3   What happens if you stop the T3 therapy abruptly?
Q4   Will the patient have to stay on the T3 therapy for life?
Q5   What is the percentage index?
Q6   Wouldn't increasing the dose of T3 every 3 days instead of every day be easier for the patients to tolerate?
Q7   What if a patient's temperature goes down with T3 therapy?
Q8   How high up on the medicine does one go on each cycle of T3 therapy?
Q9   How long should a patient stay up on a cycle before weaning back down again?
Q10 How fast does one go off a cycle of T3 therapy?
Q11 If a patient's temperature slips while they are weaning down off the T3 therapy, should the dose be increased back up an increment before continuing to wean?
Q12 When weaning a cycle of T3 therapy, does one wean part-way down, down to the starting dose, or all the way off?
Q13 How long does one stay off between cycles?
Q14 If the patient is feeling very well, but her temperature is still less than 98.6°F when measured as indicated, is it really necessary to push the temperature up to 98.6°F?

Q15 How do you wean a WTS patient who is also hypothyroid? See c11.

Q16 What if a patient's temperature and symptoms do not remain improved after the treatment is discontinued?

Q17 What are the risks of staying on T3 therapy for a long time?

Q18 How many patients can be weaned off T3 therapy?

Q19 What if the patient improves at first, but then stops feeling as well even though the temperature is holding?

Q20 What if the patient's temperature goes up to normal and the patient still doesn't feel very well?

Q21 What if the patient is feeling improved on the T3 therapy, but when the dosage is increased to bring the temperature closer to normal, the temperature drops and the patient feels worse?

Q22 What if a patient has a slump of fatigue or some other complaint at the same time each day?

Q23 How often are office visits?

Q24 If a patient starts having any side effects, does that mean that the treatment isn't likely to work out very well?

Q25 How are side effects managed?

Q26 What is a T4 test dose?

Q27 If the T4 test dose works, how often should it be taken?

Q28 Do temperatures or T4 test doses have to be taken to the minute like the T3?

Q29 What if the treatment doesn't work?

Q30 What happens if the patient's T4 and TSH levels drop while on T3 therapy?

Q31 How often does one order the thyroid blood tests?

Q32 What would the expected thyroid blood test values be after a couple of weeks of T3 therapy?

Q33 What should the patients do with the T3 dosing if they miss the dosing time?

Q34 What if the patient is up to 90 mcg BID of T3, and the temperature is still not up?

Q35 What if a patient gets a fever due to a virus or cold?

Caveats

c1   If a patient has no symptoms before treatment (just a low temperature): I do not feel that T3 therapy is necessary if a patient is not symptomatic even if the temperature runs below 98.6°F. I have been amazed at how sensitive patients are to small changes in their body temperature patterns. If their temperatures are not doing well, they can usually tell by the way they feel. So if a patient has absolutely no complaints, and feels very well, I don't feel treatment is necessary.

c2   Weigh the pros and cons of treatment (Q2): Before therapy is started, and at each step along the way, the patient and physician must carefully weighs the pros and the cons and all the alternatives to T3 therapy. If the pros of T3 therapy do not outweigh the cons, then of course T3 therapy should not be started, or if it has been started it should be gradually (not necessarily slowly – see c22) weaned.

c3   Some symptoms are more predictably responsive than others: Some of the most gratifying symptoms to treat include migraines, PMS, panic attacks, and depression. These symptoms have two things in common. First, they are among the most debilitating of complaints, and secondly, they are among the most typically responsive to T3 therapy. On the other hand, other symptoms are less predictably responsive. For example, it's harder to predict who might enjoy relief from the disturbing complaint of easy weight gain, and who will not. For instance, in some cases patients may experience an appreciable weight gain together with the onset of many other symptoms of WTS after a major stress. And, with treatment, all of those symptoms may resolve, while the weight remains. In such cases, the patients are often perplexed. They wonder why the weight didn't normalize with the other symptoms, when it clearly came on with them (I personally feel that part of the explanation for this phenomenon has to do with the change in a patient's surface area to volume ratio, which is an issue discussed in the book: *Wilson's Temperature Syndrome—A Reversible Low Temperature Problem*). At any rate, it is clear that weight is a multi-faceted issue that depends on a number of factors such as diet and exercise, among others. These observations suggest that the symptoms that are the most predictably responsive depend on factors that are the most directly influenced by body temperature patterns.

c4   The whole trick is to start with a steady level of T3 and keep it steady (Q13): If this is not the first cycle, then sufficient time should be allowed between cycles to allow the T3 levels to steady down **(p105)**. If this is the first cycle, then the T3 level should be endogenously steady **(p102)**; or the patient may be taking a T4-containing medicine, which should be weaned prior to initiation of T3 therapy.

c5   Use the percentage index to get a quick start on clinical assessment: The percentage index is useful in giving one a general idea of how well the patient is doing on the treatment protocol. Patients usually determine their complaints to be symptoms of some problem when they consider them to be inappropriate given the circumstances. To get a feel for how abnormal a patient judges his or her collection of symptoms to be, I will frequently ask him/her, "Compared to a normal person, all things taken together, would you say you feel 20, 40, 60, or 80 percent normal?" Or, "Compared to the way you felt before developing all these symptoms, all things taken together, would you say you feel 20 percent normal, 40 percent, 60 percent, or 80 percent?" It is often helpful to get this overall subjective assessment of a patient's clinical status initially and at each office visit. The symptoms often worsen and improve together in a group and this assessment helps give one an idea of a trend.

c6   Slow compensators tolerate rapid increases better than rapid compensators tolerate slow ones (Q7): If you don't increase a patient's T3 dose quick enough, then you may not give her enough T3 to get her temperature up, but only enough to make it unsteady. Her temperature will still be as low as it ever was, but now not only will it be too low, but also it will be unsteady, and her symptoms may actually become worse than they were when she started T3 therapy **(p105).**

c7   If the patient's symptoms resolve completely with a temperature less than 98.6°F (which is very seldom the case), it is not necessary to push the temperature higher: Patients may feel very well with temperatures less than 98.6°F, but they usually feel better when their temperatures are averaging 98.6°F when measured as indicated **(p83, Q14).** The whole reason therapy is being implemented in the first place is in the hope of resolving the patient's symptoms. So if the symptoms are gone, even if the temperature is a little less than 98.6°F, then that goal has been achieved.

c8   The word sufficiently pertains to the present cycle, and may or may not also pertain to the treatment in general: The higher the dose of T3 therapy, the harder it is to keep T3 levels steady. So at some point during treatment, it may be felt that the current degree of symptom resolution is sufficient for now, and that it might be best to leave well enough alone for the time being, rather than to risk destabilizing things while attempting to further resolve the symptoms. To illustrate, I will review briefly an analogy I often give patients:

Let's suppose a person traveling to a distant city stopped along the way in an intermediate city, and really liked it there. He could stay there for 3 weeks if he wanted to. But he is not going to get to his final destination of the distant city until he gets back on the road and continues his journey. Likening this to the progress of T3 therapy, the distant city represents the ultimate goal of the patient's body temperature patterns remaining more normal and the patient's symptoms remaining resolved even after T3 therapy has been discontinued. If on the way to that goal the patient notices a remarkable improvement (and not necessarily complete improvement) in his clinical status at a certain level in a particular cycle of T3 therapy, then he may remain at that level and in that cycle of T3 therapy for a period of time if he prefers, and if he is without complaints. He may even remain at that level and in that cycle indefinitely (for as long as a year or more). However, the patients that do accomplish the ultimate goal of T3 therapy usually accomplish it by going up and down on the T3 therapy, getting closer and closer to normal on less and less medicine until the ultimate goal of being normal off medicine is accomplished.

So even though a patient being maintained at a certain level in a certain cycle may be maintained in that way indefinitely, he will not be able to obtain the ultimate goal (when possible) until he "gets back on the road" by continuing to increase and decrease the medicine through the process of cycling until he gets closer and closer to normal on less and less medicine until the process is complete. Thus, as long as a patient is not having any problems or complaints, when a patient goes up and when a patient goes down on T3 therapy is largely a matter of preference according to the doctor's and patient's priorities.

c9   The full benefit of a cycle, in terms of resetting the system, is obtained once the temperature has been "captured" (p101, Q9): Patients are much more likely to need less medicine on subsequent cycles, if their temperatures are captured on previous ones. If it's the first dosage increment, and the patient hasn't "compensated" before, then you may have to wait 3 weeks to see if the patient is going to compensate, because if the patients haven't compensated within about 3 weeks, they're probably not going to compensate. If this is not the first dosage increase of the first cycle, and the patient has compensated before, then you can wait to see if the patient will compensate again in about that same time period. If the patient does not compensate back down, then the patient's temperature has been "captured".

c10   The closer patients' temperatures are brought to 98.6°F, the less medicine they'll need on subsequent cycles (if such cycles are needed)(Q14).

c11   If the patient may be hypothyroid (low thyroid gland function), it may be necessary to support the patient with T4 as she is being weaned off a cycle of T3 therapy: However, just because a patient presented taking a T4-containing medicine does not necessarily mean she is hypothyroid. If it is felt that the patient may not be hypothyroid, she may be challenged by gradually weaning her off the T3 therapy without T4 support to see if she can maintain her temperature and clinical status on her own. When challenged, if her temperature begins to drop as soon as the weaning process begins, she is probably being weaned too quickly. However, if her temperature holds well through several decrements in T3 dose (and it doesn't seem that the patient is being weaned too quickly), and then hits a "wall" where the T3 dose cannot be decreased any further without the temperature dropping, the patient probably is hypothyroid and cannot make sufficient T4 on her own to provide for sufficient levels of T3. When it is felt a patient should be supported with T4, add back a small amount of T4 (0.0125–0.05 mg) even if the patient presented on 0.2 mg, because after cycling on T3 therapy, patients can often do much better even on much less T4 medicine. Continue the process above, and add back more T4 if another "wall" is encountered. It's best to have patients remain on the smallest amount of T4 possible (the taller the tree, the harder it falls; I believe patients on the smallest dose of T4 needed to do the job are less susceptible to a relapse of WTS). If she can stay off T4, then she is probably not hypothyroid and may be cycled on and off the T3 therapy in the usual fashion (and watching her expectantly for 1–2 months after the last cycle of T3 has been weaned to see if her symptoms relapse or if low T4/high TSH appear). If T4 is added back, and another T3 cycle is to be started, go through **Module 1** first.

c12   When weaning, the goal is to wean slowly enough that the patient's temperature doesn't drop: I usually start by weaning the patients by one 7.5 mcg decrement of T3 per dose, every 2 days. For example, if the patient is now on 30 mcg BID, then I would recommend that the patient go down to 22.5 mcg tomorrow, and then down to 15 mcg BID 2 days later, and so on. However, if the patients' temperatures are clearly trending downward, then I would decelerate the weaning process to one decrement every 4 days. And if that's still too fast, I would decelerate the wean to one decrement every 6 days. The less a patient's temperature drops during the weaning process, the less medicine (often many multiples less – one fifth, one tenth, one twentieth, etc.) will be needed to get the temperature up during the next cycle. If one weans too quickly off a cycle, and does not give the body a chance to take over again, then one can squander much of the benefit of a cycle. If there has been any improvement with a given cycle, much if not all of it is retained if the T3 is weaned slowly enough and the patient is not under a great deal of stress (**Q10**).

c13   T3 therapy can be used as symptomatic, therapeutic, or prophylactic treatment: In some cases, it can be a symptomatic treatment in that it may be used to improve a patient's symptoms, when other treatments fail, even if for some reason the symptomatic improvement does not persist after the T3 therapy has been discontinued.

In some cases, it can be a therapeutic treatment in the sense that the symptoms remain improved even after the treatment has been discontinued.

It can also be used as a prophylactic treatment in that some patients have noticed that small doses of T3 can be used to ward off relapses of WTS. Some patients (especially those with hereditary predispositions to WTS) have learned to predict when their symptoms are likely to relapse. Upcoming conditions of emotional stress can cause relapses in patients who are remaining well after the T3 therapy has been discontinued. For example, one susceptible patient was required to give an important presentation every 3 months. She noticed her symptoms relapsing after her first "post-T3" presentation. She was able to quickly nip her symptoms "in the bud," by starting back up on a small cycle of T3 therapy once her symptoms reappeared. She found she was able to predict a relapse with almost every quarterly presentation she was required to make. She also found that she was able to ward off relapses by taking the lowest dose of 7.5 mcg BID (lower doses can be made for more sensitive patients, but it is rarely necessary) the day before, the day of, and the day after her presentations. And thus she was able to see her presentations come and go without the first onset of symptoms. Likewise, some such patients feel more comfortable just staying on the lowest dose of T3 therapy as maintenance to more continually exert the slightest pressure against a relapse, but such cases are exceptional.

c14   The more corrected a patient's WTS, the less likely it is to relapse: Even though patients can often hold a subtotal improvement indefinitely, the more complete it is, the easier it can be held. The more complete the improvement, the further back the vicious cycle is turned, and the more reserves the patients have.

c15   Once people have been successfully treated, and are doing well off treatment, it is usually much easier to correct their symptoms, should they relapse, than it was the first time around: This is especially true when it is caught early. When a person is first treated for WTS, the process ideally involves the patient getting better and better, a step at a time, on less and less medicine until the process is complete. When such patients then relapse, their condition doesn't typically relapse immediately back to "square one." Their symptoms tend to start getting worse step by step, especially under stressful circumstances. So if a person needed three cycles of T3 therapy with dosage levels as high as

82.8 mcg p.o. BID when initially treated, that same person might only need one cycle with doses up to 15 mcg/dose to easily treat a relapse. Relapses can often be much more easily treated when caught early (within days or weeks, as opposed to months or years), the earlier the better.

c16 **Patients' symptoms can often improve in stages that stick, just as they often have worsened in stages that have stuck (p106).**

c17 **Subsequent cycles are promising if there is a net clinical improvement from a previous cycle:** When a patient retains a net (albeit subtotal) clinical improvement from a cycle of T3 therapy, this is the first strong indication that the therapeutic trial of T3 therapy has been a success. At that point, it becomes quite likely that the patient has "made it over the hump," and has a good chance of being able to retain more and more net improvement as the cycling process continues, until the process is complete (especially if the patient is not under tremendous stress, and can employ reasonably good habits of diet, exercise, sleep, etc).

c18 **Periods of great stress and/or stringent dieting are not generally the best times to wean cycles of T3 therapy:** When weaning T3 therapy, it is best to give the patients every opportunity for their systems to come back up to give their bodies every opportunity to maintain naturally the temperature and clinical status that has been re-established artificially. Of course stress and fasting can decrease the conversion of T4 to T3. So, if patients are under a lot of stress that is likely limited to a week or two, it is often better to wait until then before weaning. If the patients are under chronic stress that does not appear likely to change any time soon, then it is best to just proceed with the therapy as well as possible. Likewise, stringent dieting while the T3 therapy is being weaned, or after the therapy has been discontinued, might cause the patients' systems to slow back down again. So, if patients are planning to diet to achieve some much needed weight loss, it is generally best for it to be done before the T3 therapy has been weaned (while on T3 therapy the "T4/rT3-preponderance-generating" effect of fasting on 5'-deiodinase is muted because the patients' T3 is largely being supplied directly by mouth, essentially bypassing the function of the deiodinating enzyme) **(p93)**.

c19 **Any side effects indicate less than optimal management and should be addressed:** T3 therapy is not a "no pain, no gain" approach. Patients should not have any complaints and should only feel better. Any complaints, even if mild, simply indicate that the T3 levels are not sufficiently normal and steady, so the T3 therapy should be adjusted to eliminate them. Also, a patient with mild complaints is that much closer to having more severe complaints, and it is best to stay as far away from such complaints as possible.

c20 **It is best to address side effects early so that they can be easily nipped in the bud.**

c21 **Patients should check their pulse rates daily and call if they go above 100 bpm at rest.**

c22 **The best treatment of severe side effects of T3 therapy is prevention, but...:** Severe side effects rarely, if ever, come on all at once, without warning. Side effects tend to appear and worsen gradually, progressively. The major cause of side effects with T3 therapy is unsteady T3 levels.

Two major factors contribute frequently to unsteady T3 levels. The first is patients not being very compliant with the treatment (especially in terms of taking their medicine very much on time **(p103)**. The second is not taking deliberate control of a person's thyroid system, by increasing the T3 dose quickly enough, especially in rapid compensators. **(p104)**. The secret is to start the T3 therapy steadily, in patients with steady T3 levels, and to keep the T3 therapy and T3 levels as steady as possible from the start. At the first sign of any potential side effects, a T4 test dose can be considered, as well as weaning the patient gradually off the T3 therapy **(p112)**. A difficult situation arises when the T3 dose is increased in the face of unaddressed potential side effects. The higher the dose of T3 therapy, the harder it is to keep T3 levels steady, and the greater the potential of side effects from unsteady T3 levels. It is not wise to decrease the T3 therapy too quickly or to stop it abruptly, lest the patients' own thyroid systems are not given enough time to come back up and support their metabolisms. If the "rug is pulled out from under their feet," by dropping the T3 abruptly, then patients can have low blood pressure, which can lead to lightheadedness and palpitations; they can have severe fatigue, headaches, and other complaints (also, if no thyroid support of any kind is given, these complaints can last as long as 3 weeks). Thus, the difficulty, in circumstances of very severe side effects, is this: the person is having severe side effects, which suggest the patient should be weaned off the T3 rather quickly; but, severe side effects can in some cases be worsened by decreasing the T3 therapy *too* quickly. This is especially difficult should the patient be experiencing any severe cardiovascular complaints such as chest pain, left arm pain, nausea, sweating, that would raise concerns about the patient being close to having a myocardial infarction. The best way to deal with this difficult situation is to avoid the circumstances that lead to it in the first place. It is best not to implement the T3 therapy in older patients who are frail and/or very much at risk for having a myocardial infarction; and it is best to address side effects very early, when they first appear.

But should this difficult circumstance develop, it is probably best to err on the side of going down quickly on the T3 therapy, perhaps even faster than one decrement per day, or perhaps even faster than one decrement per dose. The plummeting T3 levels would at least reduce what is likely to be a major factor in the side effects: T3 unsteadiness. If the T3 therapy is decreased very quickly, a commensurately supportive dose of T4 therapy should be considered. For example, if the T3 was being decreased from 75 mcg/dose down to 37.5 mcg/dose in one day, a supportive dose of 0.025–0.05 mg of T4 should be considered. If that 37.5 mcg/dose was reduced to zero the next day, the T4 dosage could be continued or perhaps increased slightly. Remember, T4 is four times less potent than T3, less than half of the T4 prescribed will be converted to T3, and it will take a week for half of what will be converted to T3 to be converted. But it will be a steady source, and it will help to give the patient's own thyroid function time to come up.

c23 **Side effects can be caused by T3 levels that are too high, too low, or unsteady:** The side effects of T3 levels that are too high, too low, or too unsteady are very similar. It is assumed by many that if a patient on T3 therapy begins having symptoms of shakiness, increased heart rate, and increased awareness of the heartbeat, then that patient is necessarily suffering the effects of excessive T3 levels. But actually, patients can develop these same symptoms if there is a sudden *drop* in their T3 levels (due to compensatory increased sympathetic tone to maintain blood pressure) due to the patients missing doses of the T3 for instance. In such a circumstance, *adding* T3 can help resolve the complaints. Also, such side effects often respond to a stabilizing T4 test dose in those patients with *unsteady* T3 levels due to, say, decreased dosing compliance.

The distinction can easily be made by the patient's average body temperature. If it is too low, and the clinical picture would correlate to a drop in T3 levels, then the side effects are likely to be due to T3 levels that are too low. If the temperature is averaging normal, but the temperature and clinical story would correlate with unsteady T3 levels, then the side effects would likely respond to a T4 test dose. If the temperature is too high, then it may be that the patient is on too much T3. However, in patients being treated with the T3 therapy protocol described in this manual, it is very rare that such side effects are due to excessive T3 levels. This is because patients are not to increase the T3 therapy unless their temperatures are below 98.6°F on average. And by following this guideline, it is very unusual to overshoot the needed level of T3. If patients are having these types of side effects, yet their temperatures are not above 98.6°F, then they are not on too much T3 (except perhaps in the sense that it is difficult to keep their T3 levels steady on their current doses; see c24).

c24 **The higher the dose of T3 therapy, the harder it is to keep T3 levels steady:** Nevertheless, by cycling off the T3 therapy and starting another cycle, patients are often able to get their temperatures up on much lower doses (which are easier to keep steady) on subsequent cycles than they were on previous ones, until they are able to wean off the T3 therapy completely, staying normal off therapy **(see p111, c8, c22, and c28).**

c25 **Steadiness is everything (p95, p103, and p110).**

c26 **Unsteady T3 levels are the most common cause of side effects, and poor clinical results (p102, p103, and p105).**

c27 **It is not wise to stop the T3 medicine abruptly (see p107, p125, and c22).**

c28 **T3-level unsteadiness can result in decreased clinical improvement before it results in side effects:** Sometimes, when the patient's temperature is averaging normal, and the patient is still not feeling as well as one would hope, it is due to unsteady T3 levels. This is evidenced by such a patient's appreciable clinical improvement (within about 45 minutes) with a T4 test dose **(p112)**, and/or over a week or two of increased compliance with the dosing times. And sometimes patients can notice not feeling quite as well on a given dose than they were previously, even though their temperatures are still averaging normal. Such patients can often associate the slip in their clinical status with a time that they were having trouble taking their doses on time, or during a time of destabilizing stress (e.g., significant emotional stress or mental pressure). Increased compliance with dosing times and/or a T4 test dose might restore their clinical improvement, but sometimes it doesn't. It is easier for T3 levels to get unsteady, and also to stay unsteady, when the patients are on higher doses of T3 therapy. When clinical improvement cannot be restored in the present cycle, then it is usually best to wean off the T3 therapy (to let things steady down), and start again **(Q13).**

c29 Side effects from T3 therapy are dependent mainly on how well the molecule is delivered: To illustrate: If the T3 levels were to be kept steady enough, even people who don't need T3 therapy would not have side effects from exogenous T3 (provided their temps were kept close to 98.6°F). When people are given T3, their own systems compensate (through negative feedback inhibition of the pituitary) by making less T3 of their own. If enough T3 were given by mouth to healthy people, their own systems would be completely suppressed and their T3 levels would be completely replaced with exogenous T3. If their temperatures were not too high or too low, then how they would feel while replaced on the exogenous T3 would mainly depend on how close to endogenously steady the T3 levels could be kept.

Questions

Q1 How do you know it's thyroid?

You don't. It's a therapeutic trial. There are several reasons, however, that it should be considered first, not last. Many people respond well to the treatment, it doesn't take long to see if you're on the right track, it's simple (there are few variables to manage), when it works it often works very well, the symptoms often remain improved even after the treatment is discontinued, T3 therapy is not foreign, and proper T3 is generally well tolerated. The therapeutic trial can help distinguish between WTS and other problems. It is not a cure-all.

The T3 therapy can be tried in conjunction with other approaches, but doing so can sometimes add variables that confuse the therapeutic trial. It may be difficult to see how much of the patient's response, or lack thereof, is due to one approach or the other, or the combination of them. Because one can usually tell within about 2 weeks how well a patient is responding to T3 therapy, I usually like to start T3 therapy by itself at first, to more easily gauge the patient's response to it. Encouraging good health habits such as proper nutrition, exercise, and rest is always a good idea. Discouraging harmful habits such as smoking, drug and alcohol abuse, and others is also in order.

To be sure, a lot of other problems can cause symptoms similar to WTS, which can be affected in various ways. For instance, it is interesting that many diabetic patients notice that when their blood sugars are higher, their temperatures are higher; and when their blood sugars are lower, their temperatures are lower. When hypoglycemic patients have their hypoglycemic episodes, they usually if not always experience a drop in their temperatures when their blood sugar drops. I have seen the symptoms of "WTS" respond sometimes to hypoglycemic diets alone; and I have seen the symptoms of "hypoglycemia" respond sometimes to T3 therapy alone. The same could be said about antidepressants, female hormones, adrenal hormones, yeast-free diets, and a number of other approaches. So it's certainly not the only approach, it's just that in a lot of cases it's the approach to try first not last.

Q2 What are the substantive risks of T3 therapy (c22)?

T3 is a molecule that is present from birth in every human's body, and is absolutely necessary for good health. There is nothing inherently bad about the molecule – our lives depend on it. It can't and hasn't directly damaged the tissue of heart, brain, or other tissues. There is not a shred of evidence that suggests that thyroid hormones, when used properly, can damage the body in any way. But T3 is not candy, and T3 therapy is not completely without risk, as nothing is. The major consideration in terms of risk is cardiovascular. Cardiovascular disease is a major problem in our country. Every day many people who are not on thyroid medicine have heart attacks, strokes, and develop arrhythmias. The whole trick to T3 therapy is keeping the T3 levels steady. Unsteady T3 levels can increase a patient's chances of increased heart rate and palpitations. And if a patient is already on the verge of having a heart attack or a stroke, these cardiovascular side effects could aggravate the situation (p120). In some cases it is difficult to avoid unsteady T3 levels, and so it might not be advisable to implement T3 therapy in those patients who may not have the cardiovascular reserve to tolerate unsteady T3 levels very well (for example, certain elderly patients) (Q17). T3 therapy is not addictive, and does not necessarily need to be taken for life. With proper T3 therapy, one does not expect drastic problems, because one does not make drastic changes, and any side effects are addressed early. The T3 should be taken as well on time as possible to minimize the chance of side effects.

Q3 What happens if you stop the T3 therapy abruptly (c22)?

It is usually not wise to decrease the T3 therapy too quickly or to stop it abruptly, lest the patients' own thyroid systems are not given enough time to come back up and support their own metabolisms. If the T3 is stopped abruptly, patients may experience low blood pressure, which can lead to lightheadedness and palpitations. They can also experience severe fatigue, headaches, and other complaints and if no thyroid support of any kind is given, these complaints can last as long as 3 weeks (see also c22).

Q4   Will the patient have to stay on the T3 therapy for life?

No. The advantage of T3 therapy is that patients' symptoms often remain improved even after they have discontinued T3 therapy. Sometimes the symptoms do not remain improved after the treatment has been discontinued **(Q16)**, but it is extremely unlikely that any patient's symptoms will be persistently worse after T3 therapy than they were prior to T3 therapy.

Q5   What is the percentage index (c5)?

The patient's estimate (in percentage form) of how good the patient feels as compared to what the patient imagines a normal person to feel like.

Q6   Wouldn't increasing the dose of T3 every 3 days be easier for the patients to tolerate?

Increasing the dose of T3 every 3 days or longer is tolerated well by 9 patients out of 10. Most patients tolerate the dose being increased every 3 days very well. But if you increase the patients' dosages every 3 days, you must be willing to accept the 10% chance that the patient is a 1-day compensator, and will have less chance of tolerating the T3 therapy well, and it is likely that she will be more difficult to manage than she would have been if her dosage had been increased every day. It is easier to prevent people from becoming a management problem than it is to stop them from being management problems once they are.

Q7   What if a patient's temperature goes down with T3 therapy?

This is your first clue that the patient may be a 1-day compensator **(p103)**. Such patients' negative feedback inhibition of the pituitary gland may be so rapid that the patients can actually over-compensate, such that their temperatures can temporarily go lower than they were prior to T3 therapy. Such patients' symptoms can worsen at such a time as well. These patients are more likely to experience side effects of unsteadiness from the T3 therapy than others. It is more difficult to keep the T3 levels steady of such patients, and so extra care should be taken to keep T3 levels as steady as possible from the start. If the patient's T3 levels become too destabilized to proceed with the T3 therapy, the patient should be weaned off the therapy. The pros and cons of the T3 therapy should be reconsidered in light of it being likely that the patient is a 1-day compensator. If the T3 therapy is re-initiated, it should be done after the patient's T3 levels have had a chance to steady down very well (off T3 for 5–14 days), and the T3 therapy should be increased rapidly enough to take deliberate exogenous control of the thyroid system to make the transition of control as smooth as possible or it should not be done at all (remember – it is important that everything be done gradually, but not necessarily slowly).

Q8   How high a dosage of the medicine does one go on each cycle of T3 therapy?

Rather than to go much higher than 90 mcg BID, it is usually best to wean off the present T3 cycle in preparation of beginning another cycle **(p99, c12)**. This is because the temperature can often be brought up to normal on much lower doses in subsequent cycles, when it never could be on much higher doses in previous cycles. Also, if the temperature has not been brought up to normal with the 90 mcg/dose, it very often will not be even with much higher doses. This is especially true when doses close to 90 mcg have seemingly no effect on the patients' temperatures. However, when a patient's temperature is responding to each incremental dosage increase, only to predictably drop back down again each time (within about the same period of time, each time – the patient's compensation time), then it may be productive to go up higher than 90 mcg/dose (a step at a time, as needed, up to several increments higher, if there are no side effects or complaints).

Compensation is not an infinite process, and the hope is that the patient's temperature is very close to being captured **(c9)**. When there is a cause–effect relationship that is being demonstrated with each increase, the use of slightly higher dosages is more clearly justified.

Q9   How long should a patient stay up on a cycle before weaning back down again?

It depends on whether or not the patients' temperatures are yet up to normal. If the patients' temperatures are up to normal, then the cycle should not be weaned until the patients' compensation times have passed by at least a day or two (in other words, until their temperatures have been captured). This is to ensure full benefit of the cycle **(c9, Q8)**. Patients who have gotten their temperatures up but who have not demonstrated a predictable compensation time, however, may need to stay up on that cycle for 3 weeks to see if their temperatures have been captured (because the longest compensation times are around 3 weeks, and if the patients don't compensate within 3 weeks they're probably not going to compensate). Now if the patients' temperatures haven't come up to normal, and the maximum dosage **(Q8)** has been reached, the patients may begin weaning the cycle right away. There is no added benefit in staying up on the cycle for 3 weeks in this circumstance. There's no point in waiting to see if their temperatures are captured when they aren't even normal (remember if the patient's temperature isn't up within a few hours of an increased dose, it probably isn't going up on that dose no matter how many weeks it's continued). It's important that progress not be delayed unnecessarily.

Patients do not necessarily need to be weaned off a cycle immediately after it is clear their temperatures have been captured. In fact, usually if the patients are feeling very well they do stay up on that plateau for a time depending on the circumstances (c8). Not uncommonly patients will say: "This is the first time that I have felt well in 20 years, so if it's all the same to you, I'd rather not wean down off the medicine right now." They are often concerned that they will start feeling badly again. But there is often so little breakthrough of the patients' symptoms that after a few months they seem to forget what it feels like to have those symptoms, and begin to gain confidence that they will be able to wean off the medicine and stay normal. This confidence is bolstered by them getting tired of taking the medicine every 12 hours, and tired of paying for it, and so the treatment is usually self-limiting with the patients becoming motivated to wean off. Of course, if a patient begins having side effects or complaints, it may be necessary to wean the T3 at that time, even if the temperature hasn't come up.

Q10   How fast does one go off a cycle of T3 therapy?
It depends on how far along a patient is in treatment. For example, if you were tuning a radio by turning a knob, and you wanted to tune in a station that was on the other end of the dial, you would probably turn the knob more quickly at first, more slowly as you got closer to the station's frequency, and most slowly as you were fine-tuning the radio to bring the station in without static. Sometimes, patients' histories suggest that it may take several cycles of T3 therapy to return a patient's temperature patterns to normal, if at all. Each cycle can take over 4 weeks. At best, such patients may be looking at 3 months' worth of therapy before doing very well, so it is usually best not to dillydally. And, whereas, it is good to get as much benefit out of each cycle as possible, the preceding cycles can often be thought of as "coarse-tuning," with subsequent cycles being thought of as "fine-tuning." There is little point in fine-tuning a coarse-tuning cycle, it is usually more productive to move on to a more productive cycle. If it is likely that this is not the last cycle, it is usually best to simply decelerate the rate of wean (c12) rather than go back up a dosage increment if the temperature starts to slip a little (also see Q11).

However, if there is a good chance that this may be the last cycle, and the patient is not in a hurry to wean off the medicine, it may be best to wean down by 7.5 mcg/dose/7–10 days to give the patient's body every opportunity to come back up on its own again.

Finally, in cases where patients go up to about 90 mcg/dose of T3 and notice no changes whatsoever, good or bad – as if they were only taking water – I will frequently try going down a 7.5 mcg dosage decrement every day if the patient has no complaints. It is usually more effective to wean off such a cycle and to start another than it is to continue increasing the dose. This is because sometimes a patient can keep increasing the dose and the temperature still doesn't go up. But interestingly, when the cycle is weaned and another one is started, the temperature can frequently go up on less T3 when it never did on more. Also, it is usually better to wean off a cycle that has demonstrated no effect (in preparation for starting another), than it is to stay on that cycle for weeks hoping it will demonstrate more effect (p105). See also Q9.

Q11   If patients' temperatures slip while they are weaning down off the T3 therapy, should the dose be increased back up an increment before continuing to wean?
Usually not (c12, Q10). However, if there is a good chance that this may be the last cycle it may be worth going back up an increment (or perhaps two if necessary) for a day or so to bring the temperature back up before decelerating and continuing the wean as suggested in c12. If the patient begins to feel any worse when his/her temperature slips, and for some reason (usually because of things becoming destabilized) increasing the T3 back up one or two increments is not successful, it may be necessary to go back to the **Cycling Up module** (increasing the T3 according to its rules), and perhaps to give a stabilizing T4 test dose to recapture the patient's temperature and clinical status.

Q12   When weaning a cycle of T3 therapy, does one wean part-way down, down to the starting dose, or all the way off?
If it is decided that it is time for a patient to wean the T3 therapy, then it is usually best for the patient to wean all the way off. Imagine having a pile of dirt in your front yard that you want to move with a wheelbarrow to the back yard. Yes, you could wheel a full load to the back yard, dump it only halfway, and then return to the pile in the front yard for another load. But when you wheel a full load to the back yard and you dump it completely before returning for another load, you could accomplish twice as much work with much less effort. By weaning off the T3 therapy completely, the patient does not waive her chance at being able to get her temperature up on the smallest dose she

can. This is no small opportunity. Generally, the lower the dose of T3 therapy, the easier it is to keep it steady, the better the patient feels, the less the chance of side effects, the less the expense incurred, and the closer the patient is to being finished with the treatment.

Q13   How long does one stay off between cycles?
This depends on where one is in the therapy, and why the cycle was being weaned. If a cycle was being weaned because of side effects: if the side effects resolve while the patient is weaning down off the medicine, then one can stay off the treatment for 2–3 days before starting back up again. If the side effects only begin to resolve while the patient is weaning down off the T3 therapy, and resolve completely only after the patient is off the therapy for a couple of days, then the patient should stay off the T3 therapy for another couple of days after that to allow the T3 to steady down further to provide a better start with a steadier foundation for the next cycle.

Theoretically, if someone wanted to let the T3 level steady down as much as possible, one could argue that the patient should remain off the T3 for about 2 weeks. Even so, most of the steadying is probably accomplished within about 10 days, so there is probably not much added benefit in staying off the T3 for much longer than that. This approach is indicated when one would like to eliminate the unsteadiness as much as possible to see if the patient will respond well to treatment. It also underscores the importance of not taking a steady start for granted, because if the T3 levels are destabilized (muddying the water, so to speak) right from the start, it would take quite a bit of time to reproduce another opportunity with that patient at so steady a start.

Q14   If the patient is feeling very well, but her temperature is still less than 98.6°F when measured as indicated, is it really necessary to push the temperature up to 98.6°F?
No it isn't, but patients usually feel their best when their temperatures are 98.6°F. Also, a patient may be less likely to relapse after the treatment has been discontinued if his/her temperature has been "punctuated" up to 98.6°F before weaning.

Q15   How do you wean a WTS patient who is also hypothyroid (see c11)?

Q16   What if a patient's temperature and symptoms do not remain improved after the treatment is discontinued?
If patients' temperatures begin to drop right away as soon as they start weaning, then it is likely that the T3 therapy is being weaned too quickly **(c12)**. If the patient is able to wean down several decrements without a drop in temperature, but cannot go below a certain level without the temperature dropping, then it may be that the patient does not have a sufficient supply of endogenous or exogenous T4 available for conversion to T3 to maintain the present level of thyroid stimulation to the cells (the patient may be hypothyroid, see c11). If the patient is able to wean all the way off the cycle and stay well for a period of days before the symptoms return, it indicates that the patient was almost able to maintain well off the treatment, and might not have because the treatment was weaned just a little too quickly. Or the worsening of the symptoms again may be due to an actual relapse due to some precipitating factor (such as a big stress). On the other hand, if the patient's temperature and symptoms worsen as the T3 is being weaned even though it is being weaned slowly enough, and there is a sufficient supply of T4 for conversion to T3, then this suggests that there may be some unaddressed factor(s) that are preventing the patient from staying improved (e.g., continuing stress, environmental toxin, nutrient deficiency, etc.). If the patient is not under a lot of stress, then some other factor may be preventing the improvement on T3 therapy to persist after the treatment has been discontinued. In such cases, one might consider adjusting some other medicines a patient may be taking (such as female hormones), and look to see what other changes can be made in other areas **(Q10, Q29)**.

Q17   What are the risks of staying on T3 therapy for a long time?
There was a boy who was born with congenital hypothyroidism and was raised on traditional T3 (Cytomel™). He was never treated with a T4-containing medicine, and so essentially never had a molecule of T4 in his body. By age 26, he had developed normally with no problems. This underscores the fact that the importance of T4 lies very much in that it is "T3 waiting to happen." Nevertheless, duration of treatment may be limited by risks of longer-term treatment (>1 year or so). The potential of increased osteoporosis should be considered (especially in patients at risk). The studies that link increased osteoporosis with long-term thyroid therapy have been done with thyroid therapy managed much differently than discussed here. The studies involve patients managed with suppressive doses of T4-containing medicine, without regard to their body temperature patterns or clinical well-being. This textbook should make it clear that a good many of these patients are perhaps being "pushed too far in the wrong direction with the wrong medicine." I would not be at all surprised if the vast majority of the patients involved were clinically hypothyroid with low body temperature patterns. Perhaps if the patients in these studies had been treated with T3 instead that normalized their temperatures

and lessened their symptoms they might have enjoyed increased bone densities. T3 therapy usually lasts on the order of months, and the osteoporosis studies involved patients treated for years (e.g., 10 years). I am not concerned about increased osteoporosis in patients who are treated for months. Circumstances have been such that I have treated a few patients for more than a year, and some for a couple of years. I have done serial bone scans in a couple of these patients who I felt were at higher risk for osteoporosis. I was able to see no decreased bone density in this tiny cohort, and I wondered if it might have actually increased. But because osteoporosis is a serious condition, the potential should be seriously considered and weighed and managed accordingly. Of course, these long-term studies did not address the need to ensure optimal calcium, vitamin D, and vitamin K2 nutrient status.

Q18   How many patients can be weaned off T3 therapy?
They all can. The question is: Will all of the patients who do improve remain improved, as compared to the way they were before treatment? Even though many patients do enjoy persistent improvement, some of the patients will go back to feeling as they did prior to treatment. Much less than 1%, if any, will have symptoms that are persistently worse after T3 therapy than they were prior to T3 therapy **(Q16)**.

Q19   What if the patient improves at first, but then stops feeling as well even though the temperature is holding?
If the T3 therapy improves a patient's symptoms at all, it is because it has increased the patient's body temperature patterns. This is a very good sign because it suggests that the patient's symptoms are at least to some extent temperature-mediated. During T3 therapy, it is not uncommon for a patient's temperature to drop back down again (due to compensation, see **p100**), or for it to become unsteady **(c24)**, and therefore for the patient's symptoms to return. When a person first starts the T3 therapy, it is easier to keep the T3 level steady because one is building on a steady endogenous foundation of T3. For this reason, the beginning of a cycle often provides the best opportunity to see if the symptoms are temperature-mediated and T3-responsive. At that point of the cycle, if the temperature can be raised close to normal, it has a better chance of being steady also. And a temperature that is sufficiently normal and steady is what is required for clinical improvement. Of course, as a cycle wears on, and as the doses of T3 increase, the chances of "muddying the water" (making the T3 level unsteady) also increase. If the T3 therapy improves a patient's symptoms to any degree, it is likely that the symptoms are to some extent temperature-mediated. It becomes less of a question as to whether the T3 therapy is on the right track, and more of a matter of whether or not the T3 therapy can be adjusted (e.g., with increased compliance, T4 test dose, cycling the patient on and off therapy) to cause the patient's temperature to become and stay sufficiently normal and sufficiently steady for the symptoms to improve and remain improved **(c28)**.

Q20   What if the patient's temperature goes up to normal and the patient still doesn't feel very well?
Patients' hypothyroid symptoms not improving at all with normalization of their body temperatures strongly suggests unsteady T3 levels. The purpose of going on T3 therapy is to reset the thyroid system. It is nice when T3 levels can be held steady enough in the meantime for the patient to notice an improvement clinically while on a given cycle **(p95, p95)**. If a patient's temperature goes up to normal but the patient is still feeling no improvement, it is very likely to be because of unsteadiness of the T3 level. This is one instance in which a T4 test dose might be illustrative. If the patient's symptoms improve within an hour or so of the test dose, then that is a good indicator that it's just a matter of the patient's T3 levels not being quite steady enough. If the patient responds tremendously well to the T4 test dose, then one could consider continuing the present T3 cycle, and using the T4 test dose Please Repeat as Necessary (PRN) (as needed). But if the symptomatic resolution with the T4 test dose is not sufficient, then it would be best to wean the present T3 cycle. As patients wean off the T3 therapy, their own T3 production comes back up, and their T3 levels become more and more endogenously steady. And as they do, the patient's symptoms often begin to resolve if their temperatures hold while weaning. If their temperatures don't hold, and the patients notice no symptomatic improvement while weaning off the T3, then they will often be able to get their temperatures up on less medicine on the next cycle. With the patients on less medicine, it is easier to keep T3 levels steady, and they are much more likely to notice an improvement in their symptoms. This is why I often refer to the first cycle as a "reset cycle," and why I consider a therapeutic trial of T3 to be at least two cycles **(p112)**.

Q21   What if the patient is feeling improved on the T3 therapy, but when the dosage is increased to bring the temperature closer to normal, the temperature drops and the patient feels worse?
If this occurs at a time consistent with a patient's compensation time, then it may just be due to compensation **(p100)**. However, if this occurs after a patient's usual compensation time has clearly passed, at a time of severe stress, it may due to a reduction of remaining endogenous T4 to T3 conversion. Finally, if it occurs after a patient's usual compensation time has clearly passed, and the patient is not under significant stress, it may be due to a "crumbling effect" from an unsteadying of T3 levels **(p110)**. This is very unusual but does occur.

If it is due to compensation or reduced T4 to T3 conversion as mentioned above, then one may continue cycling the patient up on the T3 therapy if there are no complaints. If it seems due to crumbling, then a T4 test dose may be helpful in steadying the patient's T3 level, and the patient's temperature may come back up. If it doesn't come back up with the T4 test dose, but the patient does notice an improvement, then continue cycling the patient up on the T3 therapy in an effort to raise the temperature back up, with T4 doses taken PRN indications of unsteadiness. If the temperature cannot be raised with this approach without the T3 level steadiness getting more and more out of control, then it may be necessary to wean off the current cycle of T3 to recapture the patient's T3 level steadiness, and then begin another cycle. This may be necessary to get the patient's temperature back up to normal, and to keep it normal, often on less medicine than the previous cycle.

T3 dosage level does not always equate, for some reason, with T3 stimulation of the cell. It is clear that the effectiveness or degree of stimulation of a certain amount of T3 has something to do with its steadiness. For instance, I had one patient misunderstand the directions for taking the T3. She continued to increase the dose of T3 she was taking until she was on 800 mcg per day. Yet her temperature was still low, and she wasn't having any complaints. When the error was discovered, she was gradually weaned off the T3, and after a time another cycle was started. On that cycle, she was able to get her temperature up on 150 mcg per day when she never could on 800. In some cases, the T3 could be increased "until the cows come home," and the patients' temperatures never would come up (this is particularly the case when there are indications of unsteady T3 levels).

Another example was a case of a young woman who accidentally took massive doses of T3 (1000-fold the usual therapeutic dose, for 8 days). She had cardiovascular and central nervous system symptoms that required intensive care support, but she didn't die. She made a satisfactory recovery.

Q22 What if a patient has a slump of fatigue or some other complaint at the same time each day?

If a patient has fatigue that comes and goes at the same time each day, it may be that the T3 level is "resonating" in such a way that the T3 level is lower at that time of day. Frequently the patients report that their body temperatures drop at such times. This problem is often alleviated by shifting the dosage times in relation to when the patient awakens. For example, have the patient try taking the T3 doses at 8 am and 8 pm, instead of 7 am and 7 pm. Or one could try moving the doses up 1 hour instead, say to 6 am and 6 pm.

It is helpful to determine if the slumps can be correlated to any other factors (such as meal times, diet, or sleep cycle), and making adjustments as indicated. For example, it is interesting that many diabetic patients notice that when their blood sugars are higher, their temperatures are higher; and when their blood sugars are lower, their temperatures are lower. When hypoglycemic patients have their hypoglycemic episodes, they usually if not always experience a drop in their temperatures when their blood sugar drops. I have seen the symptoms of WTS respond sometimes to hypoglycemic diets alone; and I have seen the symptoms of "hypoglycemia" respond sometimes to T3 therapy alone. The same could be said about antidepressants, female hormones, adrenal hormones, yeast-free diets, and a number of other approaches.

Q23 How often are office visits?

When patients are first started on the treatment, it is best for them to be educated well, with 2 weeks' worth of instructions, and to be prescribed at least 2 weeks' worth of medication. This prevents them from having to make extra phone calls and extra trips, which can be inefficient for both them and the staff. After patients are started on the T3 therapy, they should be seen back in the office in 2 weeks (Note: If a patient presents taking a T4-containing medicine and, at the start of treatment, the patient is instructed to wean the T4-containing medicine before/during the T3 therapy is being initiated, it may be best to schedule the following visit for 3 weeks instead of the usual 2). After 2 weeks of being on a therapeutic trial, it is much easier to predict what course a patient's treatment is likely to take, because the patient's initial response greatly narrows the scope of likely scenarios. Predictable parameters include: projected length of treatment, number of cycles that may be necessary, range of T3 dosages that may be necessary, expected outcomes, etc.

At that 2-week appointment, if the patient is doing well and it seems that the patient is on a predictable course, then the next appointment might be scheduled for 4 weeks (this is true for ≥85% of patients). If at that 2-week appointment, it is not as easy to predict the patient's likely course, or how the patient is likely to do, scheduling the next appointment for 3 weeks would be better (very rarely, one may want to schedule the next visit less than 3 weeks out). Thereafter, the return visits might be scheduled for every 4 weeks (extending to every 6 weeks, and then perhaps every 8 weeks as indicated).

This rate of office visits is in contrast to the every 6 months to every year appointments that are often scheduled for patients being treated with T4-containing medicines. Thyroid therapy need not be so static as many people consider it to be. T3 therapy is very dynamic. With T4 therapy, it takes over a week for half of the T4 given to be converted to the active hormone T3. But with T3 therapy, all of the active hormone is available immediately. That changes everything. That puts the therapy on the order of minutes, hours, days, and weeks; not months, and years. If the treatment is well managed, a lot can happen in a short period of time.

Q24   If a patient starts having any side effects, does that mean that the treatment isn't likely to work out very well?
Not necessarily. The first thing that side effects suggest is an unsteady T3 level. The whole trick to T3 therapy is keeping the T3 level steady. Granted, if the level is steady but is too high or too low, then a person may have side effects. But if patients' temperatures are not above 98.6°F, then their T3 levels are not too high. And if their temperatures are not lower than they were before treatment, then any new complaints are not likely to be from the T3 levels being too low. If a patient is having side effects from the T3 therapy, it is usually because of T3 unsteadiness **(c24, c25)**. This suspicion can be confirmed with a T4 test dose **(p112)**.

The most common side effects in order of appearance with increasing levels of T3 unsteadiness
Fluid retention
Achiness
Dull headache
Edginess
Increased awareness of heartbeat and/or increased heart rate

With T3 therapy, it is important to start with steady T3 levels **(c4)**, and then to keep the T3 levels steady thereafter with good patient compliance. When a patient begins having any side effects, the first question to be addressed is: Has the patient been able to take the medicine very much on time as directed? Although unsteady T3 levels can develop even with good compliance, it's important to rule out poor compliance, which is a likely cause that is easy and important to address **(c29)**. Stress can also contribute to unsteady T3 levels.

Q25   How are side effects managed?
Side effects can be caused by T3 levels that are too low, too high, or unsteady. The body temperature patterns are useful in helping one make the distinction. The most common cause of side effects are T3 levels that are unsteady. Unsteady T3 levels are most commonly generated by not getting a good, fresh, steady start on a cycle; or by not taking the T3 compound very well on time every 12 hours **(p108)**. Improved compliance to dosing times may be all that is necessary to alleviate the side effects. If side effects are more severe, then one should consider a T4 test dose **(p112)**. If that doesn't work, then it would probably be best for the patient to wean gradually off the T3 therapy. If it is decided that another cycle will be started, then one should make sure that the patient remains off the T3 therapy long enough to get a good, fresh start on the next cycle **(p105)**.

Q26   What is a T4 test dose? (see p112)
The T4 test dose is a small dose of T4 given to a patient suspected of having unsteady T3 levels. The T4 is four times weaker than T3 and three times longer acting and competes with T3 at the level of the thyroid receptor. The dose is usually half of a 25 mcg tablet of levothyroxine. Patients taking WT3 therapy that are experiencing symptoms consistent with unsteady T3 levels such as shakiness, jitteriness, fluid retention, achiness, and palpitations often notice improvement in about 45 minutes of a T4 test dose. It is called a test dose because a lessening of the symptoms suspicious of unsteady T3 levels by a T4 test dose tends to confirm the suspicion. T4 test doses help so often in such cases that a lack of improvement with T4 test dosing suggests that they symptoms are probably not due to the T3 but may be due to some other cause. If half of a 25 mcg tablet of levothyroxine does not improve the symptoms, the dose may be repeated in about 90 minutes to see if that will help.

Q27   If the T4 test dose (p112) works, how often should it be taken?
Now that the patient knows the clinical difference between better and worse, if she ever feels worse again, she can take another dose of T4 (PRN similar side effects or decreased symptom resolution). If she doesn't feel worse again, she shouldn't take it because it goes against what we're trying to accomplish. On a certain level of T3, if the patient ends up needing to take the T4 more than once, it commonly will be needed in a recurring interval of time (e.g., every 3 days, every 5 days, every 7 days). Also, so long as the patient remains on that level of T3, the amount of T4 that is

effective as a test dose shouldn't change. But if a patient is on a higher dose of T3, it may be necessary to increase the T4 test dose in a roughly proportionate manner **(p113)**.

Q28 Do temperatures or T4 test doses have to be taken to the minute like the T3?
No. Temperatures should be taken about every 3 hours, 3 times a day, starting about 3 hours after waking, but the timing is not critical. Likewise, the T4 test doses are taken only as needed according to the clinical situation, and exact timing is not critical. Some people may find that they need a T4 test dose about every 3 days, but that T4 wouldn't have to be taken every 72 hours precisely.

Q29 What if the treatment doesn't work?
In well-selected candidates for treatment, the most common reason for difficulty is unsteady T3 levels **(c25)**. But I'll address this question, based on the assumption that the T3 therapy has been administered as well as possible, and still does not work for a patient as hoped. Briefly, the human body is a complexly interrelated system. By affecting one area, many other areas may be affected in turn. For example, getting enough exercise, getting enough sleep, and eating well can each, individually, cause significant changes in the entire body (from bowel movements to headaches). There are a great many influences that can have widespread effects, even to the recalibrating of the system, as it were. Such as: T3 therapy, female hormones, adrenal hormones, and other medicines. When combined, these influences can be synergistic or antagonistic. If a patient seems to be progressing nicely on T3 therapy, and that progress is inexplicably halted, it may be that there is an opposing influence that is not allowing endogenous recalibration in a certain area (see "ropes and rings" analogy in book: *Wilson's Temperature Syndrome—A Reversible Low Temperature Problem*). For example, if a patient is taking 0.625 mg of Premarin each day, it may be helpful to see how well the patient does on 0.3 mg each day. By changing the "tension" in a potentially oppositional influence, progress can often be resumed (see end of Q22). Other examples of such influences include certain blood pressure medicines and antidepressants.

Nevertheless, T3 therapy is no more a panacea than any other medical treatment. Even though it works exceptionally well for a large number of people who previously were unable to find relief, it, sadly, does not work for everyone. When it is decided that an adequate therapeutic trial has been given, and the patient's symptoms have not responded, the patient will be back in a similar spot he/she was in before hearing of WTS: square one, looking for a solution for his/her frustrating situation. As far as leads go, if the patient's symptoms are classic for WTS, they are classic for abnormal body temperature patterns. If the patient has an abnormal body temperature pattern that does not respond to T3 therapy (very rare), then perhaps there is some other temperature-mediating factor involved. If the treatment failed because for some reason the patient could not tolerate T3 therapy (usually because of unsteadiness), then the patient may want to look toward the not-too-distant future. Because although T3 compounded with a sustained release agent in a capsule is a great approach, it's not perfect. The technology is already available and the application will certainly come that provides for more steady, better controlled, and better tolerated administration of T3 therapy (e.g., infusion pumps, patches, etc.).

It is important to be as supportive as possible towards patients for whom the treatment doesn't work. They can easily feel despair. I feel it is important that the patients cope as well as they can with their complaints, but I don't feel that it is warranted to tell them: "You'll have to live the rest of your life feeling the way you do." Many of the people who respond fabulously well to T3 therapy have been told that same thing in the past. But it wasn't true. Such a comment is without basis and should be avoided. It can be very destructive, and accomplishes very little. More than one patient with such symptoms has mentioned suicide. Things change and new answers come every day, and probably will more so all the time. WTS is a precedent for such simple answers.

Q30 What happens if the patient's T4 and TSH levels drop while on T3 therapy?
A decrease in TSH and T4 levels is exactly what one would expect in a patient receiving exogenous T3 therapy. In fact, the resetting phenomenon is often not seen unless there is a decrease in T4 levels for a time **(p92)**. It is not alarming if their T4 levels and TSH levels are suppressed even to essentially zero, for a time (provided the patients are feeling very well without any side effects, and their temperatures are not above 98.6°F). Such low levels are not always necessary, but decreased T4 and TSH levels are an indication that T4 and rT3 levels are being well depleted (which is often the point of T3 therapy).

Hyperthyroidism often causes very low TSH levels and symptoms of hyperthyroidism. Yet proper T3 therapy often causes very low TSH levels without symptoms of hyperthyroidism while providing normal temperatures and a decidedly euthyroid clinical state. This shows that very low TSH levels do not necessarily equate with a hyperthyroid state. Also, there is no evidence that low TSH levels alone necessarily equate with increased osteoporosis (because some have concluded that very suppressive doses of T4 given over many years without regard to patients' clinical status or body temperatures is associated with increased bone loss, does not mean that the same can necessarily be concluded about suppressive doses of T3 given over a period of months, that are associated with normal body temperatures and a clinically euthyroid state). There is no evidence that endogenous hyperthyroidism has ever been generated in a euthyroid patient with suppressive exogenous thyroid medicine. And there is no evidence that endogenous hypothyroidism has ever been generated in a euthyroid patient with exogenous thyroid medicine.

Q31   How often does one order the thyroid blood tests?
The thyroid blood tests are not so much to diagnose WTS as they are to rule out thyroid gland dysfunction before treatment. Also, they provide a baseline against which to compare future thyroid blood tests. It is reassuring to have this baseline, because with it and post-treatment blood tests it can be demonstrated that the T3 therapy has not adversely affected endogenous thyroid gland function. Once T3 therapy is initiated, the thyroid blood tests do not significantly affect management decisions. They more reflect the changes that are occurring in the thyroid system than they are useful in directing the therapy that brings about those changes. Therefore, it is not necessary to get the thyroid tests often, if at all. But that's not to say that they are completely without value, because it is sometimes helpful to see how the blood tests reflect the effects and progress of the therapy. The thyroid tests do sometimes show some interesting trends. For example, a symptomatic patient may have a temperature of 97.8°F before treatment with a T4 of 7.2 mcg/dl, a TSH of 4.1 mIU/ml, and a rT3 of 247 pg/ml; and yet feel very well having a temperature of 98.6°F with a T4 of 7.1 mcg/dl, a TSH of 4.2 mIU/ml, and a rT3 of 85 pg/ml after treatment. Granted, rT3 levels can change quickly and readily under various circumstances, but that doesn't mean the averages can't be lower. Such interesting trends are what have led to the paradigm upon which the T3 therapy has been designed.

Q32   What would be the expected thyroid blood test values after a couple of weeks of T3 therapy?
One would expect the TSH, T4, and rT3 levels to be lower, and the T3 to be higher than when the patient started T3 therapy. One would expect the T3 resin uptake test to be lower than it was, because the T3 resin uptake test is low when total T3 by RIA is high, and it is high when total T3 by RIA is low. Depending on the dose the patient is taking at the time of the blood tests, the TSH, T4, and rT3 levels may be quite low (approaching zero). But suppressing T4 levels by suppressing TSH levels for a time appears to be very important in resetting the system. In other words, the suppression of T4 levels for a time is the whole point of the treatment, and in no way comes as any surprise.

Q33   What should the patients do with the T3 dosing if they miss the dosing time?
If patients discover that they have missed a dose by an hour or so, it is usually best for them to go ahead at that time and take the missed dosage, and to get back on schedule as quickly as possible (by taking the next dosage at the same time they would have had they not missed the time) so that there is only one aberration rather than several.

However, if the patients discover that they are very late (e.g., 5 hours), then one might consider having them go ahead and take the medicine at that time, and then take a number of subsequent doses at equal intervals that are less than 12 hours until the patients are back on schedule. If the patients are without complaints, one might consider having the patients eliminate the missed dose completely, while staying on schedule by taking the next dose at the same time they would have had they not missed the dose. Generally, the former alternative is better in patients who are less clinically stable.

Q34   What if the patient is up to 90 mcg BID of T3, and the temperature is still not up? (see p99, c12, and Q8)

Q35   What if a patient gets a fever due to a virus or cold? (see p103)
If a patient is doing well on a set dose of the T3 then the dosage is usually not changed if the patient gets a fever from illness. Whenever the dosage of T3 is changed, the T3 level can become a little destabilized for up to 2 weeks. Since a fever due to a viral illness usually only lasts less than 3 days, the dosage of T3 is not changed because it is usually best not to take a chance on destabilizing the T3 levels for 2 weeks while trying to manage an aberration that will likely only last a few days.

Case Studies

Case Study 1

A 43 year old (y.o.) mother of four presents to the office complaining of fatigue, listlessness, fluid retention, irritability, PMS, and easy weight gain. These symptoms came on 8 months ago after the birth of her fourth child. All of her blood tests are normal, and her body temperature averages 97.8°F during the day. She is started on 7.5 mcg BID of T3 compound **(p108)**, and is instructed to increase the dose by 7.5 mcg/dose/day until her temperature is 98.6°F on average during the day. Her temperature goes up to 98.6°F when she reaches 22.5 mcg BID. Her symptoms respond dramatically.

She does very well for several days on 22.5 mcg BID, until on the fourth day on that dose her average temperature drops to 98.0°F. At this time, some of her symptoms return. The dose is increased to 30 mcg BID, and her temperature goes to 98.6°F again and she again does exceptionally well until her temperature drops back down 4 days later. She is increased then to a dose of 37.5 mcg BID. Her temperature and symptoms respond for 4 days, then slip again. However, when her dose is then increased to 45 mcg BID, her temperature rises to 98.6°F again, with her symptoms resolving, and remaining resolved even longer than 4 days.

About 7 days after her temperature and symptoms remain resolved on the dose of 45 mcg BID, it is felt that her temperature has been "captured." **(p101)** At this time, the patient is instructed that she is likely to do well weaning off the T3 therapy, and has a good chance of remaining normal off the treatment. She feels completely well, but is a little reluctant to wean off the T3 therapy right away for fear of feeling badly again. She has also noticed that she has lost 5 pounds without changing her exercise or eating habits and wonders if it would be all right for her to stay on the 45 mcg BID T3 for about a month or so longer while she works with good diet and exercise to get off the other 15 pounds.

She is without complaints of any kind, so the regimen is continued, and a month later she is doing well. The following month she is ready and confident to wean off the T3 therapy. She is able to decrease her dose by 7.5 mcg/dose every 2 days without her temperature dropping, and in a couple of weeks she has successfully weaned off the T3 therapy. Her temperature has remained 98.6°F with her symptoms remaining resolved, even off T3 therapy.

Case Study 2

A 43 y.o. businessman presents to the office complaining of severe fatigue, difficulty sleeping, and headaches. The symptoms first started about 10 years ago when his business went into bankruptcy. The symptoms persisted to roughly that same degree until about 5 years ago when he became divorced, at which time his symptoms worsened considerably. His symptoms worsened yet again about 6 months ago when his brother died. To him, his symptoms are inexplicable because he feels that he has gotten over the loss of his brother, and he now is very happily remarried and the business he now owns is exceptionally successful. All tests are normal, but his temperature averages a degree low during the day.

He is started on a cycle of T3 therapy. He is started on 7.5 mcg p.o. BID and is instructed to increase the dose 7.5 mcg/dose/day if he is without complaints until his temperature is 98.6°F by mouth on average, and to call the office if he does develop any complaints, and to return to the office in 2 weeks. At the 2-week visit, the patient relates that he is taking 90 mcg BID and his temperature is still not up. Because his temperature did not budge at all during the first cycle and he has noticed no difference at all in the way he feels since starting the treatment, he is instructed to try weaning off the T3 therapy by 7.5 mcg/dose/day if he remains without complaints. This is done so that the treatment will not be unnecessarily delayed. He is able to decrease the dose every day without complaints.

The patient is then started on a second cycle, with the same instructions as the first. This time his temperature goes up to 98.6°F on 75 mcg BID. His symptoms begin to improve, but after about 3 days his temperature drops back down again. The dose is increased to 82.5 and his temperature returns to normal. After about a week on that dosage, his temperature starts to go down again and he loses some of the clinical improvement that he gained. The dose is increased to 90 mcg/dose, and his temperature goes up again, restoring some of his clinical improvement.

His temperature went down again after an undetermined time (because he wasn't taking his temperatures very well). Since he had been showing a definite response to each recent increase, and he was without complaints, he was increased above the usual maximum dose of 90 mcg BID to see if his temperature could be captured **(p101)** with one or two more increases. The temperature responded and dropped again on the 97.5 mcg dose. Then his temperature went up and stayed normal on 105 mcg BID and did not drop again.

Because he did not demonstrate any clear compensation time **(p100)**, he was left on 105 mcg BID for at least 3 weeks to help make sure that his temperature was indeed captured. During that 3 week period of time, he wasn't able to take his medicine very well on time for a few days, and he began to notice feeling a little headachy, tired, and more on edge. His temperature log revealed that his temperature had become a little more unsteady at that same time. His temperature was ranging more widely across his three daily temperatures **(p83)**. He was then given a T4 test dose of half a 0.025 mg tablet (0.0125 mg) of levothyroxine, and within 45 minutes his complaints resolved completely.

Anxious to see if he might be able to capture his temperature with a smaller dose of T3 on the third cycle **(p96)**, he was weaned off the second cycle. Because unsteadiness of the T3 level had been demonstrated in the second cycle with the T4 test dose, and because the patient was wondering how well the T3 therapy was going to end up working for him (even though he had gotten a fairly good response to treatment so far), it was decided to let him remain off for 10 days between cycles to let the T3 level steady down as much as possible so that he could get as fresh a start as possible **(p105)**. He tried weaning down off the T3 every 2 days, but with the third decrease his temperature started to drop a little. Because it looked as if he might have a cycle or two more to go, he did not increase his dose back up, but simply decelerated his wean to going down a 7.5 mcg decrement every 4 days **(c12)**. He was then able to wean off without much of a drop in his temperature.

On the next cycle, he was able to capture his temperature on 60 mcg BID. His symptoms were all but completely resolved at this point. He was without complaints. After a few weeks he was ready to proceed with the therapy and be weaned off the T3 to see if he could capture his temperature with less medicine on a subsequent cycle for complete resolution of his symptoms. He decreased the dose by one decrement every 4 days without any drop in his temperature.

On the fourth cycle, his temperature was captured with 15 mcg BID, and his symptoms resolved completely. He was later able to wean off the T3, and remain improved even after the T3 had been discontinued. His temperature remained normal as well.

Case Study 3

A 36 y.o. real estate agent presents to the office complaining of PMS, depression, fatigue, and admits to a peculiar throat sensation (she says it feels as if someone is pressing his thumb against her trachea toward the base of her neck). Her symptoms came on about a year ago. The only thing she can remember about that time, is that's when she was having some problems with her 12 y.o. daughter, and that's also when she received increased management responsibilities at the brokerage.

After evaluation, she was started on a cycle of T3 therapy with the usual instructions. The day after starting the T3 therapy, she called the office to point out that her temperature had gone down instead of up. Her temperature was lower the day after starting than it was before she started. She was also experiencing a little bit of tightness in the rings on her fingers, but no other complaints. It was explained to her that she may very well be a 1-day compensator **(p103)** and that she was going to need to be extra careful to take the medicine exactly as possible on time, and to call the office at the first sign of any complaints. It was explained that her chances of developing side effects might be a little higher than usual, and she needed to consider whether or not she wanted to proceed. Also, if she did want to proceed then she would have to increase the T3 very deliberately **(p105)** and carefully, or not at all.

She opted to proceed, and because it was agreed that the potential benefits outweighed the risks, her T3 dose was increased by 7.5 mcg/dose/day. Her temperature reached 98.6°F on 30 mcg BID, but dropped back down again later that day so her average was below 98.6°F. She stated feeling noticeably better when her temperature had gotten up to normal. She went up to 37.5 mcg and her temperature went up, and then back down again in one day. This same thing occurred when she increased to 45 mcg and 52.5 mcg BID. After a weekend, she called to say that she was feeling more irritable, bloated, and achy, almost as if she had the flu. Her complaints had started over the weekend. As it turned out, she had gone to the store with her daughter on Saturday morning and missed taking her dose by about an hour and a half. She denied any irregular heartbeats, increased awareness of her heart beat, shortness of breath, or any other complaints. Her side effects resolved completely within 45 minutes of a T4 test dose **(p112)**. She was able to get a timer and organize herself such that she was then able to make sure and take her T3 very much on time thereafter.

She proceeded with treatment and was able to capture her temperature on 60 mcg BID. Her symptoms began to resolve, and continued to get better and better over the next 2 weeks or so **(p103)**.

She did well on that regimen for about a month or so, until she had a bout of missing several times her dosage an hour here and two hours there. She began noticing feeling a little jittery, achy, bloated, and tired. Her temperature had also dropped about half a degree **(p110)**. She responded fairly well to a T4 test dose, but when it was repeated an hour and a half later, her complaints had not resolved sufficiently enough to comfortably allow any further T3 increase in this cycle. She was weaned off the T3, so that her system could settle down, and to see if she could get on less medicine on the next cycle, which would be easier to manage (easier to keep the T3 level steady) **(p110)**. She was able to wean down off the T3 every 2 days without her temperature dropping. Her side effects diminished more and more as she went off the T3, but did not disappear completely until after she had been off the T3 for about 3 days, so she was left off the T3 for another 3 days after that (for a total of 6 days) to give her T3 level more time to steady down very well **(p114)**. On her own, she opted to stay off a couple of days more (for a total of 8 days between cycles) to get a nice fresh start **(p105)**, because she wanted to see if she could get as much correction as possible out of the upcoming cycle.

On the second cycle, she was able to capture her temperature on 30 mcg BID, and she felt far better than she ever had on the first cycle. Her symptoms were almost completely resolved. About a week after her temperature was captured, she wanted to see if she could wean off and stay improved off T3 therapy. To her amazement, her temperature held as she weaned off the T3 therapy, and her symptoms actually got better and better. This continued until it got to the point that her symptoms only resolved completely after she had been off the treatment for a few days. It was only after the treatment had been discontinued that she felt completely normal; she felt better after the treatment than she ever had during the treatment **(p95)**. And after treatment, she felt as good or better than she did before she ever got sick in the first place.

Case Study 4

A 50 y.o. woman presents to the office with a long history of "thyroid" trouble. Her symptoms of decreased energy, decreased ambition, listlessness, dry skin, fluid retention, and cold intolerance began in her late twenties. She also remembers a distinct down-turn in her condition after a series of cortisone shots she received when she was 32 y.o. When she was 33 y.o., her family doctor felt her symptoms were characteristic of low thyroid function, even though her blood tests were just within the limits of normal. He started her on half a grain of dessicated thyroid (e.g., Armour Thyroid) to see how she'd do. Her symptoms responded dramatically well to the Armour, so it was felt his suspicion of low thyroid was confirmed.

Unfortunately, her symptoms started to return about 3 months later. Her dose was increased to 1 grain, and she improved again. Again, 3 months later, her condition slipped back downward. He did not increase her dose at that time. She took that same dose for many years, and did fairly well. She didn't complain of any side effects. Occasionally, she wondered if she needed more thyroid medicine but her doctor didn't agree. Over the years she has been to several doctors, but none of them felt she needed to take more thyroid medicine because her tests showed a TSH near the lower limits of normal. About a year ago, a doctor she was seeing agreed to increase her dessicated thyroid to 1.5 grains to see if that would help any.

Her symptoms improved markedly, and both patient and doctor were well pleased. She became disappointed when the symptoms started coming back again about 3 months later. Her doctor, who was somewhat surprised when her symptoms returned, was even more astonished when he increased her dose to 2 grains only to see her symptoms of hypothyroidism get even worse!

To remedy the situation, a doctor knowledgeable about WTS instructs her (after evaluation) to decrease her dessicated thyroid to 1 grain for 2 days, and then to discontinue it (she is otherwise in good health, and she hasn't noticed too much of a change in the way she feels when she skips a day here or there of her Armour). She is concerned, however, when she's told she is to stay off all thyroid (if without complaints) for 10 days before starting the T3 therapy **(p116)**. She feels she needs more thyroid stimulation, not less, and can't picture how she might feel if she goes off her thyroid treatment. She is reassured that she may start on the lowest dose of the T3 therapy before the 10 days are up, should she notice any worsening of her symptoms, and that she may increase the T3 as much as one 7.5 mcg increment/day to prevent any worsening of her hypothyroid symptoms during those 10 days. Furthermore, she is counseled that she'd be better off not to start or increase the T3 therapy at all for those 10 days if she doesn't worsen **(p116)**.

She is able to remain off all thyroid without discomfort for 10 days, and then begins a cycle of T3. She gets to 90 mcg BID without a noticeable difference in her temperature or the way she feels, so she is weaned off the first cycle, or reset cycle **(p111)**. She is able to wean off by 7.5 mcg/dose/day without complaints.

With the second cycle, her temperature and condition still do not improve in spite of her reaching 90 mcg BID. The second cycle is weaned as the first.

On the third cycle, her temperature begins to go up, and she begins to feel better on 67.5 mcg BID. On 75 mcg BID, her temperature reaches 98.6°F and she feels even better. Two days later, her temperature slips back down a little, and so her dose is increased to 82.5 mcg BID. Two days later it slides back down again, and she is increased to 90 mcg BID. She is without complaints. Her temperature does not drop back down in 2 days, so the patient begins to wonder if her temperature is captured. Three days after that (a total of 5 days), her temperature still has not dropped so it is felt her temperature is pretty well captured. She subjectively felt about 40% of what she imagined a normal person to feel like when she started T3 therapy, and now she feels about 60% normal.

She begins having some stress at work, on top of getting the flu, and missing some of her dose times (she missed one dose entirely), and begins noticing some lightheadedness, shakiness, and palpitations when she stands up quickly. Her side effects respond partially to a T4 test dose. Because she is having some side effects, and since this is a reasonable time to wean anyway, it is determined that it would be best for her to wean off the present cycle at this time. Her side effects resolve when she has weaned about half-way off the present cycle, so she is kept off the T3 therapy for only 2 days between cycles **(p114)**. On the next cycle, she is able to capture her temperature on 52.5 mcg BID, and feels 80% normal.

After a time **(Q9)**, she is weaned off the present cycle, to start another. On the next cycle (her sixth overall), she is able to capture her temperature on 15 mcg BID and she feels 100% normal, subjectively. This cycle ends up being her last because she is able to wean off the T3 and stay normal even after the treatment is finished.

Case Study 5

A 48 y.o. college administrator presents with extreme fatigue and listlessness, as well as difficulty sleeping at night, cold hands and feet, and irritable bowel syndrome. Twenty two years ago she developed hypothyroidism, with a low T4 and a high TSH. She is well acquainted with some of her symptoms, as she has had them to varying degrees for the last 22 years. Her symptoms are severe enough now, that she "just knows there's something wrong," in spite of the fact that her thyroid blood tests are normal. She is currently taking 0.2 mg of levothyroxine (e.g., Synthroid™, Levothroid™).

After evaluation, she is instructed to decrease her T4 dosage from 0.2 mg to 0.1 mg for 2 days and then to discontinue it. She is instructed that she should try to remain off all thyroid medicine for 10 days, but that she should start and increase the T3 therapy as is necessary (and only as is necessary) to prevent a worsening of her symptoms. After the 10 days are over, she may then increase the T3 by 7.5 mcg/dose/day if without complaints until her temperature is 98.6°F or until she reaches 90 mcg BID, and to call the office if she has any questions or problems, and to return to the office in 3 weeks.

At her next visit, she relates that after she was off all T4 for 2 days, her hypothyroid symptoms started to worsen, and her temperature dropped from averaging 97.8°F to about 97.5°F, so she started taking 7.5 mcg BID. Her symptoms did not continue to worsen, so she did not increase the dose any further, until 3 days later (fifth day of being off T4) when her symptoms started worsening again. At that time, she increased her dose to 15 mcg BID, and with that she was able to hold her own until the rest of the 10 days had passed.

At that point, she began increasing the T3 therapy by 7.5 mcg/dose/day in an effort to bring her temperature up to normal. Her temperature normalizes at 52.5 mcg BID, and her symptoms improve markedly (she feels 80% normal when she had been feeling 20%).

After a time, it is determined that she should proceed with treatment to see if she can completely resolve her complaints and go back on T4 therapy **(p120)**. She begins to wean down by 7.5 mcg/dose/2 days (and she is further challenged by not adding back any T4 at first). Her temperature begins to slip after the second decrease, so it is felt that she may be weaning the T3 dose too quickly. This suspicion is confirmed by going back up one increment of T3, waiting 4 days before the next decrease (instead of 2 days), and seeing her temperature hold this time. She continues to be able to decrease the T3 by 7.5 mcg/dose/4 days without a drop in her temperature until she gets down to 22.5 mcg BID. She finds that she cannot decrease the dose past this "wall" without experiencing a drop in her temperature, so it is felt that she probably is not producing sufficient T4 to support endogenous T3 production sufficient to replace the exogenous T3 being weaned. So, 0.025 mg/day of levothyroxine is begun. After a day or so, she is then able to finish weaning off the T3 therapy without problems. At this point, she is still feeling about 70–80% normal **(Q5)**.

Two days after the first cycle of T3 therapy has been discontinued, the levothyroxine dose is discontinued. She again is instructed to wait up to 10 days without starting the T3 if possible between cycles (because she is only on 0.025 mg of T4, 5–7 days would probably be sufficient, but in cases of being on 0.1 mg or so, patients should wait the full 10 days). This time, she is able to remain off the T3 until she decides to begin the next cycle on the sixth day (which she has permission to do).

With this cycle, she is able to get her temperature up on 30 mcg BID, and she enjoys complete resolution of her symptoms. When she is weaned off the T3 therapy, she weans down every 4 days, and again needs 0.025 mg T4 to be added back when she gets down to 22.5 mcg BID. When she gets down in the cycle to 7.5 mcg BID, it seems that she could use a little more T4 (based on her symptoms and temperature), and so her dose is increased to 0.05 mg/day. She remains very, very well off T3 therapy, and finds herself 6 months later, with normal thyroid blood tests and doing far better on 0.05 mg/day than she ever did on 0.2 mg/day!

Case Study 6

A 38 y.o. woman had been fine until about 3 years ago when she developed signs of hyperthyroidism. Her T4 was very, very high, and her TSH was extremely low. She had lost 10 pounds in less than a month, was experiencing a rapid heart rate, and feeling quite ill. She underwent ablative radioactive iodine treatment, and her symptoms of hyperthyroidism gradually abated. She began gaining her weight back, and also felt more fatigued, with difficulty concentrating. A low T4 and an elevated TSH revealed that she had been rendered hypothyroid, which was no surprise. She was started on levothyroxine, and after some adjusting, her blood tests were normalized with her being on a dose of 0.1 mg/day. The only problem was that she was still suffering from the symptoms she had developed after the ablative therapy. She was still gaining some weight and she was still exhausted. She also noticed she was retaining more fluid, and was losing some hair; she was also developing very dry skin and dry, brittle hair. Because the thyroid tests were normal, her doctors felt that she was normal, and that if anything her complaints were from something else if not from simply getting older. They did not feel that increasing her dose would be indicated or helpful.

She had lived for 37 years previously without any trace of such a complaint, and she knew she felt nothing like the way she felt prior to developing hyperthyroidism. The symptoms she was experiencing were just like the ones she began to have after the ablative therapy, which had partially responded to levothyroxine to the satisfying of blood tests. Her temperature was running 97.0°F on average.

After evaluation from a WTS perspective, it is determined that she should decrease her T4 to 0.05 mg/day for one day, and then discontinue it. She is instructed to start and increase the T3 therapy only as is necessary to prevent a worsening of her symptoms for 10 days (staying off T3 completely for 10 days if possible) and then to increase the T3 by 7.5 mcg/dose/day if without complaints until her temperature is 98.6°F or until she reaches 90 mcg BID, and to call the office if she has any questions or problems, and to return to the office in 3 weeks.

She is able to stay off the T3 comfortably for 10 days after discontinuing the T4. She is able to capture her temperature on 45 mcg BID. Her symptoms of hypothyroidism almost completely resolve, but not quite.

She is feeling well enough, that she would like to stay on the 45 mcg BID for a time, because it has been a while since she's felt very well. After about a month on that dosage, she comes down with the flu. Although her temperature had been running normal before the flu, her temperature is now running close to 100°F. Since her temperature had been normal for a while on 45 mcg BID, she is instructed not to decrease her dose of T3. She is advised to treat this fever the way anyone else would treat a fever when they would get with a flu, and to call the office if she develops any unusual complaints. After 4–5 days her flu abates, and her temperature returns to normal, as does her previous level of well-being.

After a time **(Q9)**, it is determined that she should wean off the present cycle in favor of the next cycle of T3. It is also hoped that she can avoid having to wean T4 before the next cycle, by not having to go on T4 after this cycle. She is instructed to wean off the T3 by 7.5 mcg/dose/2 days if without complaints, and to remain off for 2 days before starting another cycle. It is explained to her, that should her temperature begin to drop, and should she begin to feel significantly worse that some T4 will be added back.

As she weans off the present cycle of T3, her temperature slips a few tenths, and she feels a little more tired, but is sufficiently comfortable that she doesn't need to add back any T4 between cycles.

On the second cycle her temperature is captured on 30 mcg BID, and she enjoys complete resolution of her symptoms. She states that she feels the way she did before any of this ever started (before getting hyperthyroidism). She is allowed to remain on 30 mcg BID for 2 months because she does not have any complaints, and she is afraid she would not feel as well with the T4. Over that time, she begins to forget what it was like to feel badly, and becomes confident that she will be able to wean off T3 therapy. Because she is in no hurry to wean off, and because she wants to stay on the smallest amount of T4 that is effective, she weans down off the T3 by one 7.5 mcg every 10 days. As she weans down off the T3 therapy, her temperature slips some when she decreases the T3 dose to 15 mcg BID, so she is given 0.05 mg of T4. She is then able to wean off the rest of the way without difficulty. Her thyroid blood tests 6 weeks out are within normal ranges. She feels back to normal, and maintains a normal temperature on 0.05 mg/day of T4 (levothyroxine). These are two things she didn't have prior to T3 therapy even though she was on 0.1 mg/day of T4.

Case Study 7

A 34 y.o. woman who is part Irish and part American Indian presents complaining of fatigue, panic attacks, migraine headaches, and irregular menstrual cycles. She has a fair complexion and some freckles, and naturally has reddish highlights in her hair. She has been more tired than she thinks is normal, for as long as she can remember. Over the years, she has seemed to pick up more and more complaints. She remembers no obvious correlation between the onset of any of her symptoms with any identifiable stressful event, or identifiable change. Her temperature has run between 97°F and 98°F for as long as she can remember. "I have to get sick to get a temperature of 98.6°F, and my doctor used to tell me that if I ever did get a temperature of higher than 98.6°F, that for me it was a fever and to treat it as such."

After evaluation, she is started on 7.5 mcg p.o. BID and is instructed to increase the dose by 7.5 mcg/dose/day if she is without complaints until her temperature is 98.6°F by mouth on average (or until she is up to 90 mcg BID), and to call the office if she develops any complaints, and to return to the office in 2 weeks. The patient is very apprehensive about increasing the medicine every day because she has a history of being very sensitive to medicines. It is explained to her that she may go up on the medicine by 7.5 mcg increments every 3 or 4 days if she prefers, but that 10% of patients don't tolerate that very well, and that she might be one of them **(p105)**. It is decided that she will increase the T3 every 3 days instead of every day, but that a careful eye will be kept on her to watch and make sure that she is not a 1-day compensator **(p103)**.

Her temperature first reaches 98.6 on 37.5 mcg BID. She feels significantly improved (from 30% normal to 60% normal). After 5 days on that dose, her temperature drops back down again, and so her dose is increased to 45 mcg BID. About 5 days later, her temperature begins to slip again, and so her dose is increased to 52.5 mcg BID. Her temperature again goes up, and she again feels well until about 3 days later, when she missed a couple of dose times by an hour or so (she admits that she has been having a little trouble getting her doses on time all along). At this time, she doesn't haven't any complaints or side effects, but she is just not feeling as well as she was. She is given a T4 test dose **(p112)** and within 45 minutes of the dose she returns to feeling as well as she ever has during the T3 therapy. Two days later (her fifth day of being on 52.5 mcg BID), her temperature slips down again. She is increased and compensates again in 5 days, and then when she is increased to 67.5 mcg BID, her temperature appears to be captured (because more than 5 days have passed, and the temperature hasn't dropped back down again).

After being on 67.5 mcg for about 3 weeks, she again has some trouble getting her doses on time, and her temperature slips a little and some of her symptoms return. She improves a little with a T4 test dose but not as well as before, and no further improvement is obtained when the T4 test dose is repeated in 1 and 1/2 hours. Her temperature is raised back to normal when her dose is increased to 75 mcg BID, but she still is not feeling as well as she had been previously on 67.5 mcg BID.

It is determined that it would be best to wean her off the present cycle in favor of the next cycle, and she begins to wean off the medicine by 7.5 mcg decrements every 2 days. Her temperature starts to slip, so her wean is decelerated to one decrement in her dose every 4 days, which works out well.

After remaining off T3 for 3 days between cycles, she begins the second cycle. She is able to capture her temperature on 30 mcg BID this time. She now feels what she considers to be 80% normal. She is satisfied for now and would like to stay on this dose for a month or so, because she has some stressful weeks coming up and doesn't want to take the time to change her dosing, or take the chance of not feeling as well.

Two months later, she weans off the 2nd cycle as she did the first, and 3 days later begins the 3rd. She captures her temperature on 15 mcg BID, and feels now what she considers 100% normal. After a couple of months, she weans off the treatment and remains well off therapy.

Three months down the road, she makes a stressful presentation, and notices herself starting to slip clinically, over the next several days. Her temperature has slipped as well. She finds that she is able to get her temperature back up on only 7.5 mcg BID, which she discontinues successfully after about a week. She now uses small doses of T3 to quickly catch relapses. She has even noticed that if she takes 7.5 mcg BID the day before, the day of, and the day after a presentation she knows will be stressful (and would typically cause a mild relapse for her), she can often prevent the relapse from occurring at all.

Case Study 8

The patient is a 45 y.o. woman who is complaining of severe fatigue, headaches, depression, decreased memory, irritability, and easy weight gain. Her symptoms first appeared 10 years ago after the birth of her second child. Her symptoms tend to worsen each time she goes on a strict diet to lose weight (she often gains the weight back, and then some). They did seem to improve somewhat when she was treated on a clinical basis with some thyroid medicine for several months about 4 years ago. But she moved to another state, and could not find a doctor who would treat her with thyroid medicine, because her tests were normal.

Upon evaluation, it was determined that her temperature averaged 97.3°F during the day, and her blood tests were normal. Also, her EKG revealed her heart rate to be very slightly irregularly irregular, so slightly that most doctors would probably say that she had normal sinus rhythm. In the history she admitted to having noticed some skipped beats from time to time. She was counseled that she had a higher than normal risk of having cardiovascular side effects such as palpitations, skipped beats, or increased heart rate (p83). But all involved felt that her potential benefit outweighed her risks.

She is started on 7.5 mcg p.o. BID and is instructed to increase the dose by 7.5 mcg/dose/day if she is without complaints until her temperature is 98.6°F by mouth on average (or until she is up to 90 mcg BID), and to call the office if she develops any complaints, and to return to the office in 2 weeks. Her temperature first reaches normal on 15 mcg BID. Six days later, it drops back down again. Her dose is increased to 22.5 mcg and then the next day to 30 mcg BID, which brings her temperature back up to normal. About 6 days later, her temperature drops back down again, and her dose is increased again. Finally, her temperature is captured on 60 mcg BID. She feels very well. In fact, she is incredulous that she can feel so well after so many years of feeling so badly, and especially that the treatment was so simple. She finds it hard to believe/understand that this treatment wasn't thought of sooner.

She stays on 60 mcg BID for almost 3 months before wanting to proceed with the treatment's course. She has not had any complaints on the T3 therapy. Unfortunately, she misunderstood or forgot the instructions and weaned off the T3 therapy by 7.5 mcg/dose/day in spite of the fact that her temperature dropped after the third decrease. Some of her symptoms returned as she weaned off, and she was discouraged. It was explained to her how she should have weaned off more slowly, to give her own system a chance to come up and maintain her temperature.

She was started on a second cycle and was able to capture her temperature on 52.5 mcg BID (when she might have been able to on much less had she not squandered so much of the benefit from the first cycle by weaning off too quickly). After a month or so on that dose, she was ready to try weaning off again. This time, she began by decreasing the dose by 7.5 mcg/dose/2 days. However, when her temperature started to slip on the second decrease, she went back up an increment (because there was a good chance this could be her final cycle), and then decelerated the wean to 7.5 mcg/dose/4 days. After a couple of decreases, her temperature started to slip again, so she went back up an increment and decelerated the wean to 7.5 mcg/dose/6 days. She was then able to continue weaning off the T3 until she was off completely, and her temperature remained normal off the treatment.

She did very well for over a year, until her sister died in a car accident. Her temperature dropped and her symptoms began to return. She was started back on a cycle of T3 and after about one week, she was able to capture her temperature on 22.5 mcg BID. She stayed on that dose for about 2 months and then was able to wean off the T3 therapy again, without any difficulty in maintaining her body temperature on her own.

Same Principles Applied Differently

There are certain principles of T3 therapy that I think every doctor using this protocol should understand. The principles described in this chapter are based on the physiology of the thyroid system and its hormones. They are essential for obtaining amazing results and avoiding side effects, but may be implemented using a variety of methods. I've included below some methods other doctors are using.

For example, the importance of letting the T4/rT3 preponderance dissipate before increasing T3 to unnecessarily high levels is explained on page 118. This principle is used to explain why it makes sense to allow the T4 from T4-containing medicines to dissipate before chasing patients' temperatures with T3. Dr. Leighton's approach below applies this same principle in patients who aren't weaning off T4-containing medicine. When the patients' pulse rates increase but their temps don't come up, he sees that as an indication that there is enough T3 to decrease the patients' T4/rT3 backlog, but perhaps too much of a backlog for it to be appropriate to chase the patients' temps with T3. So he leaves them on that dose as a plateau for at least 4 weeks. On the other hand, when patients' temps come up normally without much increase in pulse rate, Dr. Leighton believes this is indicative of the fact that there is not too much of a backlog problem. I like Dr. Leighton's variation because although it is more conservative, it may not be giving up much benefit, and may even gain benefit, depending on how long it takes for the T4/rT3 preponderance to wash out. I think you may find the methods of each of the doctors below useful in the treatment of some of your patients.

In addition, every method carries with it a different risk versus benefit consideration. More conservative approaches may be better suited for some patients but may not provide all the same benefits quite as quickly, if at all. You may find other methods on our web site: wilsonssyndrome.com

Dr. Leighton

I think that heart rate is often a more sensitive indicator of thyroid stimulation than body temperature. If patients' heart rates rise on the order of 20 points during the taper-up phase of the treatment cycle, or after establishing on a plateau dose (e.g., rising from 65 bpm before treatment to around 85 bpm while on the T3), this is clearly a thyroid effect. I cycle patients up on the T3 therapy until one or more of 5 criteria are met:

1. Their temperature rises into a "normal" range of 97.8°F to 98.6°F
2. Their heart rate rises from 15–25 beats per minute (taken at the same time each day)
3. Their symptoms clearly improve (no sense in going beyond the point of symptomatic improvement)
4. They reach the maximal level of 90 mcg of T3 Q12h, or
5. They develop signs or symptoms of excessive thyroid stimulation (tremors, palpitations, anxiety – similar to drinking too much caffeine).

It is not uncommon for these signs to be delayed until after the patient has been at the maximal dose of 90 mcg Q12h for 1–3 weeks. Then, it seems as though a "light switch" has turned on, and suddenly they develop evidence of too much thyroid stimulation. This makes sense when considering this from the aspect of clearing the rT3 from the receptor sites [which may sometimes take 3 weeks]. At that point, we taper back down to a lower level where the signs of excess thyroid effect disappear again. Then, as in all of the 5 situations above, I usually put patients on a plateau dose for at least 4 weeks to give more time for the rT3 to be cleared out. It appears that patients are more likely to progress on the subsequent cycle(s) with this approach.

Stephen L. Leighton, MD
Family Care Health & Wellness Center, Inc.
Winston-Salem, NC 27101
USA

Dr. Resseger

I judge total replacement by normal body temperatures and pulse below 92 bpm. One frustration has been that about 5% of patients do get symptoms of hyperthyroidism when on enough T3 to get their body temperatures normal. The symptoms include rapid pulse and elevated body temperatures. In these people, what I've done is dropped to just below the toxic level and stayed there for 6–8 weeks and then tapered them off. Most of these patients will maintain their normal temperature as you taper them off. I have had a few patients that I have left on T3 (sometimes combining the doses into one daily dose) because they do so much better on the sustained T3 than they do on any other method of treatment.

Dr. Charles Resseger, DO
Past President, AAEM
Norwalk, OH
USA

Dr. Nesbit

If I see that patients' temperatures do begin to rise but are slow coming all the way back up to normal, and they're starting to manifest side effects or problems, then I'll wean them off the T3. On the next cycle, I will increase them to the dose where I started to see the rise in the previous cycle and leave them on that dose for a month, sometimes longer. In some cases, I have seen patients' temperatures come back up to normal after being on that same dose for several months. Once they get to 98.2°F almost universally they start feeling really good.

Dr. Ian Nesbit, ND
Billings, MT
USA

Dr. Hunninghake

Although the results may take longer, many patients can still benefit from a conservative low dose T3 therapy approach. Although there are some patients who feel better fairly soon with such an approach, it's normally a longer haul, which is characteristic of a more naturalistic approach. In some patients, I use a "mini cycling" approach where I give them a 7.5 mcg dose of sustained release T3 once a day. In a sense, they "wean on" during the day, and "wean off" at night. I have seen several patients who have seemed to do quite well with that over time. I'm often less interested in quick results and getting people off T3 therapy than I am with wanting to help people feel better as safely and conveniently as possible. Therefore, I often start patients on 1/2 grain of Armour thyroid, which contains T4. But if the 1/2 grain is not enough, instead of increasing the Armour, I'll add low dose sustained-release T3. I'm kind of giving them a low dose T3 therapy, with Armour as the stabilizing influence. It is important to pay attention to their adrenal systems as well. To me, when patients don't do well on thyroid treatment that's almost diagnostic of adrenal fatigue. However, on low-dose hydrocortisone, such patients almost never have side effects to the thyroid. They start much more smoothly on the thyroid when they already have adrenal support going. I often give patients an ACTH challenge test and give them cortisol as described in the book *Safe Uses of Cortisol* by William Jefferies, MD. Conversely, sometimes low doses of thyroid can improve adrenal function (as reflected in adrenal saliva testing) as well.

Ron Hunninghake, MD
Wichita, KS
USA

Dr. Denton

I find monitoring the pulse more beneficial than monitoring the temperature, especially in women, where there is so much fluctuation. While cycling the patient down, I feel it's also important to have patients notice any changes for the worse and stop before proceeding further down. I then step it up one dose and park there for a while before trying to wean them totally off the T3. Some patients stay at this dose for 2 or 3 weeks before I try to go to the next dose. About 10% of patients continue to need T3 indefinitely and demonstrate good health while taking it and poor health when they attempt to stop it. These patients are no longer willing to try to wean off and are faithful in taking their dose 12 hours apart.

Dr. Sandra Denton, MD
Anchorage, AK
USA

1   Schimmel M, Utiger RD. Thyroidal and peripheral production of thyroid hormones: review of recent finding and their clinical implications. Ann Intern Med 1977;87:760–8.

2   Steinsapir J. Type 2 iodothyronine deiodinase in rat pituitary tumor cells is inactivated in proteasomes. J Clin Invest 1998;102:11.

3   Christoffolete M. Atypical expression of type 2 deiodinase in thyrotrophs. Endocrinology 2006;147(4):1735–43.

4   Lam KS, Lechan RM, Minamitani N, et al. Vasoactive intestinal peptide in the anterior pituitary is increased in hypothyroidism. Endocrinology 1989;124(2):1077–84.

5   Kales A, Heuser G, Jacobson A, et al. All night sleep studies in hypothyroid patients, before and after treatment. J Clin Endocrinol Metab 1967;27(11):1593–99.

6   Eisinger J, Plantamura A, Ayavou T. Glycolysis abnormalities in fibromyalgia. J Am Coll Nutr 1994;13(2):144–48.

7   Mackowiak P, Wasserman S, Levine M. A Critical Appraisal of 98.6°F, the Upper Limit of the Normal Body Temperature, and Other Legacies of Carl Reinhold August Wunderlich; JAMA 1992;268(12):1578–1580.

8   Caldwell KL, Makhmudov A, Ely E, Jones RL, Wang RY. Iodine status of the U.S. population, National Health and Nutrition Examination Survey, 2005–2006 and 2007–2008. Thyroid 2011;21(4):419–27.

9   Crawford BA, Cowell CT. Iodine toxicity from soy milk and seaweed ingestion is associated with serious thyroid dysfunction. Med J Aust 2010;193(7):413–5.

10   Nishiyama S, Mikeda T, Okada T, Nakamura K, Kotani T, Hishinuma A. Transient hypothyroidism or persistent hyperthyrotropinemia in neonates born to mothers with excessive iodine intake. Thyroid 2004;14(12):1077–83.

11   Zimmermann M, Delange F. Iodine supplementation of pregnant women in Europe: a review and recommendations. Eur J Clin Nutr 2004;58(7):979–84.

12   Aghini-Lombardi F, Antonangeli L. The spectrum of thyroid disorders in an iodine-deficient community: the Pescopagano survey. J Clin Endocrinol Metab 1999;84(2):561–6.

13   Teodoru V, Nicolau GY. Iodine-enriched milk in goiter endemics. Rom J Endocrinol 1992;30(3–4):165–7.

14   Lightowler HJ, Davies GJ. Iodine intake and iodine deficiency in vegans as assessed by the duplicate-portion technique and urinary iodine excretion. Br J Nutr 1998;80(6):529–35.

15   International Programme on Chemical Safety (IPCS), http://www.inchem.org/documents/jecfa/jecmono/v024je11.htm.

16   Kessler JH. The effect of supraphysiologic levels of iodine on patients with cyclic mastalgia. Breast J 2004;10(4):328–36.

17   Ghent WR, Eskin BA. Low DA, iodine replacement in fibrocystic disease of the breast. Canadian J Surg 1993;36(5):453–60.

18   Roti E, Uberti ED. Iodine excess and hyperthyroidism. Thyroid 2001;11(5):493–500.

19   Premawardhana L, Parkes A, Smyth P, et al. Increased prevalence of thyroglobulin antibodies in Sri Lankan schoolgirls–is iodine the cause? Eur J Endocrinol 2000;143(2):185–8.

20   Xu J, Liu XL, Yang XF, et al. Supplemental selenium alleviates the toxic effects of excessive iodine on thyroid. Biol Trace Elem Res 2011; 141(1–3):110–8.

21   Chen X, Liu L, Yao P, et al. Effect of excessive iodine on immune function of lymphocytes and intervention with selenium. J Huazhong Univ Sci Technolog Med Sci 2007;27(4):422–5.

22   Zagrodzki P, Ratajczak R. Selenium supplementation in autoimmune thyroiditis female patient–effects on thyroid and ovarian functions (case study). Biol Trace Elem Res 2008;126(1–3):76–82.

23   Liu L, Heinrich M, Myers S, et al. Towards a better understanding of medicinal uses of the brown seaweed *Sargassum* in Traditional Chinese Medicine: A phytochemical and pharmacological review. J Ethnopharmacol 2012;142(3):591–619, doi: 10.1016/j.jep.2012.05.046. Epub 2012 Jun 6.

24   Reinhardt W, Luster M, Rudorff K, et al. Effect of small doses of iodine on thyroid function in patients with Hashimoto's thyroiditis residing in an area of mild iodine deficiency. Eur J Endocrinol 1998;139(1):23–8.

25   Papanastasiou L, Vatalas IA, Koutras D, Mastorakos G. Thyroid Autoimmunity in the Current Iodine Environment. Thyroid; August 2007, 17(8):729–739.

26   Delange F, Lecomte P. Iodine supplementation: benefits outweigh risks. Drug Safety 2000;22(2):89–95.

27   Dillman E, Gale C, Green W, et al. Hypothermia in iron deficiency due to altered triiodothyroidine metabolism. Regulatory, Integrative and Comparative Physiology 1980;239(5):377–81.

28   Smith SM, Johnson PE, Lukaski HC. In vitro hepatic thyroid hormone deiodination in iron-deficient rats: effect of dietary fat. Life Sci 1993;53(8):603–9.

29   Eftekhari MH, Keshavarz SA, Jalali M. The relationship between iron status and thyroid hormone concentration in iron-deficient adolescent Iranian girls. Asia Pac J Clin Nutr 2006;15(1):50–5.

30   Zimmermann MB, Köhrle J. The impact of iron and selenium deficiencies on iodine and thyroid metabolism: biochemistry and relevance to public health. Thyroid 2002;12(10):867–78.

31   Beard J, Tobin B, Green W. Evidence for thyroid hormone deficiency in iron-deficient anemic rats. J Nutr 1989;119:772–8.

32   Arthur JR, Beckett GJ. Thyroid function. British Medical Bulletin 1999;55:658–68.

33   Ertek S, Cicero AF, Caglar O, Erdogan G. Relationship between serum zinc levels, thyroid hormones and thyroid volume following successful iodine supplementation. Hormones 2010;9(3):263–8.

34   Yan X, Chuda Y, Suzuki M, Nagata T. Fucoxanthin as the major antioxidant in *Hijikia fusiformis*, a common edible seaweed. Biosci Biotechnol Biochem 1999;63(3):605–7.

35   Jimenez-Escrig A, Jimenez-Jimenez I, Pulido R, Saura-Calixto F. Antioxidant activity of fresh and processed edible seaweeds. J Sci Food Agric 2001;81(5):530–4.

36   Nagataki S. The average of dietary iodine intake due to the ingestion of seaweeds is 1.2 mg/day in Japan. Thyroid 2008;18(6):667–8.

37   Noge K, Becerra JX. Germacrene D, a common sesquiterpene in the genus *Bursera* (Burseraceae). Molecules 2009;14(12):5289–97.

38   Tripathi YB, Malhotra OP, Tripathi SN. Thyroid stimulating action of Z-guggulsterone obtained from *Commiphora mukul*. Planta Med 1984;50(1):78–80.

39   Singh AK, Tripathi SN, Prasad GC. Response of *Commiphora mukul* (guggulu) on melatonin induced hypothyroidism. Anc Sci Life 1983;3:85–90.

40   Wu J, Xia C, Meier J, Li S, Hu X, Lala DS. The hypolipidemic natural product guggulsterone acts as an antagonist of the bile acid receptor. Mol Endocrinol 2002;16(7):1590–7.

41   Panda S, Kar A. Guggulu (*Commiphora mukul*) potentially ameliorates hypothyroidism in female mice. Phytother Res 2005;19(1):78–80.

42   Tripathi YB, Tripathi P, Malhotra OP, Tripathi SN. Thyroid stimulatory action of (Z)-guggulsterone: mechanism of action. Planta Med 1988;54:271–7.

43   Antonio J, Colker CM, Torina GC, Shi Q, Brink W, Kaiman D. Effects of a standardized guggulsterone phosphate supplement on body composition in overweight adults: a pilot study. Current Therapeutic Research 1999;60:220–7.

44   Frances D. Botanical approaches to hypothyroidism: avoiding supplemental thyroid hormone. Medical Herbalism 2002;12:1–5.

45   Szapary PO, Wolfe ML, Bloedon LT, et al. Guggulipid for the treatment of hypercholesterolemia: a randomized controlled trial. JAMA 2003;290(6):765–72.

46   Ulbricht C, Basch E, Szapary P, et al. Guggul for hyperlipidemia: a review by the Natural Standard Research Collaboration. Complement Ther Med 2005;13(4):279–90.

47   Panossian A, Wikman G, Kaur P, Asea A. Adaptogens exert a stress-protective effect by modulation of expression of molecular chaperones. Phytomedicine 2009;16(6–7):617–22.

48   Gaffney BT, Hugel HM, Rich PA. The effects of *Eleutherococcus senticosus* and *Panax ginseng* on steroidal hormone indices of stress and lymphocyte subset numbers in endurance athletes. Life Sci 2001;70(4):431–42.

49   Gaffney BT, Hugel HM, Rich PA. *Panax ginseng* and *Eleutherococcus senticosus* may exaggerate an already existing biphasic response to stress via inhibition of enzymes which limit the binding of stress hormones to their receptors. Med Hypotheses 2001;56(5):567–72.

50   Deyama T, Nishibe S, Nakazawa Y. Constituents and pharmacological effects of *Eucommia* and Siberian ginseng. Acta Pharmacol Sin 2001;22(12):1057–70.

51   Aicher B, Gund H, Schultz A. *Eleutherococcus senticosus*: therapie bei akuten grippalen infekten. Pharm Ztg 2001;41:11–8.

52   Facchinetti F, Neri I, Tarabusi M. *Eleutherococcus senticosus* reduces cardiovascular stress response in healthy subjects: a randomized, placebo-controlled trial. Stress and Health 2002;18(1):11–7.

53   Maslov LN, Lishmanov YB, Arbuzov AG, et al. Antiarrhythmic activity of phytoadaptogens in short-term ischemia-reperfusion of the heart and postinfarction cardiosclerosis. Bull Exp Biol Med 2009;147(3):331–4.

54   Park SH, Kim SK, Shin IH, Kim HG, Choe JY. Effects of AIF on knee osteoarthritis patients: double-blind, randomized placebo-controlled study. Korean J Physiol Pharmacol 2009;13(1):33–7.

55   Jung CH, Jung H, Shin YC, et al. *Eleutherococcus senticosus* extract attenuates LPS-induced iNOS expression through the inhibition of Akt and JNK pathways in murine macrophage. J Ethnopharmacol 2007;113(1):183–7.

56   Asano K, Takahashi T, Miyashita M, et al. Effect of *Eleutherococcus senticosus* extract on human physical working capacity. Planta Med 1986;(3):175–7.

57   Dowling EA, Redondo DR, Branch JD, Jones S, McNabb G, Williams MH. Effect of *Eleutherococcus senticosus* on submaximal and maximal exercise performance. Med Sci Sports Exerc 1996;28(4):482–9.

58   Eschbach LF, Webster MJ, Boyd JC, McArthur PD, Evetovich TK. The effect of siberian ginseng (*Eleutherococcus senticosus*) on substrate utilization and performance. Int J Sport Nutr Exerc Metab 2000;10(4):444–51.

59   Niu HS, Liu IM, Cheng JT, Lin CL, Hsu FL. Hypoglycemic effect of syringin from *Eleutherococcus senticosus* in streptozotocin-induced diabetic rats. Planta Med 2008;74(2):109–13.

60   Azizov AP. [Effects of eleutherococcus, elton, leuzea, and leveton on the blood coagulation system during training in athletes]. Eksp Klin Farmakol 1997;60(5):58–60.

61   Cicero AF, Derosa G, Brillante R, Bernardi R, Nascetti S, Gaddi A. Effects of Siberian ginseng (*Eleutherococcus senticosus* maxim.) on elderly quality of life: a randomized clinical trial. Arch Gerontol Geriatr Suppl 2004;(9):69–73.

62   Soya H, Deocaris CC, Yamaguchi K, et al. Extract from *Acanthopanax senticosus* harms (Siberian ginseng) activates NTS and SON/PVN in the rat brain. Biosci Biotechnol Biochem 2008;72(9):2476–80.

63   Agrawal P, Rai V, Singh RB. Randomized placebo-controlled, single blind trial of holy basil leaves in patients with noninsulin-dependent diabetes mellitus. Int J Clin Pharmacol Ther 1996;34(9):406–9.

64   Devi PU, Ganasoundari A. Modulation of glutathione and antioxidant enzymes by *Ocimum sanctum* and its role in protection against radiation injury. Indian J Exp Biol 1999;37(3):262–8.

65   Sood S, Narang D, Thomas MK, Gupta YK, Maulik SK. Effect of *Ocimum sanctum* Linn. on cardiac changes in rats subjected to chronic restraint stress. J Ethnopharmacol 2006;108(3):423–7.

66   Singh S, Taneja M, Majumdar DK. Biological activities of *Ocimum sanctum* L. fixed oil–an overview. Indian J Exp Biol 2007;45(5):403–412.

67   Singh S, Majumdar DK. Evaluation of the gastric antiulcer activity of fixed oil of *Ocimum sanctum* (Holy Basil). J Ethnopharmacol 1999;65(1):13–9.

68   Devi PU, Ganasoundari A. Modulation of glutathione and antioxidant enzymes by *Ocimum sanctum* and its role in protection against radiation injury. Indian J Exp Biol 1999;37(3):262–8.

69   Sood S, Narang D, Dinda AK, Maulik SK. Chronic oral administration of *Ocimum sanctum* Linn. augments cardiac endogenous antioxidants and prevents isoproterenol-induced myocardial necrosis in rats. J Pharm Pharmacol 2005;57(1):127–33.

70   Gupta P, Yadav DK, Siripurapu KB, Palit G, Maurya R. Constituents of *Ocimum sanctum* with antistress activity. J Nat Prod 2007;70(9):1410–6.

71   Gholap S, Kar A. Hypoglycaemic effects of some plant extracts are possibly mediated through inhibition in corticosteroid concentration. Pharmazie 2004;59(11):876–8.

72 Maity TK, Mandal SC, Saha BP, Pal M. Effect of *Ocimum sanctum* roots extract on swimming performance in mice. Phytother Res 2000;14(2):120–1.

73 Sen P, Maiti PC, Puri S, Ray A, Audulov NA, Valdman AV. Mechanism of anti-stress activity of *Ocimum sanctum* Linn, eugenol and Tinospora malabarica in experimental animals. Indian J Exp Biol 1992;30(7):592–6.

74 Sembulingam K, Sembulingam P, Namasivayam A. Effect of *Ocimum sanctum* Linn on noise induced changes in plasma corticosterone level. Indian J Physiol Pharmacol 1997;41(2):139–43.

75 Sembulingam K, Sembulingam P, Namasivayam A. Effect of *Ocimum sanctum* Linn on the changes in central cholinergic system induced by acute noise stress. J Ethnopharmacol 2005;96(3):477–82.

76 Ravindran R, Rathinasamy SD, Samson J, Senthilvelan M. Noise-stress-induced brain neurotransmitter changes and the effect of *Ocimum sanctum* (Linn) treatment in albino rats. J Pharmacol Sci 2005;98(4):354–60.

77 Samson J, Sheela DR, Ravindran R, Senthilvelan M. Biogenic amine changes in brain regions and attenuating action of *Ocimum sanctumin* noise exposure. Pharmacol Biochem Behav 2006;83(1):67–75.

78 Sakina MR, Dandiya PC, Hamdard ME, Hameed A. Preliminary psychopharmacological evaluation of *Ocimum sanctum* leaf extract. J Ethnopharmacol 1990;28(2):143–50.

79 Mediratta PK, Sharma KK, Singh S. Evaluation of immunomodulatory potential of *Ocimum sanctum* seed oil and its possible mechanism of action. J Ethnopharmacol 2002;80(1):15–20.

80 Singh S, Rehan HM, Majumdar DK. Effect of *Ocimum sanctum* fixed oil on blood pressure, blood clotting time and pentobarbitone-induced sleeping time. J Ethnopharmacol 2001;78(2–3):139–43.

81 Joshi H, Parle M. Evaluation of nootropic potential of *Ocimum sanctum* Linn. in mice. Indian J Exp Biol 2006;44(2):133–6.

82 Jaggi RK, Madaan R, Singh B. Anticonvulsant potential of holy basil, *Ocimum sanctum* Linn., and its cultures. Indian J Exp Biol 2003;41(11):1329–33.

83 Kelly GS. *Rhodiola rosea*: a possible plant adaptogen. Altern Med Rev 2001;6(3):293–302.

84 Chen QG, Zeng YS, Qu ZQ, et al. The effects of *Rhodiola rosea* extract on 5-HT level, cell proliferation and quantity of neurons at cerebral hippocampus of depressive rats. Phytomedicine 2009;16(9):830–8.

85 Perfumi M, Mattioli L. Adaptogenic and central nervous system effects of single doses of 3% rosavin and 1% salidroside *Rhodiola rosea* L. extract in mice. Phytother Res 2007;21(1):37–43.

86 Kucinskaite A, Briedis V, Savickas A. [Experimental analysis of therapeutic properties of *Rhodiola rosea* L. and its possible application in medicine]. Medicina (Kaunas) 2004;40(7):614–9.

87 Arbuzov AG, Maslov LN, Burkova VN, Krylatov AV, Konkovskaia I, Safronov SM. [Phytoadaptogens-induced phenomenon similar to ischemic preconditioning]. Ross Fiziol Zh Im I M Sechenova 2009;95(4):398–404.

88 Maimeskulova LA, Maslov LN, Lishmanov I, Krasnov EA. [The participation of the mu-, delta- and kappa- opioid receptors in the realization of the anti-arrhythmia effect of *Rhodiola rosea*]. Eksp Klin Farmakol 1997;60(1):38–39.

89 Mattioli L, Funari C, Perfumi M. Effects of *Rhodiola rosea* L. extract on behavioural and physiological alterations induced by chronic mild stress in female rats. J Psychopharmacol 2009;23(2):130–142.

90 Qin YJ, Zeng YS, Zhou CC, Li Y, Zhong ZQ. [Effects of *Rhodiola rosea* on level of 5-hydroxytryptamine, cell proliferation and differentiation, and number of neuron in cerebral hippocampus of rats with depression induced by chronic mild stress]. Zhongguo Zhong Yao Za Zhi 2008;33(23):2842–6.

91 Olsson EM, von SB, Panossian AG. A randomised, double-blind, placebo-controlled, parallel-group study of the standardised extract shr-5 of the roots of *Rhodiola rosea* in the treatment of subjects with stress-related fatigue. Planta Med 2009;75(2):105–12.

92 Roberts HJ. Aspartame and hyperthyroidism: a presidential affliction reconsidered. Townsend Letter for Doctors & Patients 1997;May:86–8.

93 Roberts H. Aspartame disease. An ignored epidemic. West Palm Beach, FL, Sunshine Sentinel Press; 2001, p. 432.

94 Olney J. Brain damage in mice from voluntary ingestion of glutamate and aspartame. Neurobehavioral Toxicology 1980;2:125–9.

95 Sategna-Guidetti C, Volta U, Ciacci C, et al. Prevalence of thyroid disorders in untreated adult celiac disease patients and effect of gluten withdrawal: an Italian multicenter study. Am J Gastroenterol 2001;96(3):751–7.

96 "Tyrosine". University of Maryland Medical Center. Retrieved 2011-03-17. http://umm.edu/health/medical-reference-guide/complementary-and-alternative-medicine-guide/supplement/tyrosine.

97 Kelly GS. Peripheral metabolism of thyroid hormones: a review. Altern Med Rev 2000;5(4):306–33.

98 Gereben B, Zavacki A. Cellular and molecular basis of deiodinase-regulated thyroid hormone signaling. Endocrine Reviews 2008;29(7):898–938.

99 Bianco A, Kim B. Diodinases: implications of the local control of thyroid hormone action. J Clin Invest 2006;116(10):2571–9.

100 Gullo D, Latina A. Levothyroxine monotherapy cannot guarantee euthyroidism in all athyreotic patients. PLoS One 2011;6(8):e22552, doi: 10.1371/journal.pone.0022552.

101 Bernatoniene J, Trumbeckaite S, Majiene D, et al. The effect of crataegus fruit extract and some of its flavonoids on mitochondrial oxidative phosphorylation in the heart. Phytother Res 2009;23(12):1701–7.

102 Rodriguez ME, Poindexter BJ, Bick RJ, Dasgupta A. A comparison of the effects of commercially available hawthorn preparations on calcium transients of isolated cardiomyocytes. J Med Food 2008;11(4):680–6.

103 Uchida S, Ikari N, Ohta H, et al. Inhibitory effects of condensed tannins on angiotensin converting enzyme. J Pharmacol 1987;43:242–5.

104 Petkov V. Plants with hypotensive, antiatheromatous and coronary dilating action. A J Chinese Med 1979;7:197–236.

105 Ammon H, Handel M. *Crataegus*, toxicology and pharmacology. Planta Medica 1981;43:318–22.

106 Schrutka-Rechtenstamm R, Kopp B, Löffelhardt W. Studies on the turnover of cardenolides in *Convallaria majalis*. Planta Med 1985;51:387–90.

107 Lehmann HD. Effect of plant glycosides on resistance and capacitance vessels. Arzneimittelforschung 1984;34:423–9.

108 Choi DH, Kang DG, Cui X, et al. The positive inotropic effect of the aqueous extract of *Convallaria keiskei* in beating rabbit atria. Life Sci 2006;79:1178–85.

109 Nartowska J, Sommer E, Pastewka K, Sommer S, Skopin´ska-Rózewska E. Anti-angiogenic activity of convallamaroside, the steroidal saponin isolated from the rhizomes and roots of *Convallaria majalis*. Acta Pol Pharm 2004;61:279–82.

110 Ogorodnikova AV, Latypova LR, Mukhitova FK, Mukhtarova LS, Grechkin AN. Detection of divinyl ether synthase in Lily-of-the-Valley (*Convallaria majalis*) roots. Phytochemistry 2008;69:2793–8.

111 Pessah-Pollack R, Eschler DC, Pozharny Z, Davies T. Apparent insufficiency of iodine supplementation in pregnancy. J Womens Health (Larchmt). 2013 Oct 12. [Epub ahead of print].

Name: _____ Date: _____

Wilson's Temperature Syndrome
Symptom Checklist

You can use this sheet to track your progress with your symptoms by rating them before, during, and after treatment (marking the dates at the top of each column). You can rate each symptom on a scale of 1 to 10 based on how you feel, 10 being how you imagine a normal person to feel, 1 being feeling very bad.

before	during	after		before	during	after	
_____	_____	_____	(Put dates here)	( )	( )	( )	Abnormal throat sensations
( )	( )	( )	Fatigue	( )	( )	( )	Sweating abnormalities
( )	( )	( )	Headaches	( )	( )	( )	Heat and/or cold intolerance
( )	( )	( )	Migraines	( )	( )	( )	Low self esteem
( )	( )	( )	PMS	( )	( )	( )	Irregular periods
( )	( )	( )	Irritability	( )	( )	( )	Severe menstrual cramps
( )	( )	( )	Fluid retention	( )	( )	( )	Low blood pressure
( )	( )	( )	Anxiety	( )	( )	( )	Frequent colds and sore throats
( )	( )	( )	Panic attacks	( )	( )	( )	Frequent urinary infections
( )	( )	( )	Hair loss	( )	( )	( )	Lightheadedness
( )	( )	( )	Depression	( )	( )	( )	Ringing in the ears
( )	( )	( )	Decreased memory	( )	( )	( )	Slow wound healing
( )	( )	( )	Decreased concentration	( )	( )	( )	Easy bruising
( )	( )	( )	Decreased sex drive	( )	( )	( )	Acid indigestion
( )	( )	( )	Unhealthy nails	( )	( )	( )	Flushing
( )	( )	( )	Low motivation	( )	( )	( )	Frequent yeast infections
( )	( )	( )	Constipation	( )	( )	( )	Cold hands/feet, turn blue?
( )	( )	( )	Irritable bowel syndrome	( )	( )	( )	Poor coordination
( )	( )	( )	Inappropriate weight gain	( )	( )	( )	Increased nicotine/caffeine use
( )	( )	( )	Dry skin	( )	( )	( )	Infertility
( )	( )	( )	Dry hair	( )	( )	( )	Hypoglycemia
( )	( )	( )	Insomnia	( )	( )	( )	Increased skin infections/acne
( )	( )	( )	Needing to sleep during day	( )	( )	( )	Abnormal swallowing sensations
( )	( )	( )	Arthritis and joint aches	( )	( )	( )	Changes in skin pigmentation
( )	( )	( )	Allergies	( )	( )	( )	Prematurely gray/white hair
( )	( )	( )	Asthma	( )	( )	( )	Excessively tired after eating
( )	( )	( )	Muscular aches	( )	( )	( )	Carpal tunnel syndrome
( )	( )	( )	Itchiness of skin	( )	( )	( )	Dry eyes/blurred vision
( )	( )	( )	Elevated cholesterol	( )	( )	( )	Hives
( )	( )	( )	Ulcers	( )	( )	( )	Bad breath
				( )	( )	( )	**Total for both sides (out of 600)**

Referred by: _____

Comments: _____

_____

_____

WILSON'S TEMPERATURE SYNDROME

Temperature/Treatment Log

Month: _____

Directions: Mark each of the 3 daily temperatures with a '/' and the average with a 'O' (comments/symptoms may be written in vertically)

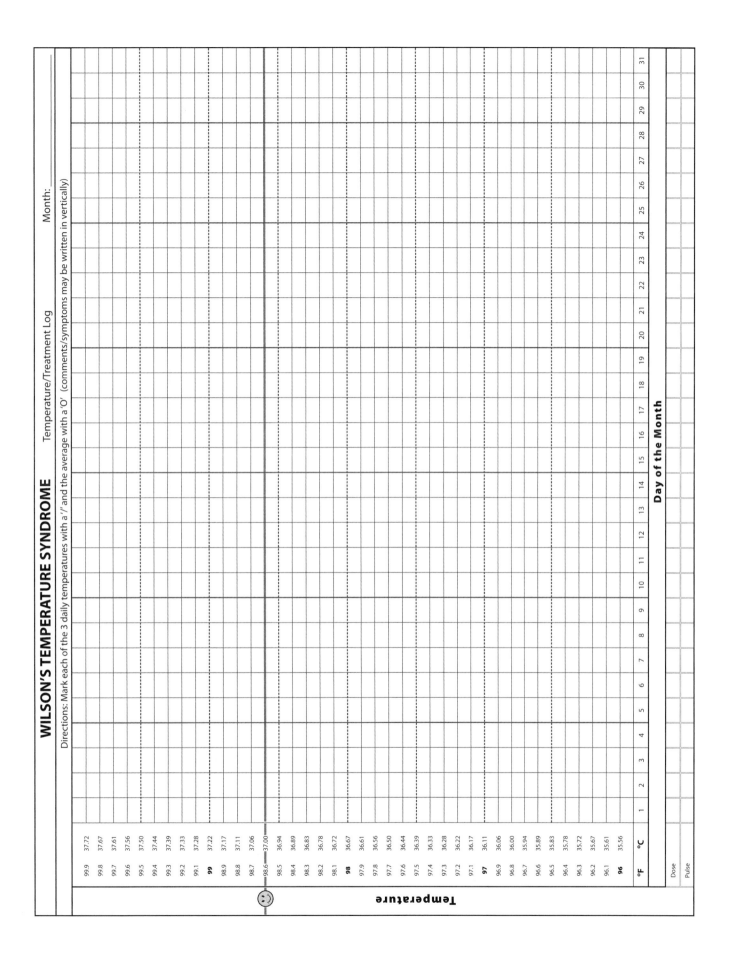

°F	°C
99.9	37.72
99.8	37.67
99.7	37.61
99.6	37.56
99.5	37.50
99.4	37.44
99.3	37.39
99.2	37.33
99.1	37.28
99	37.22
98.9	37.17
98.8	37.11
98.7	37.06
98.6	37.00
98.5	36.94
98.4	36.89
98.3	36.83
98.2	36.78
98.1	36.72
98	36.67
97.9	36.61
97.8	36.56
97.7	36.50
97.6	36.44
97.5	36.39
97.4	36.33
97.3	36.28
97.2	36.22
97.1	36.17
97	36.11
96.9	36.06
96.8	36.00
96.7	35.94
96.6	35.89
96.5	35.83
96.4	35.78
96.3	35.72
96.2	35.67
96.1	35.61
96	35.56

Temperature

Day of the Month

Dose

Pulse

Day of the Month: 1, 2, 3, 4, 5, 6, 7, 8, 9, 10, 11, 12, 13, 14, 15, 16, 17, 18, 19, 20, 21, 22, 23, 24, 25, 26, 27, 28, 29, 30, 31

Extremely low and extremely high body temperatures constitute medical emergencies. Just as a moderately high temperature can cause symptoms of a fever, so too can moderately low temperatures also cause significant symptoms. Moderately low temperatures have been ignored historically.

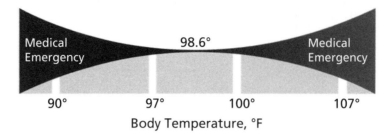

Body Temperature, °F

Index

Notes

Notes

Notes

Notes

Notes

Notes

Notes

Notes

Notes